# Geospatial Information System Use in Public Organizations

This book shows how Geospatial Information Systems (GIS) can be used for operations management in public institutions. It covers theory and practical applications, ranging from tracking public health trends to mapping transportation routes to charting the safest handling of hazardous materials. Along with an expert line-up of contributors and case studies, the editor provides a complete overview of how to use GIS as part of a successful, collaborative data analysis, and how to translate the information into cost-saving decisions, or even life-saving ones.

**Nicolas A. Valcik** currently works as the Director of Institutional Research and Business Intelligence at the University of Texas at Permian Basin. Previously, Nicolas worked as the Executive Director for Institutional Effectiveness at Central Washington University, the Director for Institutional Research for West Virginia University, and as Associate Director of Strategic Planning and Analysis for the University of Texas at Dallas. In addition, Nicolas held an academic appointment as Clinical Assistant Professor for Public Affairs for the University of Texas at Dallas. Prior to 1997, Nicolas worked for a number of municipalities, across different departments, as well as for Nortel. Nicolas received a doctorate in public affairs from the University of Texas at Dallas in 2005, a master's in public affairs from the University of Texas at Dallas in 1996, a bachelor's degree in interdisciplinary studies from the University of Texas at Dallas in 1994, and an associate's degree in political science from Collin County Community College in 1994.

# Geospatial Information System Use in Public Organizations

## How and Why GIS Should be Used by the Public Sector

**Edited by Nicolas A. Valcik**

Routledge
Taylor & Francis Group
NEW YORK AND LONDON

First published 2020
by Routledge
52 Vanderbilt Avenue, New York, NY 10017

and by Routledge
2 Park Square, Milton Park, Abingdon, Oxon, OX14 4RN

*Routledge is an imprint of the Taylor & Francis Group, an informa business*



*Library of Congress Cataloging-in-Publication Data*
Names: Valcik, Nicolas A., editor.
Title: Geospatial information system use in public organisations : how and why GIS should be used by the public sector / edited by Nicolas A. Valcik.
Other titles: Geospatial information system use in public organizations
Description: Abingdon, Oxon ; New York, NY : Routledge, 2019. | Includes bibliographical references.
Identifiers: LCCN 2019003321 (print) | LCCN 2019016697 (ebook) | ISBN 9781498767644 (E-book) | ISBN 9781498767637 (hbk : alk. paper) | ISBN 9781498767644 (ebk)
Subjects: LCSH: Geographic information systems—Government policy. | Geospatial data—Government policy. | Administrative agencies—Data processing. | Administrative agencies—Information technology.
Classification: LCC G212 (ebook) | LCC G212 .G46 2019 (print) | DDC 352.3/80285—dc23
LC record available at https://lccn.loc.gov/2019003321

ISBN: 978-1-4987-6763-7 (hbk)
ISBN: 978-0-429-27285-1 (ebk)

Typeset in Times New Roman
by Apex CoVantage, LLC

**I would like to dedicate this book to Stuart Murchison, a friend and colleague who left this world too soon.**

# Contents

# Foreword

My roots at the interface of GIS and public management are ancient, even antediluvian. In the summer of 1956, while a doctoral student at the University of Washington, I participated in a federally mandated post-nuclear survival planning exercise for the State of Washington. My contribution dealt with food supplies and was essentially spatial, but we had to do the cartographics the traditional way, by hand, using pens and ink. One of the co-investigators, civil engineer Edgar Horwood, spent time experimenting with overprinting on the line printer to enable card-fed, locationally coded images to be printed on that device via an IBM "computer". The next summer, during a time when we were busy launching geography's "quantitative revolution", I prepared an annexation plan for the City of Spokane, again a spatial exercise with hand-drawn maps and overlays on clear film to establish spatial relationships. Soon thereafter, I joined the geography faculty at the University of Chicago and was drawn by Gilbert White into his USDA and Corps of Engineers-sponsored flood plain and flood risk studies. There was need for land cover estimation, for which I developed a roster-based spatial sampling scheme that was soon adopted by the Canada Land Inventory as Roger Tomlinson began that exercise and coined the term "Geographic Information System". Soon, attempts to manipulate a 43,000×4,300 matrix of commuter flows to help the US Bureau of the Census in its rethinking of metropolitan area definition using the computers of the time led to an appeal by the Association of American Geographers' Census Advisory Committee (chair Brian J. L. Berry, Waldo Tobler, and Richard Morrill) to add latitude–longitude coordinates to their block and tract units to facilitate computerized mapping. As such coordinates began to appear, Horwood's experiments led to Howard Fisher's SYMAP project. Funded initially by Fisher, Bill Garrison, and myself, Betty Benson wrote the software at Northwestern University, and soon line-printed maps fed by row-wise interpolation began to appear. Armed with a Ford Foundation grant, Fisher took the software to Harvard University to create the Laboratory for Computer Graphics in the Graduate School of Design (later, Bill Warntz added "and Spatial Analysis"). Tobler and I gave the inauguration lectures, and a number of years later I relocated to become the Lab's director. In the first years of Lab activity, Harvard student Jack Dangermond became enthralled by computer mapping and left to start the enterprise that is now the global leader in the field of public management application, ESRI. In parallel, Carl Steinitz began his raster-based approach to substitute GIS for pen-and-ink landscape architecture. As computer-generated images began to replace the tedium, but not the artistry, of hand-drawn maps, locational coding enhanced overlay capabilities and sparked yet another revolution, in spatial statistical methodology. The rest, they say, is history.

Geographic Information Systems and Spatial Analysis have evolved into Geospatial Science, and we now see multiple real-time interacting uses in research and practice. I was pleased to lead the effort at the University of Texas at Dallas to inaugurate the first PhD degree program in the new field in the US.

But public sector usage has lagged at all levels of government, especially the state and local levels. Why should this be so? While cost barriers are abating, built-in and sometimes legally mandated practices are not. GIS training in public management programs is patchy, leading to shortages of well-trained staff—graduates who not only know how to drive ESRI's software but also know how to ask the right questions. And to be sure, there is often an upfront prime cost that is imposing: the expense of preparing and verifying the initial locationally coded base and adding the key datasets and software system. A stark contrast is emerging between those governments that have moved towards the new computer-based information systems of the fast-changing information era and those that have not, a gulf that needs to be bridged and ultimately eliminated. I therefore welcome this attempt by Dr. Valcik to show the rich variety of ways GIS can enrich and power work in the public sector, not merely by doing old things in new ways, but also by adding transformative applications to new things and radical new solutions. May their efforts to make Geospatial Science central to a broadening component of work in the public sector bear fruit.

Brian J. L. Berry
School of Economic, Political and Policy Sciences,
the University of Texas at Dallas

Richardson, TX: September 3, 2018

# Acknowledgments

I would like to thank everyone who worked on this project. A project such as this takes time and effort to perform the research and then write the chapter to a high standard for publication. I would like to thank Denis Dean for all of the work he has put into the project with recruiting the authors to two different chapters. A person who was originally going to be a co-editor on this project was Dr. Stuart Murchison. Unfortunately, Dr. Murchison passed away, and he is sorely missed. I would like to thank the reviewers for the chapters on this project, Jason Berthon-Koch, Shane Scott, and Barry Morgan. I would like to thank my co-workers and my employees at Central Washington University for support throughout this project. I would like to thank Andrea Stigdon for proofreading this book and Kerry Kunze for the amazing artwork on the cover. Last but not least, I want to thank my mother, Jo Valcik, and my wife, Kristi Valcik, for all of their love and support throughout my career. Without their support, this project would not be possible.

# About the Editor

**Nicolas A. Valcik**

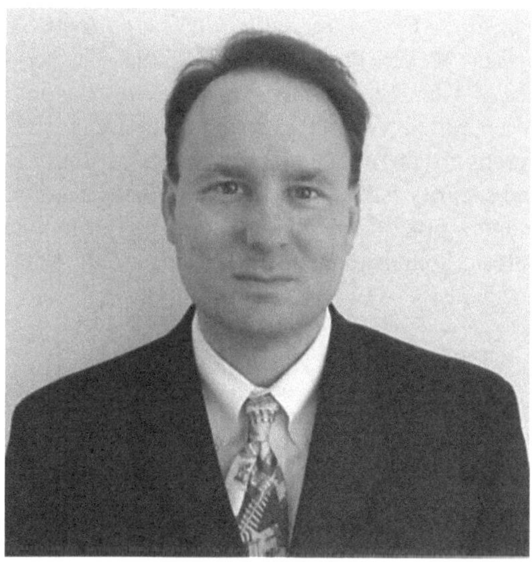

**Nicolas A. Valcik** currently works as the Director of Institutional Research and Business Intelligence at the University of Texas at Permian Basin. Previously, Nicolas worked as the Executive Director for Institutional Effectiveness at Central Washington University, the Director for Institutional Research for West Virginia University and as Associate Director of Strategic Planning and Analysis for the University of Texas at Dallas. In addition, Nicolas held an academic appointment as Clinical Assistant Professor for Public Affairs for the University of Texas at Dallas. Prior to 1997, Nicolas worked for a number of municipalities, across different departments, as well as for Nortel. Nicolas received a doctorate in public affairs from the University of Texas at Dallas in 2005, a master's in public affairs from the University of Texas at Dallas in 1996, a bachelor's degree in interdisciplinary studies from the University of Texas at Dallas in 1994, and an associate's degree in political science from Collin County Community College in 1994.

Nicolas has authored the following books for Taylor & Francis: *Institutional Research Initiatives in Higher Education* (2018), co-edited with Jeffery Johnson; *City Planning for the Public Manager* (2017), co-authored with Ted Benavides, Todd A. Jordan, and Andrea Stigdon; *Case Studies in Disaster Response and Emergency Management: Second Edition* (2017), co-authored with Paul Tracy; *Strategic Planning, Decision-Making and Practical Aspects for Public Sector and Non-Profit Organizations* (2016); *Non-Profit Organization Case Study Book* (2015), co-authored with Ted Benavides and Kim Scruton; *Hazardous Materials Compliance for Public Research Organizations: A Case Study* (2013); *Case Studies in Disaster Response and Emergency Management* (2017), co-authored with Paul E. Tracy; and *Practical Human Resources Management for Public Managers: A Case Study Approach* (2011), co-authored with Ted Benavides. Prior to 2011, Nicolas authored *Regulating the Use of Biological Hazardous Materials in Universities: Complying with the New Federal Guidelines*, which was published by Mellen Press in 2006. Nicolas has served as editor for three volumes of *New Directions for Institutional Research* (Volumes 135, 140, 14) and co-edited Volume 156 with Gary Levy, and has in addition written numerous articles and book chapters on institutional research topics and homeland security issues. Nicolas specializes in several areas as both a researcher and a practitioner: higher education, information technology, human resources, homeland security, organizational behavior, and emergency management.

# About the Authors

**Nathan F. Alleman** (PhD, the College of William and Mary) is Associate Professor of Higher Education Studies at Baylor University in Waco, Texas. Alleman studies and teaches about marginal and marginalized groups and institutions in higher education. Foci include sociological analyses of faculty sub-groups (such as non-tenure track faculty and collegiality, faculty denied tenure, and religious outsiders) and the collegiate identities and experiences of student sub-groups (among them, rural, first generation, undocumented, community college, religious minority, and food insecure). Alleman also writes about Christian higher education and the history of the YMCA student association movement.

**Greg Babinski** is Marketing and Business Development Manager for the King County GIS Center in Seattle, Washington. Previously, he was GIS Supervisor for the East Bay Municipal Utility District in Oakland, California. He holds an MA in Geography from Wayne State University in Detroit. Babinski is past president of URISA and founder of the GIS Management Institute. He has written and spoken about GIS management best practices, marketing, business development, and financial management for successful government agency GIS programs across North America, Europe, Asia, and Australia. In his spare time Greg likes hiking steep, narrow, dangerous trails that lead high above the clouds to awesome views.

**Floyd Bull** is a student in the Master of Science in Geospatial Technologies program at the University of Washington–Tacoma. He has worked in the GIS departments in the cities of Kent and Kirkland, Washington.

**Yongwan Chun** is an associate professor in the Geospatial Information Sciences program at the University of Texas at Dallas. His research interests are in GIS and spatial statistics methodology, with substantive applications in public health and urban geography. His research has been supported by multiple funding agencies, including the NIH and the NSF. He received the Emerging Scholar Award in 2017 from the Spatial Analysis and Modeling Specialty Group of American Association of Geographers. He has more than 50 publications, including 30+ journal articles, 10+ book chapters, one co-authored book (2013, SAGE), and one co-edited book (2017, Springer).

**Anthony R. Cummings** is a geographer who focuses on human–natural environment interactions and the impacts of changes in land use and land cover in Guyana on the livelihoods of forest dwelling and dependent peoples. Anthony uses GIS and remote sensing tools to argue for the development of policy that will allow stronger involvement of local-level managers, including indigenous peoples, in resource management decision-making processes. Anthony is currently Assistant Professor of Geospatial Information Sciences at the University of Texas at Dallas.

**David Donaldson** is a Clark Doctoral Fellow and graduate research assistant at the Maryland Transportation Institute located at the University of Maryland. His current research spans multiple transportation engineering projects involving traffic data analytics, simulation-based dynamic traffic assignment modeling, travel behavior modeling, and data collection for a national major transportation projects database. Originally from West Virginia, David received his bachelor's degree in civil engineering from West Virginia University. In addition to his undergraduate transportation engineering research, he worked for the West Virginia GIS Technical Center on various projects, most notably the West Virginia Trail Inventory. As the data collection lead, David field-collected, processed, and published hundreds of miles of recreation trail over a three-year period. More recently, he applied his GIS background in managing a similar trail project sponsored by the Partnership for Action Learning in Sustainability (PALS) at the University of Maryland. The project visualized eight Montgomery County recreation trails via Google Street View and developed a state-of-the-art segment-based mountain bike stress index. David expects to complete his Master of Science in Transportation Engineering in 2019.

**Kurt Donaldson** is the manager of the West Virginia GIS Technical Center, located in the Department of Geology and Geography at West Virginia University. The Center provides focus, direction, and leadership to users of Geographic Information Systems (GIS), digital mapping, and remote sensing within the State of West Virginia. Mr. Donaldson has 24 years of GIS management experience in which he has completed over 170 externally funded grants and service projects. In past years, the Center has supported the West Virginia Department of Transportation on various GIS initiatives, to include the West Virginia Trails Inventory (www.mapwv.gov/trails) and West Virginia Scanned Highway Plans projects (www.mapwv.gov/DOTplans). He is a charter member and past president of the West Virginia Association of Geospatial Professionals and in 2012 was awarded a GIS Professional Lifetime Achievement Award. In 2018, the Center received an ESRI Special Achievement in GIS Award for its significant contributions to GIS technologies.

**Warren S. Eller** is Chair of the Department of Public Management and an associate professor at John Jay College of Criminal Justice; he holds an

MPA from West Virginia University and a PhD from Texas A&M University. His research focuses on emergency and disaster management with special interest in vulnerable populations.

**Daniel A. Griffith** is an Ashbel Smith Professor of Geospatial Information Sciences at the University of Texas at Dallas, with a geography career spanning 40 years, is the recipient of many honors, including Foreign Fellow of the Royal Society of Canada. He has published 20 books/monographs and over 320 other pieces, including 167 articles in major refereed geography, economics, epidemiology, regional science, statistics, and mathematics journals. He has delivered colloquia and keynote lectures through the world, most recently at Peking University, China's premier educational institution. Part of his recent spatial statistical research focuses on space-time data analysis methodology.

**Stuart E. Hamilton** is Graduate GIS Director and Associate Professor of Geography at Salisbury University in Maryland. He is a Fellow of the Royal Geographical Society (FRGS) and a certified GIS Professional (GISP). Stuart has published numerous book chapters and peer-reviewed articles in major refereed journals, including the *Annals* of the AAG, *Nature Climate Change*, *Global Ecology and Biogeography*, and *Global Environmental Change*. In addition, he served as a Prometeo Fellow in the Ecuadorian Ministry of the Environment, examining issues of land cover change. His research interests are the human dimensions of environmental change, with a focus on coastal forests and climate change. He maintains a laboratory in Jinja, Uganda that examines the role of Lake Victoria in providing food security to the region.

**Trevor M. Harris** is Eberly Distinguished Professor of Geography at West Virginia University. He obtained his doctorate from the University of Hull, England, and specializes in Geographic Information Science. Dr. Harris has published over 60 peer-reviewed articles in leading journals and four edited books. He has made over 190 research presentations at national and international conferences. Dr. Harris's research interests focus on Geographic Information Science, including immersive GIS, 3D GIS, GIS integrated virtual reality, and 3D modeling; deep mapping, exploratory spatial data analysis, the geospatial semantic web; the spatial humanities; critical GIS and participatory GIS. Dr. Harris has undertaken numerous external funded research exceeding $18 million in awards over the past two decades, which have involved the extensive development of regional GIS databases. Dr. Harris co-directs the State GIS Technical Center, the GeoVirtual Laboratory, and the Virtual Center for Spatial Humanities.

**Jonathon D. Henderson** is Associate Director of Research at Central Washington University in Ellensburg. He holds a PhD in Education from the University of Oregon and a master's degree in conflict and dispute resolution through the University of Oregon School of Law. In addition, Dr. Henderson holds certificates in data science, instruction design, and multiple programming languages.

**L. Neal Holly** is Assistant Director of Postsecondary and Workforce Development for the Education of the States. Previously, Dr. Holly was Vice Chancellor for Policy and Planning for the West Virginia Higher Education Policy Commission and the West Virginia Council for Community and Technical College Education. Dr. Holly serves as Chief Information Officer, where his duties include managing public institution data collection and providing technical support for the distribution of state financial aid programs. Dr. Holly also advises the Commission, Council, and legislature on state and national policy issues related to higher education. In addition, he is responsible for statutory reporting, strategic planning, partnerships with other state agencies and national postsecondary organizations, and the Commission and Council's research agenda. Holly earned a BA in History from Wingate University, an MA in Higher Education Administration with a focus on student development from Appalachian State University, and received his PhD in Higher Education Administration from the College of William and Mary. His research has centered on the interaction between state higher education policy and low-income student postsecondary access and success.

**Todd A. Jordan** grew up in Kansas City and holds a PhD in Public Affairs from the University of Texas at Dallas, where he focused on qualitative and quantitative research in organizational change, public policy, and city planning. Todd joined United Way of Wyandotte County in 2015 as Director of Community Impact. For two years, Todd was responsible for monitoring and evaluating program performance and administering emergency assistance funding, as well as engaging in collaborative planning processes around health, education, and income. As of 2017, Todd is the President/CEO of United Way of Wyandotte County.

**Benjamin Kennady** is a software developer in the Texas energy industry with a Master of Science in Geospatial Information Sciences from the University of Texas at Dallas. He has worked on numerous GIS applications in North and South America. Ben specializes in using open source GIS technology to create automated workflows and web maps. His interests include the development of raster spatial solutions to better understand environmental issues impacting the world today. In his free time, Ben enjoys sailing and traveling.

**H. Franklin LaFone** is Senior GIS and Geography Applications Developer at the West Virginia GIS Technical Center. He has degrees in computer science and political science from West Virginia University and in international relations from Syracuse University. His career as a software engineer has spanned over ten years, primarily in the field of Geographic Information Science. He is currently a geography doctoral student at West Virginia University focusing upon virtual spaces, virtual and augmented reality, and new frontiers in Geographic Information Science, as well as core research areas of exploratory spatial data analysis, Internet mapping applications, and neogeography. Frank is a founding member and former president of the West Virginia Association of Geospatial Professionals. Besides his professional and research interests, Frank is Co-Founder and Co-Host of VerySpatial, LLC, a new media company that focuses on sharing information about geography and geospatial technologies. VerySpatial is the longest-running geography podcast in the world at over 13 years of continuous episodes. Frank is a past recipient of the Special Achievement in GIS Award from ESRI.

**Cheyanne Manning** is the campus cartographer at Central Washington University in Ellensburg, WA. She has a BA in Geography and a GIS certificate from Central Washington University. She uses GIS as a tool to manage the built and natural elements of the campus and to plan for future campus expansion. Her work involves collaboration across department and with other agencies and governments, and she helps to support students using GIS.

**Marco Millones** is an assistant professor in the Department of Geography at the University of Mary Washington. He has published more than 20 peer-reviewed articles and book chapters, including in the *Annals* of the AAG, *Global Environmental Change*, and the *International Journal of Remote Sensing*. His research focuses on applications of geospatial analysis for the study of human-induced landscape change, spatial accuracy, spatio-temporal modeling, and public policy. His regional expertise includes the United States, Mexico, Ecuador, and Peru.

**Benoit Parmentier** is a researcher and data scientist with the National Socio-Environmental Synthesis Center (SESYNC) based at the University of Maryland. He has published scientific articles in *Landscape and Urban Planning*, *International Journal of Climatology*, *Remote Sensing of the Environment*, and *Scientific Data Nature*. He is broadly interested in landscape change and global environmental change. Some of his research topics include tracking fire and land cover change, studying landscape changes in urban–rural transition areas, mapping flooding, producing environmental and climate datasets, studying climate teleconnections, and examining flows for sustainability studies.

**Sterling Quinn** is an assistant professor in the Department of Geography at Central Washington University. Dr Quinn researches the social influences behind the production and use of crowdsourced geographic information. Previously he worked as a software engineer.

**Rebecca Rose** is a research analyst for the Department of Institutional Effectiveness at Central Washington University in Ellensburg, WA. She holds a master's degree in experimental psychology from Central Washington

University and a Bachelor of Science in Psychology from Idaho State University.

**Daniel Servian** has been working with Geographic Information Systems for 15 years. Since 2012, he has been a GIS Analyst/Information System Specialist for West Virginia University. He focused on Geographic Information Sciences while obtaining his Master of Science in Recreation, Parks, and Tourism Resources at West Virginia University. His current research interests include exploratory spatial data analysis and indoor location analysis.

**Cy Smith** joined the State of Oregon in 2000. He is responsible for statewide coordination of all GIS activities in state, regional and local governments, helping to assure the elimination of redundant activities. He is a member of the FGDC's National Geospatial Advisory Committee. He is the past president of the National States Geographic Information Council, past president of the Urban Regional Information Systems Association, and Founding Chair of the Coalition of Geospatial Organizations, a coalition of 13 geospatial professional organizations representing over 170,000 members. Cy was GIS Manager for Olathe, Kansas for four years, Kansas State GIS Coordinator for three years, and a GIS consultant for PlanGraphics, Inc. for four years.

**Michael P. Strager** is a professor of spatial analysis in the School of Natural Resources in the Davis College at West Virginia University. His research focus is in using appropriate spatial and decision analysis techniques to aid in the analysis and management of natural resources. He has applied Geographic Information Systems, spatial analysis, and remote sensing for forestry, water quality, wildlife, recreation, and conservation planning. Much of his work has resulted in the development of spatial decision support to aid in prioritizing areas, evaluating alternatives, and examining trade-offs when managing natural resources.

# Section I

# Introduction

# 1 Introduction

*Nicolas A. Valcik*

## Goal of This Text

This book was developed to provide the profession with cutting-edge research, applied research, and practitioner uses and topics for Geospatial Information Systems (GIS). The editor of this book has recruited a variety of professionals who represent the best of the GIS field to provide research on and knowledge to the field of GIS. The number of topics that could have been included in this book were infinite, so the editors had to choose what they perceived to be the greatest need for GIS in the realm of public and nonprofit organizations. This was a difficult task for the editors, since the need for using GIS in the public and nonprofit sectors is great and the resources for those areas (e.g. funding) is usually very limited. The editors hope that the topics presented in this book can be duplicated by public and nonprofit organizations to assist those types of organizations in better decision-making by having more information through adding geospatial data to the decision-making process.

For academic and applied researchers in the GIS profession, the editors are enthusiastic about the chapters provided by the recruited authors, since those research topics will add knowledge to the profession. While compiling, developing, and editing a book for publication is a large amount of work, the editors are hopeful that the book will be used by researchers, practitioners, and students for years to come. GIS is not in the past or the present; it is the future for public and nonprofit organizations. The challenge for the profession going forward is to avoid operating in a siloed manner and to take an interdisciplinary approach not only to research, but also to training up and coming professionals who are not familiar with GIS on how to use such a powerful tool. This endeavor's success will determine how public and nonprofit administrators perceive GIS. If successful, the GIS profession has the ability to affect public and nonprofit organizations positively for decades to come.

## Birth of a Discipline

The traditional fields of geography, geology, computer science, engineering, agriculture, education, and yes, even the social sciences, as well as other fields of study, have traditionally been siloed from one another. There are few tools, mechanisms, methodologies, or research that could have unified so many fields to create much of the interdisciplinary research activities seen in current times as Geographic Information Systems, better known as GIS. Many strides in technology and innovative thought have allowed GIS to exist and progress.

While working for the government in Canada, Roger Tomlinson published the paper "A Geographic Information System for Regional Planning" in 1968, which was the birth of the modern technology of GIS (ESRI, 2012). Before Tomlinson's paper, maps were produced by hand, were labor intensive, and could not be analyzed for patterns or have data layered in a manner in which correlations in the spatial data could be discovered. Using a layering approach, data can now be layered from several different disciplines to begin analysis for correlation from one dataset to another, in order to triangulate data for accuracy and discovery purposes.

## Technology

As with any new tool or system, GIS has evolved considerably over time. In 1968, when Roger Tomlinson was initially writing about GIS, technology in the form of computers were still bulky and limited by what computers could accomplish. In terms of capability, mainframes in use in 1968 still used punch cards to input data and programming into the system, which was required for an output. These early computers, which evolved from the 1940s British Colossus computer and the United States computer ENIAC, had large hardware for storage and processing; required a considerable amount of energy to process as well as air-conditioning to reduce the heat from the computer; and had almost no memory.

In the mid-1950s to the mid-1960s, computers finally had internal memory, which ranged from 64K to 96K. While this memory by today's standards (2018) appears woefully inadequate, the memory available at that time allowed for processing of more complex data to perform different types of equations, data processing, and visual renderings. When Tomlinson wrote his paper in 1968, the first micro-computer was still six years away from being developed. It would not be until the 1980s that personal computers became capable of processing visual renderings and data, which would eventually lead to the modern GIS capabilities that are known and used currently (2018).

Until GIS was developed, the closest software with visual capability was Computer Aided Design, also known as CAD. CAD could trace its lineage all the way back to the 1960s in the United States (Coons and Mann, 1960). CAD is a visual software with limited ability to tie in large datasets for data analysis. It is highly tied to the architecture and construction of buildings, representing structures to scale in a series of line drawings. The latest versions of CAD (2018) can utilize GPS coordinates as well as conduct 3D renderings for engineering schematics. That being stated, GIS is able to layer multiple datasets that utilize a host of server platforms to interact with satellite imagery, which allows for complex analysis and mapping to be conducted over a wide region. With the advent of GIS, the field of geography has taken on new importance and relevance for interacting with scientific and academic areas of research and applied uses that could only be imagined prior to GIS's development.

## Interdisciplinary Approach

With the introduction of GIS, many fields of research suddenly had a mechanism, a methodology, and a tool to analyze different types of data in ways that, prior to 1968, could not have been foreseen or imagined. GIS has effectively added a new methodology to research with a spatial component in addition to qualitative and quantitative data. In addition to the academic disciplines working with GIS, practitioners have also expanded the use of GIS to research and resolve issues in the public arena. Practitioner areas encompassing public health, city planning, natural resources, and central appraisal districts are just a few areas that use GIS on a wide scale. To triangulate data for research, researchers have traditionally relied on essentially two methodologies: qualitative and quantitative. With the advent of GIS, spatial data should be considered a third methodology that can be used to triangulate data in a mixed methods approach.

The practitioner use of spatial data can be witnessed as early as 1854, with John Snow's mapping of a cholera outbreak in London (Kukaswadia, 2013; Science Museum, 2017). Not only is John Snow the founder of epidemiology, but one could argue he is also the founder of GIS due to his technique of using mapping with a dataset to triangulate the cause of the cholera epidemic. If Snow had simply used a dataset of addresses for the cholera cases, there is a very good chance a pattern would not have been detected for the cause of the illness. However, since Snow used not only a dataset of addresses (obtained through qualitative means) but also a map to spatially analyze the data, he could triangulate the cause of the cholera outbreak, which turned out to be the water pump located in the area (Kukaswadia, 2013; Science Museum, 2017). Using different data sources and methodologies allowed Snow to use quantitative, qualitative, and spatial analysis to triangulate the data and thereby determine the source of a public health issue.

With new public health academic programs being added nationwide (2018), GIS has proven to be an important tool for those researchers and students performing data analysis and research in the public health arena. Public health practitioners have used GIS to track outbreaks of Ebola, malaria, measles, industrial waste exposure, chronic heart problems. and river blindness caused by parasitic worms (ABC News, 2014; Hay et al., 2011; CDC, 2015; Willingham and Helft, 2012; Fitzpatrick et al., 2012; Chemical and Engineering News, 2008). Environmental professionals have been using GIS to track radioactive fallout or contaminated radioactive areas at Fukushima and Chernobyl (Krivoruchoko, 2015; Fukushima Update, 2013). Homeland security and emergency management professionals have been using GIS to determine fallout areas if nuclear reactors are breached and what areas of the population would be potentially impacted (Ayres et al., 2006). GIS has even been used recently to track shark and crocodile attacks in an effort to mitigate the possibility of attacks along certain areas of coastline and riverine areas (Tracking Sharks, 2014; Everything Dinosaur, 2013). Practitioners in agriculture and natural resources have been using GIS to track rabies outbreaks across different parts of the United States (State of Texas, 2014).

## Uses in the Social Sciences and Education Research

However, these are not the only academic fields or professional areas to use GIS. Many traditionally non-technology-based curriculum and research activities have now turned to integrating GIS for research or practitioner-based activities. Criminal justice, public administration, and higher education are all fields both academically and professionally where GIS has begun to be utilized for practitioner use and academic research. As will be seen throughout the book, practitioners and researchers alike are continuing to explore how to use GIS innovatively to accomplish certain research goals or to conduct operational analysis for public organizations. In an assessment conducted for the Kentucky College Coaching program in 2014, the use of GIS led to a discovery that not all of the success data was being captured for the program (Valcik and Scruton, 2015). This led the program to understand that there were gaps in the database, which was causing the program to underreport success when compared to the control group, which was not being college coached in those geographic areas where college coaches were located (Valcik and Scruton, 2015). Without the use of GIS, this gap in the data would not have been discovered.

## Public Sector

### *Why Is It Important?*

Throughout this book, there are sections dedicated to Academic and Theoretical Research GIS Topics at a higher level, Applied Research Using GIS, and Practitioner Use of GIS in Public and Nonprofit Organizations. Within each of these sections, the chapters discuss how GIS can be used in different areas to provide valuable information to academics, practitioners, and students in the public sector. Providing cutting-edge information to the public sector is crucial, as the public sector is involved in a wide range of areas of operation and impacts the citizenry on a large scale. If GIS can provide additional information to the decision-makers in the public sector, this will serve the public well if decisions are made by using more data to arrive at the optimum solution. In Chapters 3 and 6, the authors focus on using GIS for infrastructure purposes and discuss the issues of using crowdsourcing data, which will allow researchers and practitioners greater ability to create additional layers for the purpose of triangulating research data.

### *Municipalities, Counties, and State*

Unfortunately, the public sector has long lagged behind in using GIS. This is due to many different reasons and has negatively impacted the decision-making process. In local government, for example, GIS was not the tool of choice; for decades, city planning has largely relied on CAD. With limited funds, municipalities, for example, were slow to adopt GIS; in the 1990s, GIS was expensive and public organizations had money invested not only in equipment but also in personnel able to use CAD. Even as far back as 1996, the City of Duncanville was using GIS for a wide variety of purposes, including economic development (Valcik, 1996). During the same time period, the City of McKinney was unable to afford GIS software or personnel to use the software (Valcik, 1996), and thus still relied on CAD software; this limited the type of information available to decision-makers that could be geo-referenced or was spatial in nature (Valcik, 1996). One area where GIS usage has increased has been in police departments, where GIS provides crime statistics and intelligence for officers on patrol. This intelligence allows for the distribution of limited resources (e.g. police officers) to intervene in high-crime areas or to target specific criminal activity (e.g. burglaries). This type of intelligence allows decision-makers to use surgical precision in leveraging not only resources but also departmental policies. GIS can also produce an operational map that displays jurisdictional information, such as where police officers have arrest powers.

For economic development, GIS is invaluable, since there is a large amount of data that can be tied into the shapefiles, including central appraisal district information on property values. This allows decision-makers to visualize the locations of valuable property that are prime for redevelopment. For city planning, this type of information is critical, as how an area is zoned for construction is an important consideration for what types of economic development should be sought.

State and county public entities have a different focus than their municipal counterparts. Chapters 13 and 14 focus on using GIS at an enterprise level as well as supporting the use of GIS information for the community's benefit. In King County, Washington, there is a move to create regional data agreements with cities and counties so that efforts are not duplicated. At the state level, GIS can be invaluable for researchers and practitioners because patterns can be established to analyze data regarding the environment to demographic patterns changing throughout the state over time. An example of GIS usage at the state level is Chapter 12's topic of the creation of the trail inventory in West Virginia, which has to take into account the geography of the state where the trails are located.

### *Education*

For the education sector, GIS can be used for a wide range of purposes, which will be described in more detail in Chapters 7, 9, 10, and 15. Higher education, for example, can utilize GIS for enrollment management, alumni development, facility planning, scheduling, homeland security, and emergency management, to name just a few purposes. Since state funding has been drastically reduced for many higher education institutions across the United States, it is necessary to make decisions with as much information as possible so that upper administrators can come to fiscally sound decisions. For K–12 education areas of research, GIS can be used to detect patterns in student programs (e.g. college programs) throughout a state or a district in order for specialized pilot programs or state initiatives to determine the impact upon the student population.

### *Wildlife and the Environment*

GIS allows for tracking of a variety of flora and fauna throughout an area. For example, an endangered species of plants can be tracked to see if the habitat around those life forms needs to be protected or if the area is being encroached on by human development. This type of GIS use can also plot possible interactions between humans and animals where tensions can arise, along with diseases that can be transmitted from animals from humans (e.g. Lyme disease). The use of GIS also can provide information to project and determine if development of an area will create hazards for the environment. Chapters 2, 5, and 8 provide GIS research in relation to disasters (both natural and man-made) and consider how those disasters impacted the environment. Similar research has been conducted on the impact of radioactivity releases from nuclear reactors on the environment and residents around those incidents (e.g. Chernobyl and Fukushima).

### *Homeland Security and Disaster Response*

GIS research on homeland security and disaster response topics has only increased over the years. In Chapter 4, the authors discuss how GIS is used to gain operational intelligence to predict the most likely areas for a HAZMAT incident to take place. Using this type of GIS operational data, disaster response professionals can preposition logistics for a HAZMAT accident so that first responders can react in a shorter timeframe. Other GIS uses for homeland security and disaster response could potentially include mapping down infrastructure nationwide (e.g. electrical grid) in order to provide better protection to those types of infrastructure.

## Summary

Public organizations may have been slower to adopt GIS, but those entities are now embracing GIS and using the software in new ways to answer effectively questions that are now being raised. The broad spectrum of responsibilities charged to public organizations is staggering, especially when taking into account the different types and sizes of not only public but also nonprofit organizations. In the age of technology, the decision-makers of these types of organizations will need as much information as possible in order to make sound decisions.

As Herbert Simon stated with the theory of bounded rationality, there is only so much time an administrator has in making a decision, such that only the most likely decisions can be considered (Vasu, Stewart and Garson, 1998). There is simply not enough time in the decision-making process to consider every single option that might be workable. GIS, however, can provide an upper level administrator with intelligence to assist an administrator to make a rational and sound decision by assisting an administrator with additional information that will help on choosing an optimum decision. GIS is the future for both public organizations and practitioners to use in addressing age-old issues with cutting-edge techniques and research.

## References

ABC News, 2014. "Ebola Interactive Map Shows Virus Spread", August 5. Retrieved on June 6, 2019. https://abcnews.go.com/Health/ebola-interactive-map-shows-virus-spread/story?id=24853012

Ayres, Amy Sinatra, Blanton, Jesse D., Manangan, Arie, Manangan, Jamie, Hanlon, Cathleen A., Slate, Dennis and Rupprecht, Charles E., 2006. "Development of a GIS-Based, Real-Time Internet Mapping Tool for Rabies Surveillance", *International Journal of Health Geographics*. Volume 5, 47. Retrieved on February 10, 2015. www.ij-healthgeographics.com/content/5/1/47

CDC, 2015. "Geographic Information Systems (GIS) at CDC", *Centers for Disease Control and Prevention*. Retrieved on February 10, 2015. www.cdc.gov/gis/

Chemical and Engineering News, 2008. "Happy Birthday Love Canal", *American Chemical Society*. Retrieved on February 10, 2015. https://pubs.acs.org/cen/government/86/8646gov2.html

Coons, S.A. and Mann, R.W., 1960. "Computer-Aided Design Related to the Engineering Design Process", *Massachusetts Institute of Technology*. 8436-TM-5, October. Contract No. AF-33(600)-40604. Retrieved on March 24, 2017. http://images.designworldonline.com.s3.amazonaws.com/CADhistory/8436-TM-5.pdf

ESRI, 2012. "The 50th Anniversary of GIS", *ArcNews*. Fall. Retrieved on March 24, 2017. www.esri.com/news/arcnews/fall12articles/the-fiftieth-anniversary-of-gis.html

Everything Dinosaur, 2013. "Body Recovered After Saltwater Crocodile Attack", *Everything Dinosaur*. Retrieved on February 10, 2015. http://blog.everythingdinosaur.co.uk/blog/_archives/2013/08/27/body-recovered-after-saltwater-crocodile-attack.html

Fitzpatrick, G., Ward, M., Ennis, O., Johnson, H., Cotter, S., Carr, M.J., O'Riordan, B., Waters, A., Hassan, J., Connell, J., Hall, W., Clarke, A., Murphy, H. and Fitzgerald, M., 2012. "Use of a Geographic Information System to Map Cases of Measles in Real-Time During the Outbreak in Dublin, Ireland, 2011", *Eurosurveillance*, Volume 17, 49, December 6.

Fukushima Update, 2013. "New Map of Radioactive Iodine Released from Fukushima Daiichi", *Fukushima Update*. Retrieved on February 10, 2015. http://fukushimaupdate.com/new-map-of-radioactive-iodine-released-from-fukushima-daiichi/

Hay, Simon I., Guerra, Carlos A., Tatem, Andrew J., Noor, Abdisalan M. and Snow, Robert W., 2011. "The Global Distribution and Population at Risk of Malaria: Past,

Present and Future", *United States Library of Medicine*. National Institutes of Health. Retrieved on February 9, 2005. www.ncbi.nlm.nih.gov/pmc/articles/PMC3145123/

Krivoruchoko, Konstantin, 2015. "GIS and Geostatistics: Spatial Analysis of Chernobyl's Consequences in Belarus", *Environmental Systems Research Institute*. Retrieved on February 10, 2015. www.ncgia.ucsb.edu/conf/sa_workshop/papers/krivoruchko_old.html

Kukaswadia, Atif, 2013. "John Snow—The First Epidemiologist", *Public Health Perspectives*. Retrieved on February 9, 2013. http://blogs.plos.org/publichealth/2013/03/11/john-snow-the-first-epidemiologist/

Science Museum, 2017. "John Snow (1813–1858)", *Science Museum*. Retrieved on March 24, 2017. www.sciencemuseum.org.uk/broughttolife/people/johnsnow

State of Texas, 2014. "Zoonosis Control Branch: 2014 Vaccination Distribution Areas", Department of State Health Services, Retrieved on June 6, 2019. https://dshs.texas.gov/uploadedImages/Content/Prevention_and_Preparedness/IDCU/health/zoonosis/mapping/maps/orvp2014.jpg

Tracking Sharks, 2014. "2014 Shark Bites/Attacks 2014", *Tracking Sharks*. Retrieved on February 12, 2014. www.trackingsharks.com/wp-content/uploads/2014/01/shark_bite_2014_map.jpg

Valcik, Nicolas A., 1996. City of McKinney Intern, City Manager's Office. City of Duncanville, Intern, Economic Development.

Valcik, Nicolas A. and Scruton, Kimberly E., 2015. "Investing in the Future: Evaluating the Kentucky College Coaching Program 2012–2014", *Kentucky Campus Compact*. Retrieved on March 24, 2017. http://planning.wvu.edu/files/d/e5a18c32-0f43-4ba6-b705-a30f5c2a79c0/kcc-executive-summary-2015-revised-4-2-2015.pdf

Vasu, Michael L., Stewart, Debra W. and Garson, David G., 1998. *Organizational Behavior and Public Management: Third Edition Revised and Expanded*. Taylor and Francis/CRC Press, New York.

Willingham, Emily and Helft, Laura, 2012. "Tracking Disease Outbreaks", *PBS Nova*. Retrieved on February 10, 2015. www.pbs.org/wgbh/nova/body/disease-outbreaks.html

# Section II

# Academic and Theoretical Research GIS Topics

# 2 Hurricane Rita's Impact on Vegetation

## A Spatio-Temporal Statistical Approach to Characterizing Abrupt Change in, and Potential Disaster Management for, Target Areas

*Daniel A. Griffith, Yongwan Chun, Marco Millones, Benoit Parmentier, and Stuart E. Hamilton*

### Introduction

Millones et al. (2019) furnish a contextualization of this chapter in the existing literature, with special reference to hurricanes. Hazard events and natural disasters, such as hurricanes, can have short- and long-term impacts on socio-ecological/coupled human–environmental systems. They can disrupt the current state of a system, potentially causing visible and quantifiable human, economic, and ecological loss. Extreme events also can have longer term effects in terms of both biophysical structure and landscape functioning, as well as in the socio-economic infrastructure of a region. Standardized Earth Observation time series data produced by remotely sensed Earth Observation Systems (EOS) are now commonplace and may be used in an immediate aftermath for emergency and disaster relief management. In particular, high resolution products, suce or other disaster monitoring (Marghany and Mansor 2017). However, coarser spatial resolution EOS products with high temporal resolution (e.g. MODIS) also offer insights and opportunities to understand longer term effects by providing complementary information for characterization and impact assessment of extreme events, as well as for monitoring recovery processes in affected regions.

In this chapter, we seize an opportunity provided by EOS spatio-temporal data series in order to assess the impact of Hurricane Rita on the coastline wetlands of Louisiana. We draw on the space-beats-time (SBT) methodological framework (Parmentier et al. 2017) to exploit the following statistical principle observed after disruptive events in a spatio-temporal time series: in the aftermath of disasters and other abrupt events, past conditions, which typically provide the best predictor for present and future conditions, display substantial decline in their predictive power. During these brief post-disaster periods, geographic context (i.e. neighboring conditions) becomes a better predictor.

These brief periods (named SBT windows), during which spatial observations outperform temporal observations, can be established quantitatively in time and mapped in geographic space. These visualizations can provide promising improvements and alternatives for the identification of impacted areas, critical recovery periods that are relevant for both rapid response and longer-term post-disaster recovery management.

## A Case Study: The Coastal Louisiana NDVI Before and After Hurricane Rita

In this case study, we examine the use of the SBT framework to predict and study the normalized difference vegetation index (NDVI) before and after the arrival of Hurricane Rita, a record-breaking tropical cyclone in Louisiana (LA). This hurricane had the fourth lowest pressure of any storm ever recorded in the Atlantic Basin, reached Category 5 status within the Gulf of Mexico, and spurred at least 90 tornadoes, breaking the record for the most tornadoes ever recorded in a single event in this region (Knabb et al. 2006). Rita made landfall as a Category 3 hurricane at approximately 0740 UTC on September 24 in southwest Louisiana, between Johnson's Bayou and Sabina Pass near the Texas border (Figure 2.1). It then moved north, following a path roughly tracing the Louisiana–Texas border, and finally weakened to a tropical storm by the early hours of September 25 (Knabb et al. 2006).

Maximum sustained winds at landfall were 71 knots (kt), with peak 3-second gusts around landfall recorded at approximately 100 kt (Knabb et al. 2006). Only an extremely small portion of coastal southwest Louisiana experienced Category 3 winds, with most places experiencing Category 2 or below; due to the large size of this tropical storm (e.g. it had a 30 nautical mile eye diameter by 0740 UTC on September 23), winds extended far from its eye (Knabb et al. 2006). Accompanying storm surge was recorded at 14 feet above NAVD 88 (North American Vertical Datum of 1988), and the surge was recorded to have risen at rates greater than 5 feet per hour (McGee et al. 2006). This claim ties in well with the maximum 15 foot surge recorded by the United States (US) Federal Emergency Management Agency (FEMA) at Lake Cameron (Knabb et al. 2006). The Cameron Parish communities of Holly Beach, Cameron, Creole, and Grand Cheniere had almost total property loss, with numerous other communities, such as Lake Charles, Grand Lake, Pecan Island, and Calcasieu Lake, suffering a substantial loss of property (Knabb et al. 2006). The final estimate of property losses, both insured and uninsured, is calculated to be approximately $12 billion (2005 US dollars) (Knabb et al. 2006).

The lack of direct casualties, generally estimated at seven, is most likely attributable to the mass evacuation before the storm: an estimated more than 2.5 million people evacuated from Texas alone before the hurricane (Zachria and Patel 2006). Indeed, in Texas, over 83% of deaths were a result of the evacuation process as opposed to the actual storm (Zachria and Patel 2006), in

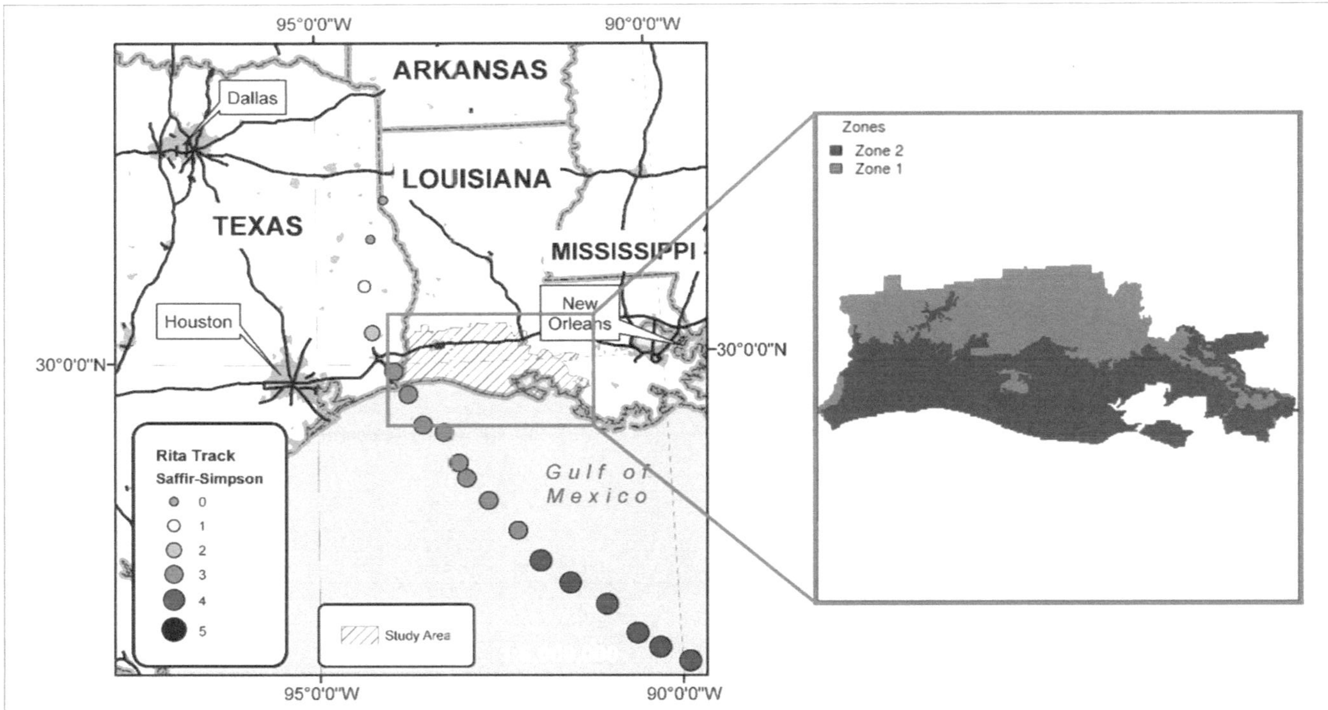


*Figure 2.1* The study area. Left: (a) the location (striped area) and hurricane path, including the Saffir-Simpson magnitude (graduated circles) of Rita's landfall in September 2005. Right: (b) the FEMA flood zones: Zone 1 was flooded; Zone 2 was not flooded.

what is reported as the second-largest ever United States peace-time evacuation. Such evacuations were likely partially driven by the events of Hurricane Katrina, which had preceded Hurricane Rita by a few weeks. Despite limited human loss, economic and ecological impacts were considerable (Morton and Barras 2011).

## Data and Methods

Following the SBT methodology (Parmentier et al. 2017), we: 1) identify the spatial and temporal footprints and path of Hurricane Rita in the Louisiana coastline (Figures 2.1a); 2) compile a dataset based on NDVI to monitor vegetation greenness change as a proxy for the hurricane's impact; 3) estimate prediction models with separate spatial and temporal components; and 4) compare each model's performance (i.e. error) and interpret results using the SBT framework (Figure 2.2). Overall, SBT can be understood as a method that measures and maps abrupt change and recovery. However, unlike other change methods, SBT does not rely on the magnitude of change in an analyzed variable; rather, it exploits the relative interplay between the spatial and temporal components of data (i.e. spatial and temporal autocorrelation).

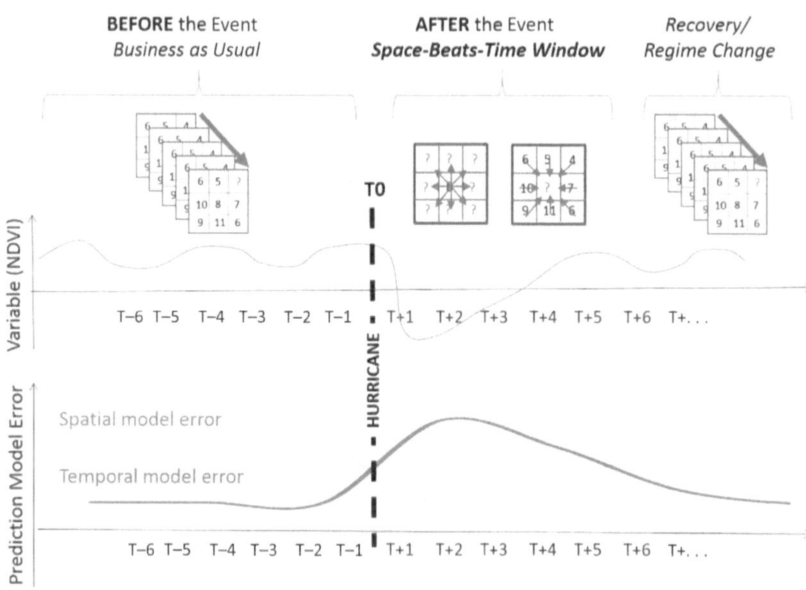


*Figure 2.2* An SBT event hypothetical trajectory based on a hurricane and the NDVI. T denotes time steps with available observations before (T−6 to T−1) and after (T+1 onward) following a disruptive event or intervention, such as a hurricane (T0). The SBT window between T+1 and T+4 corresponds to a period of time during which spatial error is substantially lower than temporal error.

***Data***

The NDVI is a commonly used EOS derived index that serves as a proxy indicator variable for vegetation change. NDVI measures the greenness/health levels of vegetation based on the difference between near-infrared and red reflectance. It has been used numerous times to assess vegetation damage produced by hurricane winds and flooding (e.g. Rogan et al. 2011; Parmentier et al. 2017), including assessments of Hurricane Rita destruction (e.g. Rodgers et al. 2009).

We compiled a spatio-temporal data series collected by the Moderate Resolution Imaging Spectroradiometer (MODIS) sensor using the 1-kilometer (km) vegetation product corresponding to MOD13A2 (Huete et al. 2002). NDVI tiles matching the study area (h09v05, h09v06, h10v05, h10v06) were mosaicked and cropped into a single raster stack for the 2002–2010 time period. We removed low quality and cloud-affected observations using MODIS quality control flags. The processed dataset has 34,568 pixels per time period, and 230 16-day time steps.

***Methods: Temporal and Spatial Prediction Models***

We created two separate prediction models: one model based on preceding observations in time to generate temporal-only predictions and another model based on neighboring observations in space to generate spatial-only predictions (i.e. interpolation). Neither model used covariates. NDVI was the single variable utilized. The temporal-only model is based on a variant of the time series autoregressive integrated moving average (ARIMA) model specification that includes seasonal terms. The temporal model generates predictions by leveraging the temporal correlation present in neighboring points in time (autoregressive regression [AR]) as well as temporal autocorrelation in residuals and trends (Griffith 2010). The spatial model relies on spatial autocorrelation via a geographic lag variable to include geographic neighborhood effects (Cliff and Ord 1981). General model formulations are described by the following two equations:

$$y_{t+1} = \alpha y_t + e_t \quad (1)$$

where $y_{t+1}$ is NDVI, α is a temporal autocorrelation parameter, and $e_t$ is an error term, with $t$ indexing the month of an image; and

$$y_i = \lambda \sum_{j=1}^{n} w_{ij} y_j + e_i \quad (2)$$

where $y_i$ is NDVI, $\lambda$ is a spatial autocorrelation parameter, $w_{ij}$ is the spatial weight contained in the spatial weight matrix **W**, and $e_i$ is the error term, with $i$ and $j$ indexing location in an image.

We used the R computing software to process data and perform estimation. The *raster* and *sp* packages were used for data wrangling, and the *spdep* package provided specific implementations of the spatial regression model. We relied on the *xts* and *zoo* packages to manipulate time series and performed ARIMA estimation using the *forecast* package (Bivand 2006; Hyndman and Khandakar 2007).

### *Model Performance Assessment*

We computed the mean absolute error (MAE) quantities separately for both temporal and spatial models, in order to compare their performance via MAE trajectory graphs. The MAE is easy to interpret and is model independent (Pontius et al. 2008; Willmott and Matsuura 2005). We identified an SBT window in which the temporal model MAE is substantially higher than the spatial model MAE. In addition, we used flood zones based on FEMA post-hurricane analysis (Figure 2.1b) to stratify the study area and calculated the MAE separately for each flood zone and for each model. Our expectation was that SBT effects would be stronger where flooding was present (i.e. Zone 1).

### *Interpretation of Prediction Performance and Residual Maps*

Using the SBT framework (Figure 2.2, lower panel graph), we identified the SBT window as the time period during which the MAE in temporal-only predictions (dark gray line) surpasses the MAE in spatial-only predictions (light gray line). Our expectation was that the MAE plots initially would show the temporal MAE below the spatial MAE prior to Hurricane Rita's landfall. In the immediate aftermath of this hurricane, the temporal MAE would increase sharply, surpassing the MAE for the spatial model. Given the nature of the environmental conditions in Louisiana and the sensitivity of NDVI to capture any green up in vegetation, we expected the temporal model to return to dominance (i.e. the spatial MAE surpasses the temporal MAE) a few time steps after the hurricane experience, marking the closing of the SBT window.

Residual maps from spatial- and temporal-only model predictions (Figure 2.4, bottom panels) provide a visual identification of areas where the SBT effect is stronger and its window is more conspicuous. These two features are the geographic counterparts to MAE plots (Figure 2.3). The expectation was that areas identified with stronger SBT effects would coincide with the flooded areas of Figure 2.1b (Zone 1), and that this effect would weaken over time (i.e. a closing of the SBT window). More substantially, these high residual areas of strong SBT effects can be thought of as potential areas to be targeted for disaster management. We derived potential target areas from the SBT residual maps by computing the difference between temporal and spatial residual maps and then standardized them. Next, these standardized difference maps were thresholded, using one and two standard deviations, to generate potential target areas such as those shown in Figure 2.5 (Area 2 is a higher priority for targeting).

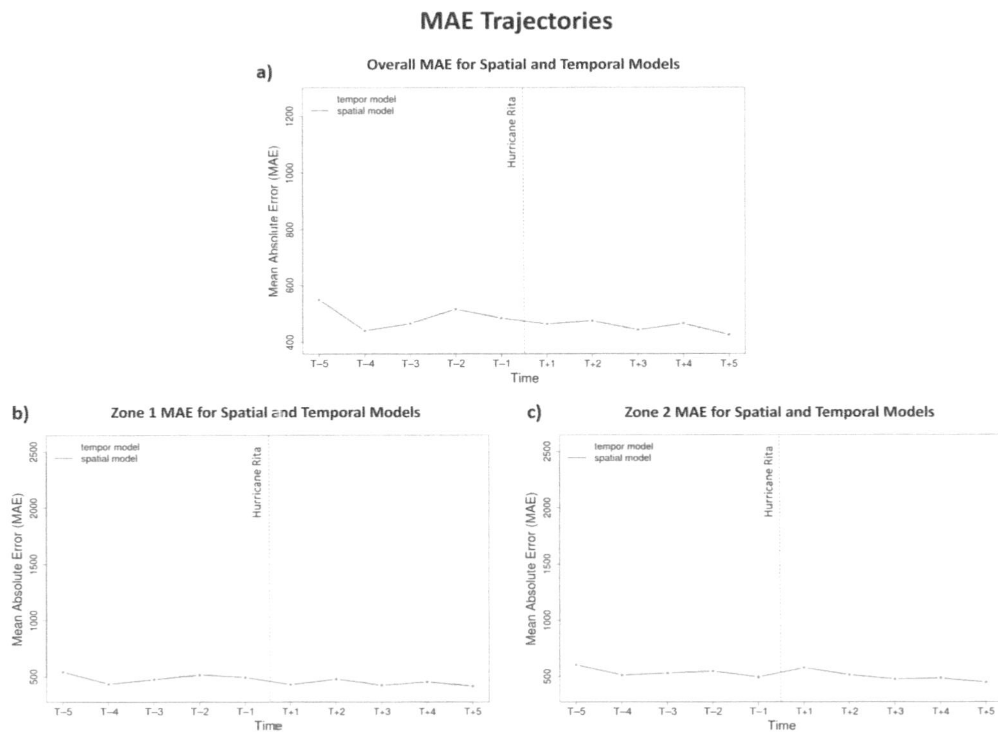


*Figure 2.3* Model performance based on MAE trajectory plots for the spatial (dark) and the temporal (light) models. A higher MAE implies a higher error and therefore lower model performance. The horizontal axis corresponds to time (16-day steps). The vertical axis corresponds to NDVI units. Top: (a) the overall MAE for the study area before and after the hurricane. Bottom: The MAE by FEMA flood Zones; (b) Zone 1 and (c) Zone 2, before (T−5 through T−1) and after (T+1 through T+5) the event (dotted vertical line).

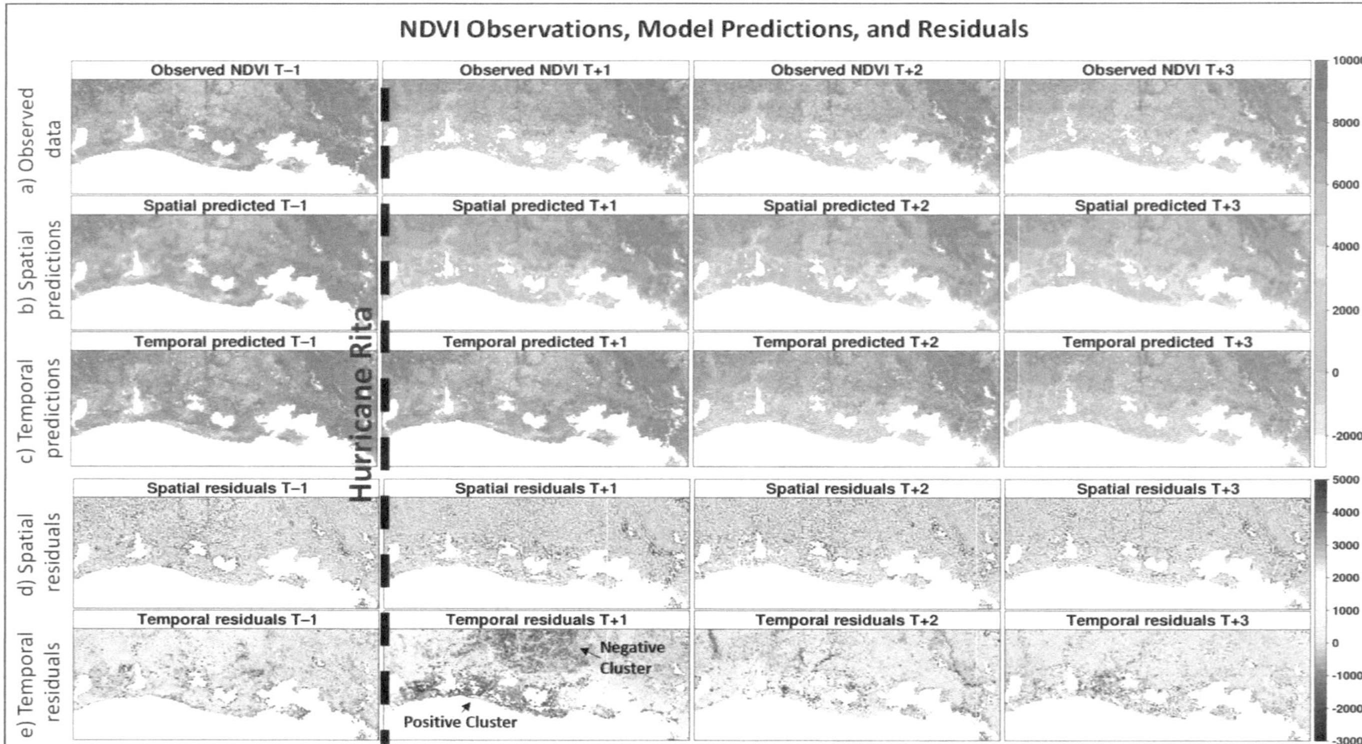


*Figure 2.4* NDVI observations (range: −10,000 to 10,000), model prediction, and residual maps before (T−1) and after Hurricane Rita's landfall (T+1, T+2, T+3). From top to bottom: (a) observed NDVI values; (b) spatial predictions; (c) temporal predictions; (d) spatial residuals; and (e) temporal residuals.

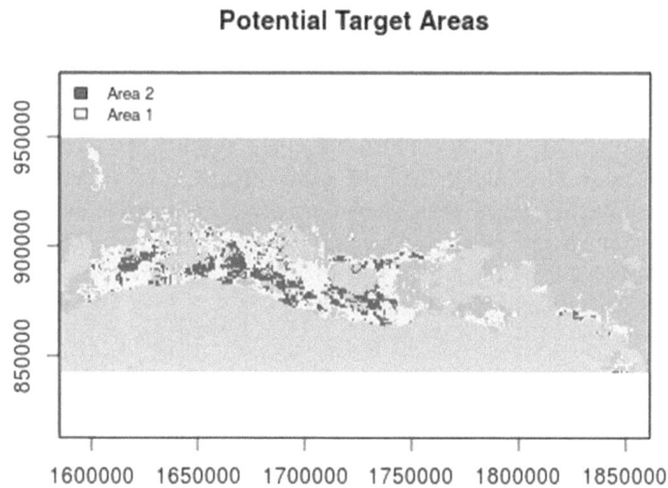


*Figure 2.5* Potential target areas to prioritize disaster management activities. Area 1 corresponds to one standard deviation from the mean of the standardized difference map between spatial and temporal residuals, whereas Area 2 corresponds to two standard deviations for the same standardized map. Area 2 can be interpreted as being of higher priority than Area 1.

## Results

Output from the prediction models and MAE plots confirms, for the most part, that pre- and post-Hurricane Rita NDVI values and spatial patterns follow SBT expectations. MAE plots (Figure 2.3) suggest that the temporal-only model performs poorly after Hurricane Rita strikes, as shown by the sharp spike in MAE in T+1 (the gray line in Figure 2.3), whereas the spatial model performs well for that time step (the dark gray line in Figure 2.3). This relationship reverses quickly 16 days after (T+2), and disappears 32 days after (T+3), marking the closing of the SBT window. We find that Figure 2.3a does not exactly follow the idealized trajectory suggested in Figure 2.2, because the temporal model MAE pre- and post-Hurricane Rita is not consistently lower than that of the spatial model. Results in Figures 2.3b and 2.3c, which depict MAE trajectories stratified for each flood zone, show a similar pattern to the average measures for the entire study area (Figure 2.3a). More critically, Zone 1 (the FEMA flood zone) shows substantially stronger SBT effects than Zone 2 (not flooded, but potentially affected by winds).

Figure 2.4 portrays results from mapping the observed NDVI over the study period and area, as well as the predicted and residual values from the spatial and temporal models. These maps also align with SBT expectations. Residual maps show the performance (and error) of the spatial and temporal models at each time step. The temporal residuals map for T+1 shows a large spatial swath from a strong SBT effect [positive and negative residuals outlined for Map (e) at T+1] that coincides with the hurricane-affected regions. This pattern is markedly distinct from the temporal residual maps for preceding and subsequent time steps (blue pixels in T-1, T+2, T+3). Spatial residual maps across all analyzed time steps remain similar overall, with relatively smaller residual values (blue pixels). T+1 maps (Figure 2.4) are a cartographic counterpart to the SBT window identified in the MAE plots (Figure 2.3).

Finally, potential target areas, shown in Figure 2.5, provide an example of how residual maps can be used to identify priority target areas. We see that the identified areas coincide with the overall affected region, as well as with the FEMA-delineated flood area (Figure 2.1b).

## Conclusion and Discussion

This chapter presents an application of the SBT framework that highlights regions of fast and abrupt change in disaster-hit areas. We show that, overall, the Hurricane Rita case study follows the expected SBT trajectory: space outperforms time as a prediction tool in the immediate aftermath of Rita's landfall, and the SBT window is clearly identifiable in both MAE trajectory plots and residual maps for T+1. Inspecting the differentiated effect in flooded and non-flooded areas, as identified by FEMA (2006), further confirms this pattern. However, its match with our expectations is not perfect: sometimes temporal MAE is higher than spatial MAE before and after the SBT window (time steps other than T+1). As reported previously (Parmentier et al. 2017), this incongruency might be the result of noise in the data, or a mismatch in temporal or spatial sampling by MODIS (i.e. 16-day, 1 km). In addition, NDVI recovers rapidly, because it detects green up from any type of vegetation cover, which is not equivalent to a full return to previous land cover types or ecological recovery. Finally, the identification of SBT events and windows also depends on the nature of a phenomenon (its speed and strength) and the properties of a dataset (the sampling frequency in time and space).

The Hurricane Rita case study results track closely with findings by the authors in other hurricane applications of SBT using NDVI as a proxy for land cover change and impact on vegetation (Parmentier et al. 2017; Millones et al. 2019). This chapter adds to this literature by using residual maps to produce potential emergency management target areas after a disaster. This use of SBT requires further research and validation, but the following features of the framework deserve additional attention in order to understand its contribution in this context:

1. The areas of abrupt change (and derived target areas) that SBT identifies may coincide with areas identified by other conventional change methods (such as image differencing, change vectors analysis) for T+1. However, they will differ markedly for subsequent time steps (T+2 onward). One important reason for this difference is that the source and interpretation of

change and recovery are quite different. SBT measures neither the magnitude of change in a variable (e.g. NDVI) per se, nor its return to pre-hurricane levels as recovery finishes. SBT measures the capacity of temporal observations (i.e. past conditions) and geographic context (i.e. neighboring observations) to predict the conditions after a hurricane strikes.

2. Change measured in T+1 is so drastic that past data are unable to yield predictions with high accuracy. In contrast, geographic context (spatial neighbors) may still produce good predictions after such a change. This prediction success can be interpreted as signaling processes of diffusion/contagion (invasive species, migration), or highlighting strengths subjacent to environmental conditions (climate, soil regions), at least for a brief period of time.
3. Hurricane aftermath (e.g. T+1) target areas also can be roughly geographically equivalent to those identified with other methods. We can see similarities in the spatial patterns appearing of the observed NDVI and temporal residuals outlined in row (e) for T+1 in Figure 2.4.
4. The subsequent maps at times T+2 and T+3 show markedly different patterns because conventional methods measure recovery of a variable (NDVI) using pre-event levels of that variable as a benchmark. SBT maps do not show recovery of a variable. Rather, they show if each pixel is still better predicted by the past or by its neighbors. This feature can be interpreted as a second-order measure of resilience. Potentially, the question being answered asks whether or not the landscape system being studied has shifted from one sociological regime to another.
5. This potential measure of resilience and potential regime change may deliver clues about the nature of new drivers in a system in transition after an abrupt change. For instance, Wernette et al. (2018) suggest that SBT is a promising approach for understanding the forces controlling the changes in shore and beach morphology, which, in turn, can provide important managerial insights.
6. In summary, while the potential target areas presented in Figure 2.5 may not appear to add any value to the identification of impacted areas in the aftermath of Hurricane Rita vis-à-vis other change methods, their real potential is in their capacity to inform about post-disaster changes that are more meaningful and transformative in the longer term.

## References

Bivand, R. (2006). Implementing spatial data analysis software tools in R. *Geographical Analysis*, 38(1), 23–40.

Cliff, A., and K. Ord. (1981). *Spatial Processes*. London: Pion.

Federal Emergency Management Agency (FEMA). (2006). Louisiana Hurricane Rita surge inundation regional overview Eastern and Western parishes. Available at www.fema.gov/pdf/hazard/flood/recoverydata/rita/rita_la_overview-e.pdf; last accessed on March 30, 2017.

Griffith, D. A. (2010). Modeling spatio-temporal relationships: Retrospect and prospect. *Journal of Geographical Systems*, 12(2), 111–123.

Huete, A., K. Didan, T. Miura, E. P. Rodriguez, X. Gao, and L. G. Ferreira. (2002). Overview of the radiometric and biophysical performance of the MODIS vegetation indices. *Remote Sensing of Environment*, 83(1), 195–213.

Hyndman, R. J., and Y. Khandakar. (2007). Automatic time series for forecasting: The forecast package for R. Monash University, Department of Econometrics and Business Statistics.

Knabb, R. D., D. P. Brown, and J. R. Rhome. (2006). *Tropical Cyclone Report, Hurricane Rita, 18–26 September 2005*. Miami, FL: National Hurricane Center.

Marghany, M., and S. I. Mansor. (2017). Three-dimensional Nepal earthquake displacement using hybrid genetic algorithm phase unwrapping from Sentinel-1A satellite. In T. Zauaghi (ed.), *Earthquakes—Tectonics, Hazard and Risk Mitigation*. London: InTech. DOI:10.5772/66636. Available at https://mts.intechopen.com/books/earthquakes-tectonics-hazard-and-risk-mitigation/three-dimensional-nepal-earthquake-displacement-using-hybrid-genetic-algorithm-phase-unwrapping-from; last accessed on March 27, 2018.

McGee, B., B. Goree, R. Tollett, B. Woodward, and W. Kress. (2006). Hurricane Rita surge data, Southwestern Louisiana and Southeastern Texas, September–November 2005. Data Series 220. Available at pubs.er.usgs.gov/publication/ds220; last accessed on March 29, 2018.

Millones, Marco, Benoit Parmentier, Daniel A. Griffith, Yongwan Chun, and Stuart E. Hamilton. (2019). Space beats time: A framework for leveraging temporal and spatial autocorrelation in prediction models for disruptive social and environmental events. *Annals of the Association of the American Geographers*. Submitted and under revision.

Morton, R. A., and J. A. Barras. (2011). Hurricane impacts on coastal wetlands: A half-century record of storm-generated features from Southern Louisiana. *Journal of Coastal Research*, 27(6A), 27–43.

Parmentier, Benoit, Marco Millones, Daniel A. Griffith, Stuart E. Hamilton, Yongwan Chun, and Sean McFall. (2017). When space beats time: A proof of concept with Hurricane Dean. In D. Griffith, Y. Chun, and D. Dean (eds.), *Advances in Geocomputation*, pp. 207–215. Cham: Springer.

Pontius Jr, R. G., O. Thontteh, and H. Chen. (2008). Components of information for multiple resolution comparison between maps that share a real variable. *Environmental and Ecological Statistics*, 15(2), 111–142.

Rodgers, J. C., A. W. Murrah, and W. H. Cooke. (2009). The impact of Hurricane Katrina on the coastal vegetation of the Weeks Bay Reserve, Alabama from NDVI data. *Estuaries and Coasts*, 32(3), 496–507.

Rogan, J., L. Schneider, Z. Christman, M. Millones, D. Lawrence, and B. Schmook. (2011). Hurricane disturbance mapping using MODIS EVI data in the Southeastern Yucatán, México. *Remote Sensing Letters*, 2(3), 259–267.

Willmott, C. J., and K. Matsuura. (2005). Advantages of the mean absolute error (MAE) over the root mean square error (RMSE) in assessing average model performance. *Climate Research*, 30(1), 79.

Wernette, P. A., C. Houser, B. A. Weymer, M. E. Everett, M. P. Bishop, and B. Reece. (2018). Directional dependency and coastal framework geology: Implications for barrier island resilience. *Chest Journal, Earth Surface Dynamics*, 6(4), 1139–1153.

Zachria, A., and B. Patel. (2006). Deaths related to HRita and mass evacuation. *Chest Journal*, 130(4_MeetingAbstracts), 124S-c-124S.

# 3 Evolving Trajectories in Public Sector Statewide Spatial Data Infrastructure

## From Data Product to On-Demand Services and GIS Apps

*Trevor M. Harris and H. Franklin LaFone*

### Introduction

Almost all states in the United States have, to varying degrees, some statewide GIS spatial data capability to provide a repository, clearinghouse, and support center for state-delineated spatial data resources. This chapter draws upon the operation and experiences of the West Virginia State GIS Technical Center at West Virginia University (hereafter Technical Center) (http://wvgis.wvu.edu) to track several significant and continually evolving trends in statewide spatial data infrastructure (SDI) initiatives over the past quarter century. The Technical Center was established under West Virginia Executive Order No. 4–93 in November 1993 and was tasked at the time with providing spatial data and technical support services to assist and promote the development and operation of GIS in West Virginia.

The initiative in West Virginia preempted subsequent statewide GIS enterprises and was part of a broader narrative coordinated by the federal government to move towards a national and global SDI that built on the pivotal role of discrete spatial datasets, spatial data standards, interoperability, and the availability and searchability of critical spatial data resources (Craglia and Masser, 2003; Kelly, 2009; Masser, 2005, 2006; Moeller and Reichardt, 2010; Williamson et al., 2003). In the United States, the Federal Geographic Data Committee (1997) (FGDC) was established by the President's Office of Management and Budget to coordinate geospatial data activities and was charged with coordinating the development of the National Spatial Data Infrastructure (NSDI, nd). This coordination involved three major activities focused on the development of a national geospatial data clearinghouse; the establishment of data standards and metadata for data documentation and exchange; and the development of policies, procedures, and partnerships to create a national digital geospatial data framework. The origins of the Technical Center sat squarely in the center of these national and state initiatives.

During the 25-year operation of the Technical Center, several trends can be discerned that reflect the evolving role of GIS and geospatial technologies; the increasing availability, accuracy, and resolution of spatial data; the changing sources of spatial data; the dramatic advances in computational and data storage capability and software development; the introduction and impact of broadband Internet; and the ever changing and growing sophistication of the GIS user community. Over its lifetime, the Technical Center has seen a paradigm shift from the early dominance of a federally sourced spatial data infrastructure to one where local, state, and private sector entities now play the major role in spatial data generation and distribution.

The Internet and Web Service Protocols such as REST services (Representational State Transfer) and SOAP (Simple Object Access Protocol) have transformed data access from a mode premised on the discovery and dissemination of specific spatial datasets through clearinghouse nodes and state–federal SDI to a near real-time distributed electronic network of connected data producers and consumers accessing spatial data on demand. The Technical Center SDI has become a web of interconnected local stewards who maintain their own spatial data, which are accessed remotely through the Technical Center by calls to real-time, on-demand services. REST software architecture and RESTful systems and interfaces are now central to supporting these distributed on-demand services and contribute significantly to underpinning a scalable spatial data web service to data consumers.

However, to imply that the only changes experienced by the Technical Center over nearly two and a half decades relate solely to spatial data and its dissemination is to ignore a number of additional and inter-related trends that have changed not only the face of geospatial technologies and spatial data processing but also, increasingly, the evolving role that the Center plays as an SDI and GIS resource hub in state GIS initiatives. This chapter, then, discusses the evolution of several trends and themes experienced by the Technical Center in its statewide enterprise over 25 years that extends well beyond its early focus on generating and distributing spatial data and SDI activities. It would perhaps be impolitic to rank these evolving trends in some semblance of prioritized order, because in reality almost all these trends are inter-related in some way and are equally significant. In reality, though, we begin with a core discussion of the evolving nature and production of geospatial data and of the methods for data dissemination, both of which have tended to dominate the mission and role of the Technical Center.

## Spatial Data, Data Dissemination, Interoperability, and Local–State–Federal Coordination

### *Spatial Data and Inverting the Pyramid*

One of the most remarkable transformations in the work of the Technical Center over the past 25 years revolves around the changing nature of spatial data. Within these changes, four themes might be identified:

1. The changing origins and stewards of the data.
2. The increasing accuracy and resolution of the data.

3. The evolving technologies employed in spatial data production.
4. The onset of a movement from standards-based authoritative data to volunteered asserted spatial data.

The early focus of the Technical Center was on providing spatial data to those state agencies who were early adopters of GIS. In the process, the Technical Center drew heavily on existing federal spatial and analog data originating from the USGS, Census Bureau, National Elevation Dataset, National Hydrography Dataset, and the National Agriculture Imagery Program. These agencies, among others, populated several critical statewide spatial datasets through an FGDC clearinghouse node established in the Technical Center. Central to this goal was an awareness of the need to reduce the duplication of multiple and costly data development efforts then ongoing among state organizations and to facilitate state–federal coordination in spatial data development and sharing. Thus, an early mission for the Technical Center was to convert USGS topographic mylar sheets that formed the base layers of 1:24,000 quadrangles into Digital Line Graphs (DLG) for the entire state. Together, these federal data initiatives contributed to the base structure of the NSDI Framework initiative (www.fgdc.gov/initiatives/framework) that sought to assemble a series of data layers commonly, if not universally, required and used by public and private organizations within the United States.

The NSDI Framework was one of the key building blocks of the national spatial data backbone of the US, and it relied heavily on spatial data generated and served by the federal government. In West Virginia, the DLG analog to digital conversion in the 1990s provided foundational GIS layers that were served through the state spatial data clearinghouse and utilized by some state agencies but only a few community and corporate entities. The Framework was designed to facilitate the production, sharing, and use of geographic data, reduce spatial data generation costs, and improve service and decision-making. Such a spatial data structure was typical of the 1980s and 1990s, whereby federal government sources formed the foundation of a pyramid-style data model and provided the bulk of the data to the GIS user community (Figure 3.1). Building on the foundation of federal data, the next level in the pyramid comprised data from private enterprise, state government, and regional agencies. At the peak of the pyramid was the spatial data garnered from local communities, local government and agencies, small groups, and individuals. Driving this framework were issues of resources, expertise, and the availability of a technologically capable bureaucracy seeking to meet administrative mandates and operational requirements. The decision not to enter into a cost recovery process greatly facilitated the early uptake and use of GIS in the United States and certainly so when compared to other nations where some form of cost recovery was imposed.

The spatial data paradigm shift over the past two or more decades and the inversion of the data pyramid reflects the diffusion of GIS technology and expertise away from the historically dominant GIS role of major government

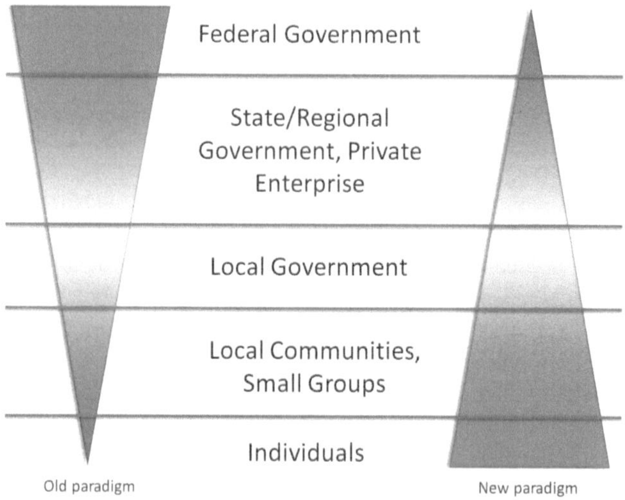


*Figure 3.1* The changing paradigm shift in sourcing spatial data.

agencies towards local, state, and regional entities as significant spatial data providers and users. This process has been facilitated by the growing availability of cost-effective geospatial data capture technologies in the form of Global Positioning Systems (GPS), Location-Based Services (LBS), and digital sensor data from aerial photographs and satellite imagery.

A second trajectory experienced by practically all users of spatial data over the past few decades has been the increasing accuracy, resolution, and availability of spatial data. The early dominant scale for most spatial data tended to adhere to the existing analog sources such as provided by the USGS and remotely sensed data. Thus, 1:24,000 for DLG products and 30m DEM were typical for much GIS data processing and were clearly related to the scale of data capture. In contrast, today several counties in West Virginia now have LiDAR derived elevation values accurate to within 0.5-meter nominal pulse spacing or 1:1,200 scale. Several of these counties have accompanying aerial imagery, and yet others have 0.3-meter resolution. However, as these data were acquired and funded by specific counties, they are not available for the entire state. Yet even the most recent NAIP aerial ortho-rectified imagery is at 1:12,000 scale (1-meter Ground Sample Distance) and is available statewide.

Thus, data resolution and accuracy have improved markedly in order to meet governmental needs, and a considerable quantity of spatial data is now generated by local entities and state–federal cooperative initiatives. Most counties in West Virginia, for example, have complete tax parcel maps generated locally to support county and state taxation code for both surface and subsurface tax parcels. West Virginia is somewhat unique in having a separation of surface and subsurface mineral rights, which may be owned by separate entities. The scale of these tax parcel maps is at 1:4,800 for rural areas and 1:1,200 for urban areas. The willingness to fund these local datasets is obviously spurred by the now widespread adoption of GIS for mapping and data analysis throughout state agencies and local agencies. This growth in spatial data availability and increased accuracy has been bolstered significantly by the greater efficiencies and cost reduction enabled by technological advances such as LiDAR, and increasingly drones, along with a competitive corporate spatial data marketplace.

A more recent trend is also emerging that reinforces the paradigm shift reflected in the inverted spatial data pyramid; this is related to spatial data generated by non-traditional sources and especially social media technologies and social media Internet databases. Volunteered Geographic Information (VGI) has forced many in GIS and SDI to rethink how to handle this new source of spatial data (Goodchild, 2007a). Using now readily available handheld Location-Based Services and GPS-enabled devices such as "smart" cell phones, digital cameras, and digital audio recorders, the layperson can now tag most personal data with a digital coordinate. Storage costs are no longer an obstacle to data collection for the layperson due to cloud computing and storage and the ability to upload data to social media sites such as Flickr and YouTube. The cumulative impact of these user-generated content (UGC) technologies is that more personal data is being spatially tagged and stored than at any other time in history, and this represents a possible watershed in spatial data generation, spatial data processing, and necessarily SDIs. Web 2.0 and neogeography make available a wealth of tools and technology infrastructure to a broad popular audience. The combination of VGI with these new generation imagery-rich geobrowsers and virtual globes, integrated through now widely available application programming interfaces (APIs), has markedly changed the structured world of traditional GIS and SDI and closes the gap between data producers and data consumers. VGI has already played important roles in contributing to fighting wildfires in California, mapping and monitoring Gulf oil spills, responding to the Haiti earthquake, responding to natural disasters such as hurricanes, riot containment or "kettling" in London, and the "Arab Spring" in Middle Eastern countries.

VGI introduces a significant challenge to traditional, standards-based SDI. Tulloch (2008) describes the rise of SDI as the "institutionalization of GIS" and is redolent of the former hierarchical pyramid structure. In contrast, VGI and UGC reflect the data contributions of local agencies, communities, and individuals. The challenge to SDI, however, comes from the unofficial nature of VGI, which does not easily conform to the standards, protocols, or verifiability of traditional "authenticated" spatial data. In this respect, VGI challenges the very core of SDI because, as Goodchild (2007a) suggests, VGI "asserts" geographic information content without citation, reference, or any other supporting authority. Metadata is rarely generated or accompanies VGI, though some geotagging devices will automatically generate some metadata content.

Furthermore, many geobrowsers, such as Google Earth, do not provide metadata about the spatial coverages they display (Goodchild, 2007a). As Goodchild (2007a, 2) noted:

> The widespread engagement of large numbers of private citizens, often with little in the way of formal qualifications, in the creation of geographic information, a function that for centuries has been reserved to official agencies. They are largely untrained and their actions are almost always voluntary, and the results may or may not be accurate.

This mismatch between authenticated spatial data and unauthenticated VGI poses major challenges to traditional providers such as the Technical Center. The distinction between "expert" created data and the non-expert layperson volunteered spatial data is a growing challenge to SDI providers. Furthermore, the inherent fluidity of VGI presents challenges to traditional providers because data points can be freely added and deleted from VGI databases by users at their will. Current systems provide no mechanism for capturing time slices or an easily transferable dataset.

### *From Data Distribution to Information Dissemination*

As GIS has evolved into a recognized and established mainstream technology, there has been considerable focus by government, industry, government, and academe on data standards, interoperability, and SDI. Data dissemination has undergone a revolution from the early inception of SDI, when physical transfer methods on transferrable disk, the so-called sneaker net, dominated data sharing. The Technical Center would often hold data swapping "parties" during key GIS stakeholder meetings in and around the state, when floppy disks and nine-track tapes would be exchanged between state entities and the Technical Center. However, among the many obvious limitations of such methods encountered at the time is that only the data stewards have access to the most up-to-date data, and other users are limited by the time stamp of the last data swapping session.

In the formative years of GIS, proprietary data formats also created considerable difficulty for sharing and reusing spatial data. Facilitated by the FGDC, an early focus of the Technical Center SDI was on data interoperability, spatial data sharing, the facilitation of data sharing portals, and the all-important spatial data standards and metadata. The USGS Spatial Data Transfer Standard (SDTS) was instrumental in facilitating the early transfer of proprietary data between systems. Subsequently, the emphasis has shifted towards establishing standards for system and services protocols. As the demand for GIS has increased exponentially, and e-government initiatives and economic pressure to recover the investments made in spatial data have grown, so the emphasis has shifted over time away from data sharing towards interoperability as a way to bridge islands of GIS resources and to share GIS services across multiple platforms, servers, institutions, and countries (Kuhn, 2005).

The Internet has revolutionized data sharing by now enabling users to access data "on demand" (Kelly, 2009). Web 1.0 data retrieval technology constrained users to downloading discrete datasets one at a time, partially with an eye to total file size and available bandwidth. While on-demand data allows more frequent data access, limitations of bandwidth meant that data still suffered from time slice issues from data stewards. Entire datasets would be stored on local user workstations even if the actual area of interest was but a small subset of the total data layer. A major limitation with these data download methods centers around the related factors of data discovery, currency, and access. Typically, these functions are ad-hoc affairs that differ widely from one another. Users discovered datasets through search engine results or even word-of-mouth and were then left to determine each SDI's unique method of data retrieval and download. The FGDCH (2004) worked hard to craft explicit standards for data sharing between SDIs, and while these efforts did not supplant existing data clearinghouses' proprietary methods, they did provide a unifying mechanism.

The advent of Web 2.0 has progressively shifted the focus from spatial data sharing and exchange towards the provision of on-demand geospatial services whereby spatial data content integration occurs simultaneously. In this regard, Kuhn (2005) has suggested that the term Geospatial Information Infrastructure is now a more appropriate description of the role of SDIs. A geospatial services SDI now includes not only spatial data but the technology, the user community, the stakeholders, and the framework elements of standards, metadata, interoperability, policies, coordination, sharing, and system architectures and interfaces necessary to serve spatial data based on distributed networks (Kuhn, 2005; Rhind, 1999). Peng (2003) foresaw that the GIS community would move away from server/client architectures to peer-to-peer architectures in which distributed GIServices would include nodes as both servers and clients according to the specific need. In Peng's (2003, 10) conceptualization, GIServices broaden

> the usage of geographic information into a wide range of on-line geospatial applications and services, including digital libraries, digital governments, digital earth, on-line mapping, data clearinghouses, real-time spatial decision support tools, dynamic hydrological modeling, distance learning modules, and so on.

In essence, top-down driven data streams now become subsumed within a cloud of data generated by officials and the public alike.

The ability to interact with and contribute to distributed GIServices is limited not by authority but by accessibility to the service. Thus, data is no longer stored locally on user machines, as was the case of Web 1.0 technology, but lives within the SDI itself. Standards such as ESRI's REST provide a method of data retrieval via common web protocols, which can be embedded either in the web or in the desktop applications themselves. Users can now access an entire dataset, make frequent micro-queries of the data, interrogate the dataset as user demands expand, or divide the data into atomic units that would more efficiently leverage available bandwidth. In reality, not all datasets lend themselves to micro data queries, and data is often compiled into final mapping products for ease of transfer but as a result may not be easily decomposed into associated data layers. As such, modern SDIs tend to use a mix of both Web 1.0 data retrieval methods and Web 2.0 micro-query retrieval methods. Computational limitations require SDIs to focus on mission-critical layers for micro-query publication, such that the Technical Center publishes, via REST services, "framework" layers common to many mapping efforts such as boundaries, roads, imagery, elevation, and hydrography. Non-framework layers reside more within legacy FTP-based download mechanisms. Deciding which layers to include as framework data is a continually shifting decision matrix based on computing power, application need, and user demand.

### *Interoperability Issues*

Tightly coupled to trends in data sharing is data interoperability, which, despite recent dramatic strides, still continues to be an elusive goal within GIS. The last three decades have seen GIS evolve from a series of distantly connected stovepipes to syntactically interoperable systems and, increasingly, a world of semantically interoperable systems. GIS operates within a broad tent of technologies, each of which has had to be adapted to GIS. Early GIS technologies featured limited or no interoperability (Open Geospatial Consortium, nd), and engagement between technological systems has often involved a complex process incurring many points of failure and inefficiency. GIS bodies to define standards emerged to construct systemic methods to achieve forms of syntactical interoperability, primarily through the publication and sharing of protocols and the adoption of official file format standards. Interoperability has thus necessarily taken an evolutionary path over the years, to the point where GIS users now think less in terms of sharing spatial data files and more in terms of the sharing of geospatial services for the support of data, systems, and users. The Open Geospatial Consortium (OGC), formed in 1994 from governmental, commercial, and research organizations, has provided a forum around which consensus on open standards for spatial data, APIs, web services, and geoprocessing have been determined. These standardized protocols now include Web Feature Services (WFS), Web Map Services (WMS), Geographic Markup Language (GML), Web Service Common (OWS), and Representational State Transfer (REST) (www.opengeospatial.org). Many of these standards have also attained ISO status under ISO/TC 211 Geographic Information/Geomatics (www.isotc211.org/).

Dominant corporate organizations such as ESRI and loose affiliations of prevailing competitors have come together to form, contribute to, and adopt those formats and approaches, such as in the case of ESRI's shapefile format. Metadata continues to provide the most basic information necessary for interoperability. The implementation of metadata standards by federal and state governments has further cemented interoperability as a critical aspect of GIS and SDI. Governments have gone so far as to use their regulatory authority to force interoperability by opening monopolistic systems to competitors, such as in the case of the European Commission versus Microsoft and the Commission Decision (nd), forcing the opening of standards for interoperability purposes. Other, new directions in interoperability have focused on semantic interoperability and the transmission of not just data, but its associated semantic meaning as well. Ontology remains the key for semantic interoperability (Schuurman, 2006). Interoperability, of course, is not limited solely to data, and hardware interoperability is discussed later in the hardware section.

### *Local–State–Federal Coordination*

An important role of the Technical Center associated with data generation and dissemination has been to act as a GIS resource and link between local groups, state agencies, and federal government. Thus, while the FGDC Framework initiative focused on data layers and spatial data development, procedures, and technology for building, using, and sharing the data, it also emphasized institutional relationships and the development of business plans and practices to grow the GIS resource base of the state. The Technical Center thus performed an important role in forming the institutional relationships between state and federal spatial data resources. Personnel in the Technical Center were also instrumental in creating the West Virginia Association of Geospatial Professionals (www.wvagp.org) and in providing training courses, serving on state boards, and providing leadership in matters of GIS in the state that extends well beyond its apparent major role as a spatial data clearinghouse portal.

## Hardware, Software, and Humanware

### *Hardware*

One would reasonably expect that hardware would have seen the greatest advances and change of any trend in the Technical Center over the last few decades, and indeed it has, though these changes have been more incremental. Having said that, changes since the inception of the Technical Center in data storage, peripherals, products, connectivity, and computing platforms have resulted in a computational network that bears little resemblance to its early computing capability. Storage is perhaps the clearest example of this incremental change, in that the cost performance ratio has improved yearly and has in general become "cheaper" per metric unit each year. The initial mass data storage for the Technical Center in the mid-1990s comprised a 4-foot square device that boasted the then impressive total of 350 GB of storage at a cost of about $1,000 per gigabyte. In 2005, data storage cost an average of $.79 per gigabyte. In 2018, storage cost less than $.02 per gigabyte. At the time of publication, a 350 GB Solid State Drive housed in a device measuring 2.5 inches costs a mere $80. Certainly, it would not be an understatement to suggest that data storage is now orders of magnitude cheaper relative to even a decade ago, let alone over a 25-year span. To take one illustrative example, the 1996 Digital Orphoimagery Quarter Quads (DOQQ) for West Virginia was one of the first large scale, 1-meter resolution, statewide imagery datasets made available through the Technical Center. The DOQQ products were delivered on 560 CDs, requiring almost four entire cabinet drawers to store them. Storage for those files occupied 265 GB at an estimated cost of $1,000 per gigabyte. Storing those same files today costs a mere $5. Currently the Technical Center data storage stands at 131 terabytes.

Yet, at the same time, it is important to recognize that the sheer size of spatial databases has equally exploded over the same time period. As camera and data acquisition technologies have evolved, storage needs have also grown, such that 1-foot aerial resolution imagery and even 4-inch resolution in urban areas are common. Current recent statewide imagery datasets require over 11 TB to store. Interestingly, even at the current cost of $.02 per gigabyte, the cost to store statewide imagery between 1995 and 2018 remains almost identical. This is a good example of Moore's Law, which predicted a doubling of computing capability every 18–24 months, meeting the Great Moore's Law Compensator principle, which predicts that data needs will grow at an equal or even greater pace. Beyond the diminishing cost of data storage, issues such speed of data retrieval have equally brought about dramatic change. Even areas such as paper printing and production methods have evolved, in terms of fidelity as well as cost. Production hardware has become cheaper over time, tracking commodified inkjet technology. Early plotters in the Technical Center were expensive ink pen plotter systems requiring special pens, papers, computing equipment, and a controlled environment for successful plotting. Today's plotter is an order of magnitude cheaper and connects via standard desktop or server interfaces. Inks and paper supplies, however, remain comparatively expensive, which has the effect of somewhat negating the lower capital investment in the equipment. In tandem with the availability of larger, high resolution monitors, paper map production has markedly decreased over the years. The explosion of broadband Internet, the expectation of interactivity, and the widespread proliferation of mobile devices have all contributed to users demanding a more robust and flexible product than a paper product can provide.

Broadband connectivity has obviously enabled additional and more effective pathways for data dissemination and sharing. Whereas previously data would be compressed as much as possible to facilitate transfer to user desktops, some datasets, such as large imagery files or LiDAR files, would be unavailable for online access in native file formats due to excessive download times. Technologies such as MrSID were required to attain maximum compression and reduced file size, despite potentially introducing data degradation and data loss. Today, the availability of always-on "fat" data traffic lanes has allowed many of these constraints to be eased. Technical Center users now expect always-on continuous connectivity to the Center's datasets without the need to download directly to their own storage devices. The impact of broadband connectivity cannot be overemphasized. Data can now be stored and transmitted continuously in native file formats, and data clearinghouses have necessarily had to become considerably more reliable and robust with greater uptime dependability, enabling user access to data at any time of day or night. Greater broadband capacity now enables the Technical Center to host dozens of datasets that formerly had to be essentially stored in "offline" mode.

The Technical Center's computing platforms have similarly had to evolve in order to accommodate continuous access to data. Depending on their specific use, servers once operated in stovepipe mode, whereby a server devoted to file serving and distribution, for example, was separated from servers used for geoprocessing. In contrast, modern servers are both more powerful and can more easily accommodate multiple simultaneous roles, which is critical, as GIS now blends the lines between these respective roles. Servers are thus no longer devoted to dedicated tasks since many GIS tasks require an increasing number and variety of subtasks to be accomplished. System interoperability is less of an issue now that systems designed on the same platform are typically compatible with one another for both physical and operating system connectivity. However, hardware still retains stovepipe characteristics and can be problematic in cross-linking different systems for data or functional interoperability. Nowhere is this more evident than in the case of operating systems, for files written in one operating system usually have limited or no compatibility with files written using a different operating system. GIS engages across many forms of hardware, each with their own machine level operating system, and yet these platforms are rarely designed with interoperability as a fundamental design goal. Initially, UNIX-based SPARC systems were necessary in the Technical Center to connect large-scale server-based storage devices to servers and mission-critical hardware such as large format plotters and drum scanners.

As GIS transitioned to Microsoft Windows desktop environments, existing storage, scanning, and output hardware remained on UNIX platforms and interoperability was gained by working locally on the desktop and crudely transferring data to and from the UNIX system as workflow and availability allowed. Each piece of hardware meets a specific need within the GIS echo system, and desktop computers have traditionally dominated GIS usage. However, within the past decade the industry has exploded in the use of server-based technologies, and as a result computing and data storage in the cloud have achieved a dominant place in GIS. Thus, desktop, server, cloud, and mobile platforms, each featuring differing hardware and software systems and allied to major vendor players, require ever increasing interoperability between computing platforms and systems. Server virtualization is now dominant in the Technical Center and allows for a smaller subset of powerful equipment to simultaneously run a large number of virtual servers. As a result, as hardware has been commodified and standardized on robust and versatile hardware standards with IP communication protocols and harmonious file sharing, interoperability has been greatly enhanced within these contemporary systems.

***Software***

In contrast to the incremental nature of hardware capacity, GIS software has experienced a more punctuated sequence of advances over the past few decades, largely associated with software version updates by ESRI. Over the lifetime of the Technical Center, ESRI has emerged to dominate the commercial off-the-shelf GIS software market. ArcINFO began life as a UNIX-based command-line suite where data manipulation, geoprocessing, and map creation were performed using a series of line commands, or tools in the ESRI nomenclature, strung together in a pseudo programming language fashion. Command-line tools quickly gave way to graphical interfaces via ArcView and ArcGIS Desktop, to now give way to ArcGIS Pro. The model of a series of connected tools has remained strong in ESRI's software into the modern age.

Into this mix, however, there are now other trends emerging in Geographic Information Science that draw upon systems outside of the more traditional GIS paradigm. In 2004, Google acquired Keyhole Inc. for their mapping product, based on Web 2.0 technologies that allowed users to interact with an online map in a fluid and dynamic way. This was quickly rebranded Google Maps. The public's interest, allied to greater accessibility to spatial information, exploded almost overnight.

Traditional GIS software was still mired in Web 1.0 call/response forms of communication, which were slow and bandwidth intensive. The powerful user interface of Google Maps raised public expectations about mapping and the data and tools available to them. The "Can I see my house?" effect dominated the public discourse on mapping. Google immediately launched parallel efforts to gather and synthesize as much publicly available GIS data as possible. The Technical Center provided several datasets to Google in its role as state GIS data clearinghouse and these high-resolution elevation datasets set the standard for elevation mapping within Google Maps for several years. Other players within the market quickly followed suit with server-based technologies that could leverage their customers' data and Web 2.0 technologies. A revamped ArcServer followed the Google Maps model, extending system capabilities by allowing customers to publish their data online for general user access. In addition to Google Map and Google Earth platforms, the Technical Center is increasingly seeing greater use made of open source software such as GRASS, which has been in use since its release by the US Army Corps of Engineers in the 1980s, MapServer, and especially QGIS.

Geoprocessing has always been at the heart of spatial analysis within GIS and in tandem with advances in hardware, software and available data has seen significant transformation. Early GIS tools were designed to be strung together for custom analysis, and programming languages such as ESRI's Arc Macro Language (AML) created walled spatial ecosystems.

Moving between ecosystems required advanced programming knowledge to create wholly customized applications developed from the ground up. Even relatively simple tasks such as importing and exporting spatial data required somewhat complex custom "helper" applications to move between these ecosystems. Although it might seem that a radical shift away from this walled spatial ecosystem to more open protocols is in progress, in reality there is evidence to suggest that this trend is in fact being reasserted. GIS software vendors quickly moved away from proprietary languages to adopt more widely accepted object-oriented languages such as Python for desktop development, Swift and Java for mobile development, and the ubiquitous JavaScript/HTML/CSS stack for web-based work. Rather than replicate the cornucopia of libraries, functions, objects, and frameworks that exist for these languages, vendors produced APIs that provided specific hooks into software system functionality. Developers now utilize these APIs to tap functionality necessary for specific custom application needs and to create mashups of different APIs to create hybrid applications with greater functionality beyond that of a single API.

While the vision for spatial data processing APIs is impressive, the reality is somewhat less promising because of the need for advanced programming knowledge to stitch together various APIs with differing storage and manipulation capabilities that are not shared between APIs. Furthermore, APIs contain shared redundancy and functions, such as performing a spatial search, which might be replicated in multiple APIs, yet the accuracy, scale, and algorithms differ between systems and often lack metadata documenting the various differences. The developer must then choose which function is most appropriate and optimal for any particular application. For these reasons, it is often more advantageous for developers to align themselves within one specific walled ecosystem, venturing to use other APIs only when necessary to meet a need not contained within the primary ecosystem. The modern trend is towards standardized languages, which are considerably more powerful than earlier GIS programmatic implementations.

Contemporary GIS software systems require advanced programming knowledge, but in GIS application development, this has led to a massive skills bottleneck. Few GIS shops can afford dedicated software engineers to construct applications. Technologies such as ESRI's ModelBuilder and advanced frameworks such as Bootstrap or jQuery do provide easier programmatic interfaces to complex code. GUI-rich development environments can help overcome these deficiencies in programing skills by providing rapid prototyping, widgets, and template-based application programming environments available to "the masses".

### *Humanware*

One area usually overlooked in the evolution of statewide systems, then, has been the evolving skillsets and knowledge required for such centers to function. The changing expectations of Technical Center personnel have been quite dramatic. In the 1990s, few GIS text books existed and only a few institutions provided GIS courses, often with an equally limited number of student enrollees. The learning curve for GIS praxis was steep, and although a few systems such as SPANS had a GUI interface, mastering the command-line driven ESRI products was challenging. Students and professionals willing to persevere through the learning process were much in demand. However, such a situation has changed markedly over the intervening years. Most higher education geography students, if not some high school students, have acquired at least some knowledge of GIS concepts and software expertise. Furthermore, GIS software and educational and training materials are now readily available and quite advanced. However, the required skillsets have also evolved, such that computer programming, database management, cartographic and mapping design, web and API development, systems management, and many related computational fields are in high demand in order for GIS enterprise operations such as the Technical Center to achieve their mission goals.

## Conclusion

Based on the 25-year experiences of the Technical Center, it has become evident that when it comes to GIS and spatial data, there is no such thing as a constant, except perhaps for constant change. The Technical Center has seen advances from the sneaker-net sharing of data to on-demand data dissemination; from the digitization of analog mylar sheets to expansive high-resolution datasets and database management systems; from producing map products to custom application development; and from a configuration of desktop computers and limited and expensive data storage to sophisticated virtual server networks and storage arrays.

Much as the nature of GIS data and computing facilities have evolved dramatically over the last few decades, and the requirements of humanware have become ever more demanding, so too has the client base of the Technical Center evolved. At the onset of the Center, GIS knowledge and expertise resided in only a few state agencies, and the role of the Center was to support these state agencies through a clearinghouse portal of available spatial data. Since that time, the Center has partnered with a growing number of state agencies, communities, and the general public. It is interesting to reflect that despite disseminating some 330 spatial data layers, a flood mapping tool (www.mapwv.gov/flood/), and a sophisticated web mapping portal (www.map.wv.gov), it is the hunting and fishing tool (www.mapwv.gov/huntfish/) that is in greatest demand by the general public. While state and county agencies are often the major clients driving data and application development, the general public represent an increasing body of consumers of Technical Center data and apps.

In many respects, the trends experienced by the Technical Center mirror those experienced by the GIS community as a whole and reflect the lifecycle of GIS enterprises. Initially, GIS activities focused heavily on inventorying the built, natural, physical, and cultural environments. Much of this inventory was based on the necessary digitization of existing analog map repositories. Subsequently, technological advances in data capture have replaced much of this burdensome manual process. Having assembled an extensive repository of spatial data, the focus then shifted to more efficient data dissemination and spatial analysis, predominantly in the form of paper map products. Finally, the Technical Center has transitioned to focus on the real strengths of GIS in creating spatial decision support systems and customized applications for managers and policymakers to bring to bear in their respective fields. Whether, as predicted, the term GIS eventually becomes absorbed within some spatial decision-making related term and the complex spatial story outlined above becomes subsumed within the underlying framework of an organization's decision-making process, it is likely that the SDI and GIS activities of the Technical Center will continue to experience comparable dramatic change as during the previous era.

## References and Further Readings

Commission Decision (nd) https://fsfe.org/activities/ms-vs-eu/CEC-C-2004-900-final.pdf

Craglia, M. (2006) Introduction to the International Journal of Spatial Data Infrastructures Research, *International Journal of Spatial Data Infrastructures Research*, 1, 1–13.

Craglia, M. and Masser, I. (2003) Access to Geographic Information: A European Perspective, *URISA Journal*, 15, 1, 51–59.

Federal Geographic Data Committee (1997) *Framework: Introduction and Guide*, National Spatial Data Infrastructure, USGS, Reston, VA.

Federal Geographic Data Committee History (2004) www.fgdc.gov/resources/whitepapers-reports/white-papers/fgdc-history

Goodchild, M. F. (2007a) Citizens as Sensors: The World of Volunteered Geography, www.ncgia.ucsb.edu/projects/vgi/docs/position/Goodchild_VGI2007.pdf

Goodchild, M. F. (2007b) Citizens as Sensors: The World of Volunteered Geography. Workshop on Volunteered Geographic Information, December 13–14, www.ncgia.ucsb.edu/projects/vgi/

Kelly, M. C. (2009). The Evolution of SDI Geospatial Data Clearinghouses, in J. Wang (ed.), *Encyclopedia of Data Warehousing and Mining*, second edition, IGI Global, Hershey, PA, 802–809.

Kuhn, W. (2005) Introduction to Spatial Data Infrastructures, online presentation, www.docstoc.com/docs/2697206/Introduction-to-Spatial--Data-Infrastructures

Masser, I. (2005) *GIS Worlds: Creating Spatial Data Infrastructures*, ESRI Press, Redlands.

Masser, I. (2006) What's Special About SDI Related Research? *International Journal of Spatial Data Infrastructures Research*, 1, 14–23.

Moeller, J. J. and Reichardt, M. E. (2010) National, International, and Global Activities in Geospatial Science: Toward a Global Spatial Data Infrastructure, in Bossler, J. D. (ed.), *Manual of Geospatial Science and Technology*, second edition, CRC Press, New York, 733–759.

NSDI (nd) www.fgdc.gov/nsdi/nsdi.html (accessed July 2018).

Open Geospatial Consortium (nd) Brief History, www.opengeospatial.org/ogc/history (accessed July 2018).

Peng, Z. (2003) GIS, Internet GIS, and Distributed GIServices, in Z. Peng and M. Tsou (eds.), *Internet GIS: Distributed Geographic Information Services for the Internet and Wireless Networks*, Wiley, New York.

Rhind, D. W. (1999) National and International Geospatial Data Policies, in P. A. Longley, M. F. Goodchild, D. J. Maguire and D. W. Rhind (eds.), *Geographical Information Systems*, Wiley, New York, 767–787.

Schuurman, N. (2006) Formalization Matters: Critical GIS and Ontology Research, *Annals of the Association of American Geographers*, 96(4), 726–739.

Tulloch, D. L. (2008) Geographic Information Systems and Society, in J. P. Wilson and A. S. Fotheringham (eds.), *The Handbook of Geographic Information Science*, Blackwell, Malden, MA, 447–465.

Williamson, I. P., Rajabifard, A. and M-E. F. Feeney (eds.) (2003) *Developing Spatial Data Infrastructures—From Concept to Reality*, Taylor & Francis, London.

# 4 Using Geospatial Information Systems to Preposition Logistics in Preparation for Hazardous Materials Incidents for Disaster Response and Homeland Security Purposes

*Nicolas A. Valcik and Warren S. Eller*

## Introduction

In the United States, driving is commonplace, due in part to robust infrastructure ranging from local gravel roads to massive interstate highways. On these roadways, regular commuters share the roads with a variety of commercial and industrial traffic, and rarely is there a day that a daily commuter does not encounter a vehicle carrying a set of labels indicating hazardous materials (HAZMAT) are being transported. In large metropolitan cities, trucks carrying HAZMAT travel through busy city intersections on a regular basis throughout the day. The sight is so common, in fact, that drivers rarely think twice about what a truck is carrying in the form of HAZMAT, which could be used for nefarious activities.

Since 9/11, a great deal of research has focused on United States vulnerabilities to terrorist attacks. While there had been previous terrorist attacks on the United States and its allies before 9/11, the magnitude of death and destruction that day dramatically increased the salience of the issue, revealed vulnerabilities in homeland security, and demonstrated how modern transportation can be employed as a weapon in an unconventional manner. The events of 9/11 fueled systemic changes in the United States, including new laws, increased regulatory enforcement of commercial transit, and the creation of a unified agency, Homeland Security, as an effort to streamline operations as well as integrate communications with several different law enforcement agencies.

Unfortunately, several agencies still operate apart from the Homeland Security umbrella, which offer ripe opportunities to would-be terrorists. These agencies oversee areas of civilian commerce and have potential vulnerabilities to terrorist attacks. For example, unconventional weapons can be developed from a wide array of sources in the form of chemicals (e.g. chlorine), radiation (e.g. U-235), bio-toxins (e.g. select agents), or waste (e.g. medical waste). Five independent federal agencies are responsible for HAZMAT and their transportation throughout the country: the Department of Health and Human Services (DHHS), the United States Food and Drug Administration (USDA),

Environmental Protection Agency (EPA), the Department of Energy (DOE), and the Department of Transportation (DOT).

In the case of transportation of HAZMAT, DHS has now inserted itself into the policymaking process in place of DOT (Schweitzer, 2007). With the large amount of HAZMAT that is transported throughout public roadways in the United States, a set of issues is created for public policy administrators to take into account when attempting to secure such materials from terrorist attack (e.g. destroyed or stolen). How do public policymakers distribute resources to prevent terrorist attacks on vehicles that are carrying HAZMAT? Additionally, what do policymakers do if there is evidence to suggest that an attack on a vehicle carrying HAZMAT is a precursor to a larger attack involving the materials in question?

## How Significant Is the Potential Threat?

Before preventative action or can be taken or resources distributed, it is necessary to determine along what routes and intersections HAZMAT is being transported on public roadways. It is also necessary to determine what types and quantities of HAZMAT are moving through those public roadways at any given time. For example, how many trucks are carrying flammable chemicals along a HAZMAT-designated route? How many communities do these vehicles pass through, and what would be the impact if a truck carrying a hazardous cargo explodes? What types of vehicles are vulnerable to having their cargos stolen and weaponized against a populated area?

## Literature Review

Current research on the transportation of HAZMAT is focused on inventory control and providing information to first responders if an incident occurs in relation to what a particular vehicle is carrying. There seems to be little effort to obtain and use data to prevent or mitigate incidents with transporting HAZMAT. One such research project is currently being undertaken at the University of Tennessee Southeastern Transportation Center, which involves HAZMAT loaded onto vehicles being inventoried and tracked in real time (Goddard, 2014). To track a vehicle and its cargo in real time would require the use of a GPS locator attached to the vehicle as well as a link to a centralized database, which could have the inventory information updated from a handheld unit. Once the handheld unit collects the information, the information is directly recorded in a database or is "batched" to a database at a certain time interval. How the information is updated depends upon the design of the software and database interface. In this particular study, the real-time tracking would actually be with the vehicles with GPS locator tags and not with the containers themselves, since the containers would be barcoded for tracking purposes.

The trucking industry appears confident that proper measures are already in place to meet Homeland Security requirements. Rich Moskowitz, Vice

President and Regulatory Affairs Counsel for the American Trucking Associations (ATA), stated that a Department of Homeland Security report on trucking indicated that adequate industry security measures are already in place (Homeland Security Newswire, 2010). Mr. Moskowitz also stated security measures had been effective because no terrorist attacks using commercially transported HAZMAT have occurred in the United States since September 11, 2001 (Homeland Security Newswire, 2010). A study released in 2011, conducted by the National Academy of Science in conjunction with the Department of Transportation, reviewed existing and emerging technologies to increase safety and security of transporting HAZMAT (Tate and Abkowitz, 2011). In the report, the researchers recommend tracking HAZMAT being transported by using technology to network RFID, GPS, and GLS technologies together in a systematic manner (Tate and Abkowitz, 2011). The researchers surmise the following:

> If these sensors are deployed on commercial vehicles carrying Hazmat, any alerts or problems with the cargo condition could be detected by fixed sensors at locations such as truck stops, or even by other vehicles. That detection capability could not only enable quicker response to an anomalous condition such as a chemical leak, but could also provide a real-time early-warning system for a wide array of chemical, biological, and nuclear threats across the United States.
>
> (Tate and Abkowitz, 2011, p. 31)

The researchers' approach should in fact improve response to an emergency that could potentially occur with a vehicle carrying HAZMAT; however, the researchers do not address the potential of collecting data to work on prevention and enhance security as well as safety along the HAZMAT routes. Texas A&M University in conjunction with Texas Southern University also has a research project to track HAZMAT when cargo is being transported throughout the state (Texas A&M University Transportation Institute, 2014). However, this research project does not mention using the data to prevent HAZMAT containers from falling into the wrong hands, nor does it mention any aspect of using the data for a unified approach with any other national effort of tracking HAZMAT (Texas A&M University Transportation Institute, 2014).

## Incidents Related to HAZMAT Transportation

There have been incidents, either through intentional actions or through accidental incidents, where HAZMAT has been released from a container or stolen en route to a destination. Between 1971 and 2013, 589 people were killed in relation to the transportation of HAZMAT on United States highways (Reilly, 2014). This does not include the number of individuals injured in the transportation of HAZMAT, nor is there any information that provides a dollar amount of how much property or infrastructure damage occurred during HAZMAT transportation.

The other issue is the security of HAZMAT during transportation. For example, on December 2, 2014, a number of containers with poisonous gas were stolen in Wilmington while a vehicle was parked (Altman, 2014). The problems with transportation of HAZMAT are not limited to just the United States. In 2013, a truck carrying Cobalt 60 was hijacked in Mexico as it was taking those radioactive elements for disposal (Rodriquez, Lopez, Corcoran, Caldwell and Jahn, 2013) In November 21, 2014, a group of bandits hijacked a truck in Guinea, which was hauling blood tainted by the Ebola virus (Diallo, 2014). In short, the possibility of HAZMAT being released through accidental means or compromised during transportation definitely exists.

## Methodology Proposed

So, how does one determine how many vehicles are on certain roadways during a given timeframe? There are companies that transport chemicals, bio-toxins, radioactive isotopes, and HAZMAT waste that use GPS locator tags on each container. Additionally, there are companies that transport HAZMAT using GPS locators on the vehicles themselves (e.g. AAT Carriers) (AAT Carriers, 2014). Other governmental agencies (e.g. DOE, CDC etc.) strictly regulate how particular radioactive isotopes, chemicals, bio-toxins, or HAZMAT waste are transported and how those items are tracked. Through these tracking mechanisms (e.g. GPS locators), it should be possible to lock down time, location, and route of vehicles carrying HAZMAT as well as the type and amount of HAZMAT throughout the United States for a given time period.

Once the data is collected, it would be possible to utilize GIS to map routes in relation to populated centers (e.g. cities). Once the information is layered onto a map of roadways in the United States, it would be possible to determine what type of incidents might occur as well as when and where these incidents are most likely to take place. After the GIS is constructed for each time-period, policies and procedures could be employed that provide resources strategically located at given locations (and possibly on given dates and time periods), to mitigate the risk of death, injury, or destruction from an incident (accidental or intentional) during the transportation of HAZMAT.

In addition, government agencies (e.g. state, county, and municipality) along major HAZMAT routes of transportation could be trained and equipped to contend with specific types of HAZMAT. For smaller government entities, a federal subsidy could provide funds and equipment to assist those organizations with a potential HAZMAT contamination event or security failure. However, this would be dependent upon the data being up to date and accurate. The DOE has strict controls in place for radioactive isotope control for organizations that use such materials for research, production, medical uses, and energy production. The controls for radioactive isotopes have evolved and been strictly in place since the Manhattan project in the 1940s (Valcik, 2013).

## Shortcomings With Current Tracking Data

While there are strict inventory control procedures at the federal level for radioactive isotopes through the Nuclear Regulatory Commission (NRC), this has not always been the case for bio-toxins, chemicals, or waste. Since 9/11, these items have begun to have greater inventory controls placed on them to assist law enforcement and first responders who respond to crises or events when they occur. After 9/11, the Patriot Act was passed in 2001, which was followed by the passage of the Bioterrorism Preparedness and Response Act of 2002, designed to provide federal oversight to a narrow group of biological elements termed "select agents" by the Centers for Disease Control (CDC) and the United States Agricultural Department (USDA) (Valcik, 2013). Passing the legislative statutes did not necessarily guarantee that all select agents were accounted for accurately. For example, in 2014 it was accidentally discovered that the Federal Food and Drug Administration (FDA) maintained a storage room at the National Institutes for Health (NIH) campus that contained not only smallpox but also 12 boxes and 327 vials containing pathogens that cause dengue fever, Q fever, influenza, and spotted fever (Dennis and Sun, 2014–1). This was preceded by the discovery of live smallpox strains in a cold storage room in the NIH facility that dated back to the 1950s (Dennis and Sun, 2014–2). In short, without accurate and complete data in a centralized database, the data cannot be used to prepare and plan adequately for security breaches and failures in bio-toxin containment. Without enforcement of current statutes, the data will continue to have gaps, and these gaps will prevent tracking of improperly identified bio-toxins. An example of this failure to track bio-toxins was when Thomas Butler, a Texas Tech professor, sent petri dishes with plague to Tanzania via Federal Express; Butler was later convicted (Williams, 2004). Federal oversight of bio-toxin identification and transportation, in the form of a national database, is necessary to prevent inattentiveness to and mismanagement of HAZMAT.

Federal statutes requiring the inventory of chemicals were mandated even later than for bio-toxins. In 2007, the federal government passed the Homeland Security Chemical Facility Anti-Terrorism Standards Act, which mandated that certain chemicals in amounts over a particular threshold must be inventoried and reported to the federal government (Valcik, 2013). Before 2007, there were certain instances where chemicals had been used to construct extremely powerful explosive devices (i.e. the Oklahoma City bombing in 1995), highlighting the damage, death, and injury these devices can inflict (Valcik, 2013). Chemicals are more numerous than select agent bio-toxins and have applications not only for military and research functions, but also in commercial and residential consumer use. For example, how much fertilizer is stockpiled for normal residential gardening use or large business campuses? How does anyone accurately know how much of those chemicals are 1) in existence and 2) how those items are secured? Obtaining an accurate depiction of what chemicals and the quantities being transported can be problematic.

The City of West in Texas is a good example of what can happen when first responders are unaware of common chemicals (in this case, ammonium nitrate) being stored at a commercial facility, despite laws that required the fertilizer plant to report how much of the chemical was on site (Sivak, 2016). The fire and the resulting explosion in the City of West cost the lives of 12 first responders along with three other individuals (Sivak, 2016). This incident also had a transport HAZMAT component, which could have had a disastrous impact upon communities or transportation infrastructure if the railcar loaded with ammonium nitrate had caught fire and exploded (Gaynor, 2013). The railcar brings up a series of thought-provoking questions: did anyone know the railcar was located at the plant? Was there a record or inventory of the ammonium nitrate that first responders or law enforcement could have accessed when it was transported to the fertilizer plant? Along the railway, were there any prepositioned first responders who could have responded adequately if the ammonium nitrate had exploded en route to the fertilizer plant? These are the questions policymakers and government agencies should ask regarding how data shortfalls will be addressed to improve public safety.

Currently in the United States (2019), various transportation companies do not track chemicals or keep an inventory using a national standard. This can obviously create issues in attempting to collect, much less use, data to analyze where resources should be deployed or prepositioned in an effort to mitigate any type of accidental or intentional HAZMAT incident. Transportation companies that transport only one type of HAZMAT in a single vehicle can easily track the vehicle and its contents with a GPS locator tag.

Tracking hazardous waste can vary state by state according to the state-specific regulations and mechanisms in place. In California, however, the difficulty of using data the state has collected for years on the transportation of waste has recently been highlighted (Garrison, Poston and Christensen, 2013). In 2011, students and teachers at Saul Martinez Elementary School became violently ill due to a company dumping waste a mile from the school (Garrison, Poston and Christensen, 2013). The company had no permit to dump waste, but state officials had not analyzed the data to reveal that shipments of waste were going to this company anyway (Garrison, Poston and Christensen, 2013). The State of California could not account for 174,000 tons of hazardous materials shipped over a five-year period (Garrison, Poston and Christensen, 2013). Transportation to out-of-state locations has made gaps in collection delivery data even more problematic (Garrison, Poston and Christensen, 2013). Gaps in this type of information could prove devastating for law enforcement and first responders if an incident were to occur. This incident illustrates the importance of not only collecting data but also being able to use the data once it has been collected.

Studies have been conducted in China on tracking vehicles carrying chemical HAZMAT (Tan et al., 2014). However, even with a nationalized, uniformed approach, these studies face the same shortfalls. While a vehicle can be tracked easily with a GPS locator tag, the contents, which might include several different containers of HAZMAT within the vehicle, could be separated from the vehicle without knowledge if the containers themselves have not been inventoried and tagged. The complexity of keeping an inventory of chemicals, biotoxins, radioactive isotopes, and harmful waste at a national level increases dramatically compared to only tracking the vehicles carrying the items. Complexity of this type would require a robust mechanism such as GPS locator tags with a central collection point to store real-time locations for all HAZMAT containers.

## Feasibility

What resources are necessary to track the transportation of chemicals, bio-toxins, radioactive isotopes, and hazardous waste via a national tracking database in the United States? Technology is only one part of the effort to collect and track HAZMAT transportation. To track all four types of HAZMAT, the federal government would need to pass statutes mandating the types and amounts of HAZMAT that would be tracked. Additionally, the manner or mechanism (i.e. GPS locator tags, RFID etc.) by which these items are to be tracked and the agency tasked to do so would have to be determined. To track all four types of HAZMAT through the transportation stage, uniform standards would be needed in terms of how data would be coded and sent to a collection point (i.e. information center) that would then allow analysts access to and utilization of the data.

Maintaining a federal database with uniform standards that can transmit inventory to a centralized collection point can lessen the risk of HAZMAT getting lost while crossing state lines. However, enforcement agencies are needed to ensure compliance by the companies and agencies that transport such materials. Penalties in the form of fines and possible criminal charges will ensure compliance with legislative mandates.

To warehouse data that will be dynamic, a robust enterprise data warehouse will be needed, one that will have the specifications for storage and the processing ability for large amounts of data. Additionally, the database should be constructed in Microsoft SQL Server, Oracle, or IBM DB2 to allow the table structure to be accessed for analysis by ArcSDE, enabling GIS analysts to work with the location data in a timely fashion. Without this connectivity present, the ability of GIS to interact with the large amounts of data being gathered will go unrealized. Analysts who use ArcGIS with SAS also have the potential to forecast where specific resources will be needed for different types of incident (i.e. security, HAZMAT accident etc.) with the highest probability.

## References

AAT Carriers, 2014. "HAZMAT and high security transport". Retrieved on December 12, 2014. www.aatcarriers.com/

Altman, Larry, 2014. "Thieves steal canisters of poisonous gas in Wilmington", *The Daily Breeze*. December 2. Retrieved on December 15, 2014. www.dailybreeze.com/general-news/20141202/thieves-steal-canisters-of-poisonous-gas-in-wilmington

Dennis, Brady and Sun, Lena H., 2014–1. "FDA found more than smallpox vials in storage rooms", *The Washington Post*. July 16, 2014. Retrieved on July 6, 2016. www.washingtonpost.com/national/health-science/fda-found-more-than-smallpox-vials-in-storage-room/2014/07/16/850d4b12-0d22-11e4–8341-b8072b1e7348_story.html

Dennis, Brady and Sun, Lena H., 2014–2. "Smallpox vials, decades old, found in storage room at NIH campus in Bethesda", *The Washington Post*. July 8, 2014. Retrieved on July 6, 2016. www.washingtonpost.com/national/health-science/smallpox-vials-found-in-storage-room-of-nih-campus-in-bethesda/2014/07/08/bfdc284a-06d2-11e4-8a6a-19355c7e870a_story.html?tid=a_inl

Diallo, Boubacar, "Suspected Ebola blood stolen in Guinea by bandits", *The Washington Times*. November 21, 2014. Retrieved on December 15, 2014. www.washingtontimes.com/news/2014/nov/21/bandits-in-guinea-steal-suspected-ebola-blood/?page=all

Garrison, Jessica, Poston, Ben and Christensen, 2013. "State fails to keep track of hazardous waste", *Los Angeles Times*. November 16, 2013. Retrieved on July 7, 2016. www.latimes.com/local/la-me-hazardous-waste-20131117-dto-htmlstory.html

Gaynor, Tim, 2013. "Rail car with ammonium nitrate didn't cause Texas blast: Fire official", *Reuters*. April 23, 2013. Retrieved on July 7, 2016. www.reuters.com/article/us-usa-explosion-texas-idUSBRE93M1I820130424

Goddard, David, 2014. "UT helps effort to take some of the hazard out of hazmat transportation", *Tennessee Today*. October 17, 2014. Retrieved on December 12, 2014. http://tntoday.utk.edu/2014/10/17/ut-helps-effort-hazard-hazmat-transportation/

Homeland Security Newswire, 2010. "Trucking industry says it is prepared for terrorism threat", *Homeland Security Newswire*. March 19, 2010. Retrieved on December 12, 2014. www.homelandsecuritynewswire.com/trucking-industry-says-it-prepared-terrorism-threat

Reilly, Steve, 2014. "Open road for hazmat trucking in NY", *Press Connects*. July 22, 2014. Retrieved on December 15, 2014. www.pressconnects.com/story/news/local/2014/07/18/hazmat-trucking-ny-fdny-regulations/12856099/

Rodriquez, Olga R., Lopez, Emilio, Corcoran, Katherine, Caldwell, Alicia A., and Jahn, George, 2013. "Radioactive material stolen in Mexican truck heist found near where truck was abandoned", *National Post*. December 4. Retrieved December 15, 2014. http://news.nationalpost.com/2013/12/04/extremely-dangerous-radioactive-material-stolen-in-mexican-truck-heist-could-be-used-to-build-a-dirty-bomb/

Schweitzer, Richard P., 2007. "Homeland security takes over regulatory role from DOT", *Gases and Welding Distributors Association*. September 15. Retrieved on December 12, 2007. www.weldingandgasestoday.org/index.php/2007/09/homeland-security-takes-over-regulatory-role-from-dot/

Sivak, Cathy, 2016. "Fire code lessons from West, Texas disaster", *Fire Chief*. Retrieved on July 6, 2016. www.firechief.com/2016/06/20/fire-code-lessons-from-west-texas-disaster/

Tan, Qiulin, Zhang, Yang, Zhang, Xiaofei, Pei, Xiangdong, Xiong, Jijun, Xue, Chenyang, Liu, Jun and Zhang, Wendong, 2014. "A hazardous chemical-oriented monitoring and tracking system based on sensor network", *International Journal of Distributed Sensor Networks*. Article ID 410476. Hindawi Publishing Corporation, New York. Retrieved on July 7, 2016. www.hindawi.com/journals/ijdsn/2014/410476/

Tate, William H. and Abkowitz, Mark D., 2011. "Emerging technologies applicable to hazardous materials transportation safety and security", *Hazardous Materials Cooperative Research Program*. Transportation Research Board, HMCRP Report Number 4, Washington, DC. Retrieved on December 12, 2014. http://onlinepubs.trb.org/onlinepubs/hmcrp/hmcrp_rpt_004.pdf

Texas A&M Transportation Institute, 2014. "Security is more than a state of mind", *Texas Transportation Researcher*. Retrieved on December 12, 2014. http://tti.tamu.edu/2010/12/01/security-is-more-than-a-state-of-mind/

Valcik, Nicolas A., 2013. *Hazardous materials compliance for public research organizations: A case study*. CRC Press/Taylor and Francis, New York.

Williams, Brian, 2004. "Butler gives up medical license amid plague case", *Lubbock Avalanche—Journal*. February 7. Retrieved on July 6, 2016. http://lubbockonline.com/stories/020704/loc_020704040.shtml#.V30U2zVELmg

# 5 Fire Disturbance and Implications for Ecosystem Services Distribution in Northern Amazonia

*Anthony R. Cummings and Benjamin Kennady*

## Introduction

The hurricanes, earthquakes, and wildfires that occurred in 2017, and the resulting hundreds of lives that were lost, are the kinds of natural disasters that capture our attention. On August 24, 2017, Hurricane Harvey plowed across the Atlantic and made landfall in the US in the states of Texas and Louisiana. While recovery efforts for Harvey were underway, Hurricane Irma arrived in the southeastern United States—especially Florida—on August 30, 2017. Before the rubble from Irma could be gathered, Jose made landfall in the already ravaged Barbuda on August 31, 2017. Not to be outdone by her predecessors, Maria made landfall in Puerto Rico on September 20, 2017, leaving destruction and damage that placed additional pressures on the island's already fragile public infrastructure system (Hester & Echenique, 2017; Lu & Alcantara, 2017; Mufson, 2017). Three earthquakes, with magnitudes of 8.1, 7.1, and 6.1, displaced the Earth's crust under Mexico within a matter of weeks (Hanna, 2017), resulting in the loss of lives (Semple et al., 2017) and destruction to property. These short-lived events (see Hidore, 1996) have created disturbances to the atmospheric and terrestrial systems, and society and science have developed tools to predict and study their impacts on arrival (see Chavez, 2017; Coren, 2017; McPhate, 2017; Walker, 2017). Much of our response, at least as measured by the dominant electronic media in the United States, has been projected through the lens of social justice, highlighting the differences in the federal government's response to mainland US cities impacted by Harvey versus the responses to cash-strapped Puerto Rico (Anapol, 2017; Lopez, 2017). The debate over whether Puerto Rico should gain more attention, and aid, will likely rage on for the foreseeable future, but the response, inadequate or not, appears to pale in comparison to the pleas for help from the island's neighbors in the Caribbean who were affected by the same storms (see Raphael, 2017; Brown, 2017; Stabroeknews, 2017). Given the timeframe and scale of destruction associated with these short-lived events, the more subtle natural disasters that affect places out of the lens of dominant news programs are often ignored.

In contrast to the storms and earthquakes across the Caribbean and the Gulf Coast of Mexico, events affecting Amazonian landscapes are less predictable in their path and potential impact, and they receive considerably less attention. Like the fires in northern California (Abramson, 2017), the natural disasters occurring within indigenous people-influenced landscapes tend to be more subtle in their occurrence. For Amazonian indigenous communities, many of which are vulnerable to climatic variability (e.g. Griffiths, 2008; Malhi et al., 2008), the types of natural disasters that dominate their landscapes take a longer time to deliver their impacts. For example, El Niño events that have unfolded over the past two decades or so, in 1997–1998, 2009–2010, and 2015–2016, were associated with droughts of various severity as felt in Brazil (Hess & Tasa, 2017), Guyana (Sutherland, 2009, 2016), and other South American nation states. While the natural disasters that occurred across the Caribbean were disruptive and noticeable, El Niño's teleconnections are more latent and gradual in their arrival. The end result of El Niño's arrival, however, while dissimilar from the visible and direct destruction of homes and businesses associated with storms and earthquakes, are similar in that food and water become scarce (Sutherland, 2009). Further complicating El Niño's arrival is the fact that some of the world's most vulnerable populations are victims to its accompanying droughts.

As a precursor to natural disasters, primarily fires in Amazonia, El Niño-Southern Oscillation (ENSO) events have global-level implications (Brown & Buis, 2017). El Niño events are triggered as the low-pressure system that exists over northern Australia (Darwin) is reversed with the high-pressure system that exists over Tahiti. The reversal in pressure causes the monsoons to fail, placing in motion drought conditions that can bring famine to places like India (see Hess & Tasa, 2017) and continental South America. In Guyana, the 2009–2010 and 2015–2016 El Niño events teleconnections were linked to reduced rainfall that triggered water shortages in coastal and hinterland areas, leading to crop failure (Sutherland, 2009, 2016). While the frequency of El Niño events appears to follow the patterns of cyclical oscillations (Hidore, 1996), their intensity is raising more questions on their impacts for indigenous peoples' livelihoods (Cummings, 2016). Among the questions currently being posed by indigenous peoples and scholars alike in Guyana are: as El Niño results in reduced water availability, what is the most appropriate variety (landrace) of cassava—*Manihot esculenta*—to grow? How will changes in weather patterns, in particular droughts, impact the distribution of plant species from which indigenous peoples derive ecosystem services such as medicines and non-timber forest products? How will the distribution and density of wildlife hunted by indigenous peoples be impacted by changes in water availability? In the context of Guyana, the crop failures associated with the 2015–2016 El Niño event attracted a high level of national media attention (Guyana Chronicle, 2015; Sutherland, 2016). Despite the attention given to their woes, however, unlike their counterparts experiencing natural disasters in the global north, the response to indigenous peoples' challenges due to El Niño have often been feeble and uncoordinated. In an effort to understanding how El Niño will impact indigenous peoples' livelihoods in Guyana, this chapter begins the process of examining potential implications for plant species distribution.

Traditionally, Amazonian indigenous peoples-influenced landscapes have been associated with a number of important processes, including hosting swidden agriculture plots and forests from which they gather products to support their livelihoods (Cummings et al., 2017; Denevan 1980, 1988, 1992, 2004, 2006; Posey 1985, 1982). Indigenous peoples derive a suite of ecosystem services from the plants located in the vicinity of their swidden plots, including food, medicines, and non-timber forest products (see Cummings, 2013; Cummings & Read, 2016; Sivasailam & Cummings, 2016). Beyond being directly associated with peoples' livelihoods, the plants found within indigenous peoples-influenced landscapes support wildlife populations that are hunted for food (Cummings, 2013). In Guyana, as is the case for swidden landscapes across the tropics, fire is an important component of the food production system.

After a farmer cuts the forest to create a new farm, the trees and stems are left to dry, and then burned (see Uhl, 1987) to facilitate the production of biochar (see also Amazon Dark Earth, ADE; Lehmann et al., 2003; Major et al., 2005). Biochar is an important part of the soil column, providing nutrients and holding moisture (see Lehmann et al., 2003; Major et al., 2005) that allows for crops to be grown. While fire is important for the production of ADE soils, Amazonian forests typically do not experience extensive burning as the moist microclimate and high rainfall create nearly nonflammable conditions (Kauffman et al., 1988; Uhl et al., 1988). However, as a result of increased land use change within the region, more fuel loads are becoming available, leading to more frequent fires (Uhl and Kauffman, 1990). The increased incidence of fire events within indigenous peoples-influenced landscapes can lead to plants that are typically ill-equipped to deal with fires (see Uhl & Kauffman, 1990) becoming vulnerable to damage. The damage of plants from which indigenous peoples derive ecosystems services and on which the wildlife they hunt rely can compromise the ability of these landscapes to support human life. In this regard, as the droughts associated with El Niño make conditions more suitable for fires, it is important to study how the distribution of plant species associated with important ecosystem services may be impacted.

Studying the distribution of fires relative to indigenous peoples' lands is not a new pursuit (see Mistry et al., 2016; Huffman, 2013; Raish et al., 2005; Welch et al., 2013; Williams, 2000). However, studying how events like El Niño may impact the number of fires within these landscapes and what changes in the number of fires may, in turn, mean for the distribution of plant species remains highly unexplored. The advent of satellites capable of detecting fires has advanced our ability to study fire impacts in a number of settings (see Liu et al., 2016; Matricardi et al., 2010; Morton et al., 2011; Roy & Kumar, 2017) and in the case of the tropics provides the opportunity to study fire's impact on plant species distribution. Data derived from the Visible Infrared Imaging Radiometer Suite (VIIRS) and the Moderate Resolution Imaging Spectroradiometer (MODIS), for example, are making studying fire impacts more accessible (Elvidge et al., 2016). In this chapter, we draw on data derived from MODIS to explore the potential impacts of fires on the distribution of plant species. Our work is positioned as a part of pre-natural disaster planning, in recognition of the fact that El Niño events themselves are not natural disasters, but that their teleconnections can lead to droughts and fires that may have disastrous outcomes. Building on the notion that El Niño's teleconnections have both global (see Brown & Buis, 2017) and local (Sutherland, 2009, 2016) impacts, we utilized fire and plant distribution data to explore the probability that fire events may impact the distribution of plant species associated with important ecosystem services. Data on the distribution of five plant species from which indigenous people derive ecosystems services were collected *in situ* from the Rupununi, Southern Guyana, and used in Maxent to develop models of probabilistic species distribution. Maxent models are widely used to determine the suitability of conditions for the presence of a species based on environmental variables (see Phillips et al., 2006; Phillips & Dudik, 2008; Phillips et al., 2017). Since Maxent models predict where conditions are suitable for a species, rather than affirming where they are found, we used suitability of conditions as a proxy for species presence. The primary objectives of this chapter are: 1) examine MODIS data of the Rupununi, Southern Guyana to determine whether El Niño events led to an increase in fire frequency; and 2) use the probabilistic distribution of plant species and the location of fires to determine the likelihood that fires may impact the distribution of the five plant species of interest in El Niño and non-El Niño years. The underlying assumption of our work is that El Niño events will result in more drought-like conditions within the Rupununi and this, in turn, would lead to increased vegetation stress, more fuel for fires, and hence more fires. The increased number of fires will make more plants vulnerable to damage. With the increasing impacts of El Niño being observed across the globe, the chapter's overarching goal is to propose methods to be used for studying the impacts of natural hazards on species distribution. In this regard, we drew heavily on publicly available data and methods to address our objectives.

## Methods

### *Study Area*

Data for assessing the potential impacts of fires on the distribution of plant species and hence the ecosystem services with which they are associated were obtained for the Rupununi, Southern Guyana (Figure 5.1). The Rupununi is a tropical forest and savannah biome that lies between 0°50′—4° 49′ N and 56°54′—59°55′ W and is approximately 350 km southwest of the capital of Guyana, Georgetown (Figure 5.1). The Rupununi's population is dominated by the Makushi and Wapishiana indigenous peoples, who rely heavily on their forests for a number of ecosystem services, including fuelwood, medicines, and non-timber forest products (Cummings, 2013). A key reason why the Rupununi indigenous peoples have maintained strong ties to their forests is because the region has had very poor road and other communication links to

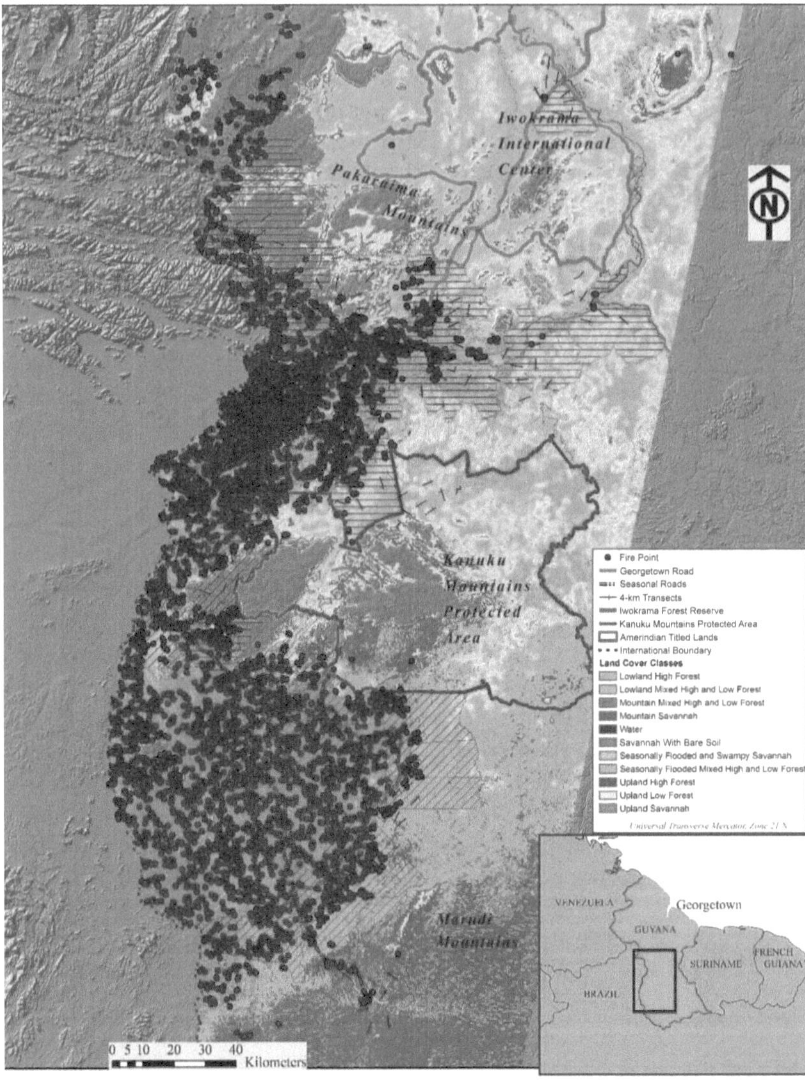


*Figure 5.1* Study area showing the Rupununi's vegetation types overlaid with the distribution of fire events used in this study.

coastal Guyana up until two decades or so ago. While the Makushi and Wapishiana indigenous peoples have been occupying the Rupununi for more than 10,000 years (Forte, 1996; Plew, 2005), the current occupants of the region have witnessed a number of changes within their homelands. As the modern-day Rupununi population observes changes within their lands, concerns are raised that their relationships to their forests could be re-shaped at the expensive of their culture. As a fair-weather road now connects coastal Guyana with Brazil (Figure 5.1), accessibility to the Rupununi has improved to the point where timber and other resources can be removed from the region. On the other hand, the addition of the road to the Rupununi landscape means that supplies of food and other materials more strongly associated with Georgetown's more westernized culture can arrive in times of need and as a matter of general commerce. The improving road connection with Georgetown is allowing for a new suite of activities that drive land-use and land-cover changes to be pursued in the area, with the area's timber and gold resources the primary focus.

The recent changes in land-use, coupled with the teleconnections associated with El Niño, are growing areas of concern for the Rupununi indigenous peoples. The changes in weather and access to the Rupununi are raising questions as to whether the ecosystem can sustain indigenous peoples' traditional livelihood activities. Many residents of the Rupununi have suggested that precipitation patterns within their homeland have changed (Cummings personal observation), but it was perhaps the 2009–2010 and 2015–2016 El Niño events (see details on the Oceanic Niño Index in Table 5.1) and their associated droughts that made some of these observations more relevant to the area. For example, as a result of the severe drought associated with the 2009–2010 El Niño event, Sutherland (2009) reported that the cassava crop in some southern Rupununi villages failed. The 2015–2016 El Niño event, more severe that the previous episode, attracted the attention of the national media (see Sutherland,

*Table 5.1* Oceanic Niño Index (ONI) for the 2009–2010 and 2015–2016 El Niño events

| *Event* | *2009–2010* | *2015–2016* |
|---|---|---|
| January | −0.8# | 0.6* |
| February | −0.7# | 0.6* |
| March | −0.5# | 0.6* |
| April | −0.2 | 0.8* |
| May | 0.1 | 1* |
| June | 0.4 | 1.2* |
| July | 0.5* | 1.5* |
| August | 0.5* | 1.8* |
| September | 0.7* | 2.1* |
| October | 1* | 2.4* |
| November | 1.3* | 2.5* |
| December | 1.6* | 2.6* |
| January | 1.5* | 2.5* |
| February | 1.3* | 2.2* |
| March | 0.9* | 1.7* |
| April | 0.4 | 1* |
| May | −0.1 | 0.5* |

Warm (*) and cold (#) periods based on a threshold of +/−0.5°C for the Oceanic Niño Index (ONI).

Source: http://origin.cpc.ncep.noaa.gov/products/analysis_monitoring/ensostuff/ONI_v5.php

2009, 2016), policymakers, and local-level managers alike. In fact, the 2015–2016 El Niño not only threatened food production and water supply in the Rupununi, but also impacted wildlife with which indigenous peoples in the Rupununi and wider Guyana (Cummings, 2016) are associated.

The Rupununi also hosts a high diversity of ground-living mammals, frugivorous primates, and birds, with 107 of the ground-living mammals, reptiles, and birds being hunted by indigenous peoples for food (Read et al., 2010). Of these species, eight (paca or labba (*Cuniculus paca*), agouti (*Dasyprocta leporina*), white-lipped peccary (*Tayassu pecari*), collared peccary (*Pecari tajacu*), red brocket deer (*Mazama americana*), white-tailed deer (*Odocoileus virginianus*), nine-banded armadillo (*Dasypus novemcinctus*), and red-footed tortoise (*Chelonoidis carbonaria*)) comprise 69% of hunted species (Read et al., 2010). Further, of these eight species, all but the nine-banded armadillo rely on the fruits of trees and palms within the study area for food (Cummings, 2013; Roosmalen, 1985).

## Study Plant Species and Their Associated Ecosystem Services

The steps taken to complete this analysis are highlighted in Figure 5.2. To examine the impacts of fires on the distribution of plants, we chose five species: four trees—baromalli (*Catostemma commune* Sandwith), bulletwood

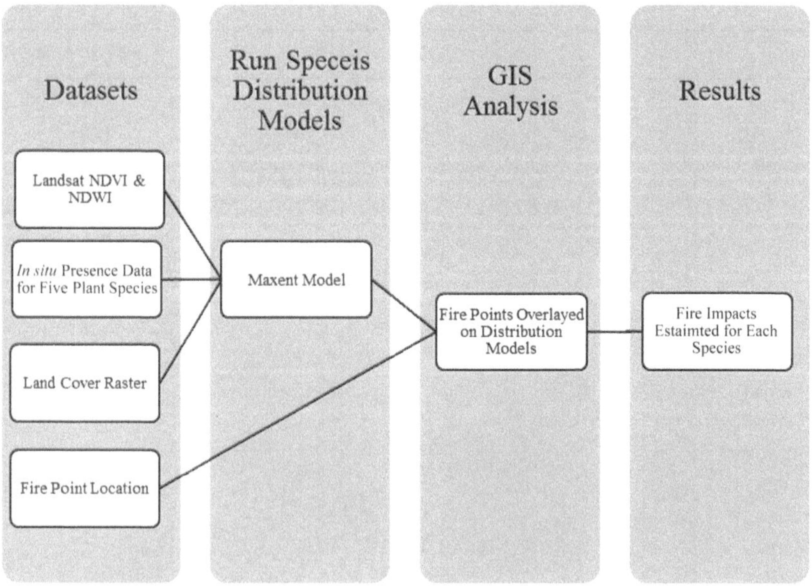


*Figure 5.2* A flow chart of the methods we used in this study.

(*Manilkara bidentata* (A.DC.) Chev.), crabwood (*Carapa guianensis* Aubl. and *C. procera* DC), locust (*Hymenaea courbaril* L.)—and one palm kokerite (*Attalea maripa* (Aubl.) Mart.) with which indigenous peoples have strong documented relationships (see Cummings, 2013; Cummings & Read, 2016; Forte, 1996). To assess how changes in fire patterns relative to El Niño may impact the distribution of these plant species and hence the livelihoods of indigenous peoples, these species were used to develop species distribution models. These five plants species are associated with a diversity of ecosystem services (see Cummings & Read, 2016), including provisioning and cultural services, as measured within the Guyanese indigenous peoples context (see Table 5.2 for the typology of ecosystem services associated with these species) and were therefore ideal to test how ecosystem services may be compromised by changes in the area's fire regime.

*Table 5.2* The five target plant species and the typology of ecosystem services with which they are associated

| *Species* | *Supporting ES (Eaten by)* | *Provisioning ES (Non-Timber Forest Products)* |
|---|---|---|
| *Catostemma commune* Sandwith<br>Baromalli | agouti, deer, tapir, howler* and spider monkeys*, bats* | Fuelwood and building materials |
| *Hymenaea courbaril* L.<br>Locust | agouti, labba, tapir, peccaries, monkeys* (saki, capuchin) | Fuelwood and building materials; fruits are eaten |
| *Carapa guianensis* Aubl., *C. procera* DC<br>Crabwood | agouti, labba, peccaries | Therapeutic oil from seeds |
| *Manilkara bidentata* (A.DC.) Chev.<br>Bulletwood | peccaries, tapir, deer, tortoise, labba, agouti, spider* and howler monkeys*, macaws* | Gum used to make utensils for storing water and beverages, figurines and toys |
| *Attalea maripa* ((Aubl.) Mart.)<br>Kokerite | tapir, agouti, labba, tortoise, deer, black curassow, marudi, macaws, parrots | Fruits eaten, used to make beverages, and leaves used for thatching roofs |

* species not hunted—data from traditional knowledge and Roosmalen (1985)

Source: data on supporting services from traditional knowledge, Roosmalen (1985), and Forget & Hammond (2005). Data on provisioning services from traditional knowledge, Forte (1996), and van Andel (2000)

Labba or paca (*Agouti paca*), agouti (*Dasyprocta leporina*), white-lipped peccary (*Tayassu pecari*), collared peccary (*Pecari tajacu*), red brocket deer (*Mazama americana*), white-tailed deer (*Odocoileus virginianus*), nine-banded armadillo (*Dasypus novemcinctus*), red-footed tortoise (*Chelonoidis carbonaria*), howler monkey (*Alouatta seniculus*), spider monkey (*Ateles paniscus*), white saki (*Pithecia pithecia*), bats (*Artibeus lituratus*, among other species), black saki (*Chiropotes satanas*), capuchin (*Cebus paella*, *C. olivaceus*), toucans (*Ramphastos toco*, *R. vitellinus*), macaws (*Ara ararauna*, *A. macao*, *A. nobilis*).

Data from Cummings (2013)

### *Sampling Plant Species*

There are 26 titled indigenous communities within the Rupununi landscape. Legal title to land means that the village has all rights over their lands, including the right to determine how their forest resources are used. We collected data on the five plants species from 14 study sites, 12 villages, and two controls, distributed across the landscape (Figure 5.1) in the period July–December 2008. The 14 study sites were a subset of the villages and control areas participating in a larger project aimed at studying indigenous peoples' influence on biodiversity (see Luzar et al., 2011; Read et al., 2010 for details). As described in Read et al. (2010), study sites were selected based on their spatial distribution throughout the study area. The study sites' location also provided the opportunity to study how these five species were distributed relative to elevation, vegetation types, and other physical environmental attributes. Sampling was completed on eight belt transects, each 4 kilometers long by 10 m wide. All trees greater than 25 cm dbh and mature palms (defined as a palm showing signs of fruiting) were included in our sample. Prior to sampling, the start and end points of each transect were mapped in a GIS, and the location of each plant of interest was then found relative to a transect and subsequently mapped in a GIS. At the time of sampling, we made a note of the local or common name of each plant so that the ecosystem services with which they are associated could be determined (see Cummings, 2013 for more details).

### *Determining Ecosystem Service Associated With Plant Species*

The process used to move from local names to common names is described in Cummings (2013), Cummings and Read (2016), and Sivasailam and Cummings (2016) and is summarized here. After sampling on transects, the common name of each plant was translated to a botanical name based on the literature (including Roosmalen, 1985; Polak, 1992; Forte, 1996; van Andel, 2000; Iwokrama, 2008), and consultation with elders and researchers within the study area. Once a botanical name was determined for each plant, it was then classified into one or more resource-use classes, or how they are used for ecosystem services, namely:

1. Commercial timber: genus or species of tree actively logged for commercial timber in Guyana.
2. Wildlife food: genus or species of tree or palm that provide food for wildlife (hunted or not).
3. Traditional uses: genus or species of tree or palm used by Amerindians for medicinal purposes, traditional weaponry, boat crafting, traditional utensils, home construction, thatching, fuelwood, making beverages, food, including utilizing same for economic purposes and other purposes.
4. No known uses: at the time of analysis no resource uses could be determined for this genus or species.

Based on the classification into the main resource-use classes, the ecosystem services of each plant species were defined as per Table 5.2. Our classification went beyond identifying which plant species provide food for hunted wildlife and also drew on traditional knowledge and the literature (e.g. Roosmalen, 1985) to identify those frugivorous primates and species that are hunted which also depend on the fruits of the plants for food. The five species in our sample (Table 5.2) therefore represented a cross-section of the ecosystem services that are associated with the plants.

## Modeling Probabilistic Distribution of Plant Species

The location of each plant was used as presence data in Maxent models (see Phillips et al., 2017). Maxent utilizes the presence data of species and physical environmental attributes to determine the probability that a location is suited for the distribution of that species. Therefore, Maxent does not determine presence but rather the suitability of the environment for the occurrence of a species. We used habitat suitability as a proxy for presence. The presence data of the five (5) species of interest along with three environmental layers—a vegetation cover map developed by Cummings et al. (2015), a normalized difference vegetation index (NDVI) layer, and a normalized difference water index (NDWI)—for the study area were used to develop Maxent models. For each species, the model was developed using 75% of the location points, with the remaining 25% of data kept for model assessment. We used the Jackknife function in Maxent to determine how each of the three environmental variables contributed to the output species distributions.

## Fire Data

To understand the distribution of the five plant species relative to fires, data were downloaded from NASA's EarthData Active Fire Dataset (https://earthdata.nasa.gov/earth-observation-data/near-real-time/firms/active-fire-data). These fire locations were derived from the Moderate Resolution Imaging Spectroradiometer (MODIS) sensor. We obtained data for the period 2007 to 2016 therefore including the 2009–2010 and 2015–2016 El Niño events. Details on the two El Niño events are presented in Table 5.1. Once the fire data were downloaded, they were imported into a GIS environment for displaying in the same spatial reference as the probabilistic distribution models of the five species of interest.

## Estimating the Impact of Fires on Species Distribution

Once the fire locations data were downloaded from MODIS and the Maxent models were developed for each species, each fire point location was overlaid on the species models to determine the probability that the fire might have impacted that species distribution. The overlay of fire on species distribution therefore returned a value between 0 and 1 such that each fire event was associated with the distribution of a species. The overlay function allowed us to populate a GIS database with each fire and the respective probability of each being associated with the five species of interest. The probability value of each fire was used to determine: 1) the average (mean) probability of each species being impacted by fires across the 2007–2016 study period; and 2) the number of fires associated with species probabilistic distribution of 50% (0.5) or greater. The data on the probabilities of species being impacted were analyzed and summarized to provide insights into how fires across the El Niño years compared with those from non-El Niño years.

## Results

Our analysis of the probabilistic distribution of the five target species relative to fire events suggested that each species was impacted differently by the changes in the number of fires across the study area and period. A species-by-species analysis showed that some distributions, as reflected through the Maxent models, and hence ecosystem services, will be impacted more than others. Over a ten-year period we found that fires could on average impact the plant species that provide ecosystem services, by up to 20%. The 2016 El Niño year showed the highest average probability of impacting the plant species, and this may have long-term implications for the plants and the people who derive ecosystem services from them. Based on the analysis of the data, it seems as though the presence and availability of plants associated with key ecosystem services may already be changing due to the increase in fires associated with El Niño.

## Target Species Probabilistic Distribution

The Maxent models suggested that with the exception of *M. bidentata*, where NDVI provided the highest predictive power of species distribution, vegetation type was the most important predictor of species distribution (Table 5.3). Overall, the species distribution models showed varying probabilities of the habitat conditions being suitable for the presence of the species of interest (Figure 5.3). It was expected that the savannah regions of the study area would not favor the distribution of the five plant species, and the Maxent models re-affirmed this point. In the case of *C. commune*, the Maxent model showed a higher probability of conditions being suitable for the presence of the species in the North Rupununi, with probability upwards of 85% in this region (Figure 5.3a). In the South Rupununi, the probability of the area favoring the species decreased markedly, with some areas, beyond the savannahs, highlighted as having unfavorable conditions for the presence of the species. Not surprisingly, in the case of *C. commune* distribution followed the forested areas. In almost a direct contrast to *C. commune*, *H. courbaril* probabilistic distribution was heavily favored towards the south of the study area, with

*Table 5.3* The Jackknife gain contribution of each environmental variable to predicting the distribution of the respective species. The approximate Jackknife gain range for each model is provided for context and appreciating the value of each variable

| *Species (Approximate Jackknife Gain Range)* | *Vegetation* | *Normalized Difference Vegetation Index* | *Normalized Difference Water Index* |
|---|---|---|---|
| *C. commune* (0.44–0.69) | 0.64 | 0.59 | 0.45 |
| *H. courbaril* (0.4–1.2) | 1.1 | 0.85 | 0.45 |
| *C. guianensis* (0.68–1.24) | 0.96 | 1.06 | 0.72 |
| *M. bidentata* (0.4–0.76) | 0.43 | 0.66 | 0.5 |
| *A. maripa* (0.45–0.76) | 0.64 | 0.59 | 0.41 |

the probability that conditions favored the presence of these species in these regions approaching 100% (Figure 5.3b). Interestingly, the Maxent model suggested that highland areas within the study area would be most suitable for *H. courbaril* distribution.

Similar to *C. commune*, the Maxent models of *C. guianensis* suggested that conditions were suitable for the presence of this species in the northern parts of the study area (Figure 5.3c). The Maxent models suggested that the lower elevations of the study areas favored the distribution of *C. guianensis*, but some higher elevations were also shown to possess favorable conditions for the species to be present. Of all the species in our sample, the conditions for the distribution of *M. bidentata* were uniformly distributed across the landscape, with slightly higher probabilities in the north than the south of the study area (Figure 5.3d). In fact, conditions were suitable for the presence of *M. bidentata* throughout the forested areas of the study area. Based on the Maxent models, the final species of interest in our sample, the palm *A. maripa* had favorable presence conditions across the study area, with a fairly uniform distribution across the forested regions. However, unlike *M. bidentata*, the Maxent models suggested conditions for *A. maripa* were more favorable in the lowland regions, primarily following the riverain areas of the study area, with a very low probability that conditions in the mountainous regions will favor this species (Figure 5.3e). The predicted probabilities for presence of each species was, therefore, slightly different across the study area.

## Distribution of Fires

Our data on fires over the period 2007–2016, as recorded by the MODIS sensor, showed that a total of 6,434 fires occurred within the study area (Table 5.4). The MODIS data showed a fluctuation in the number of fires detected over the ten years of interest with the fewest (367) in 2010 and highest (980) in 2015. The first years of the two El Niño events captured in the period, 2009 and 2015 (see Table 5.4) had the highest number of fires, with 802 and 980 respectively.

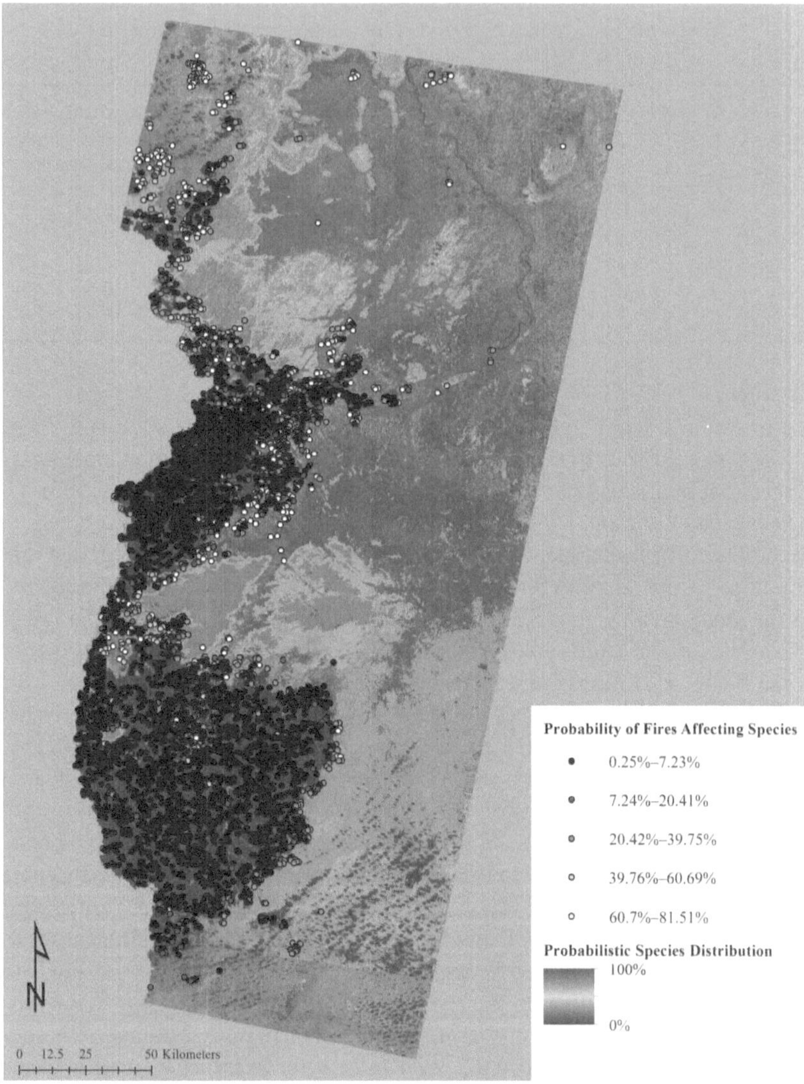


*Figure 5.3a* Maxent models and fire interactions for *C. commune*.

In contrast, the second year of both El Niño events, 2010 and 2016, had the lowest number of fires across the study period, with 367 and 452 respectively. In terms of spatial distribution, in contrast to the probabilistic distribution of the species of interest in our sample, which dominated the forested landscape, the majority of fires occurred in the savannah regions of the study area (Figure 5.1), with only 16.5% occurring in forests. In fact, most fires occurred in the

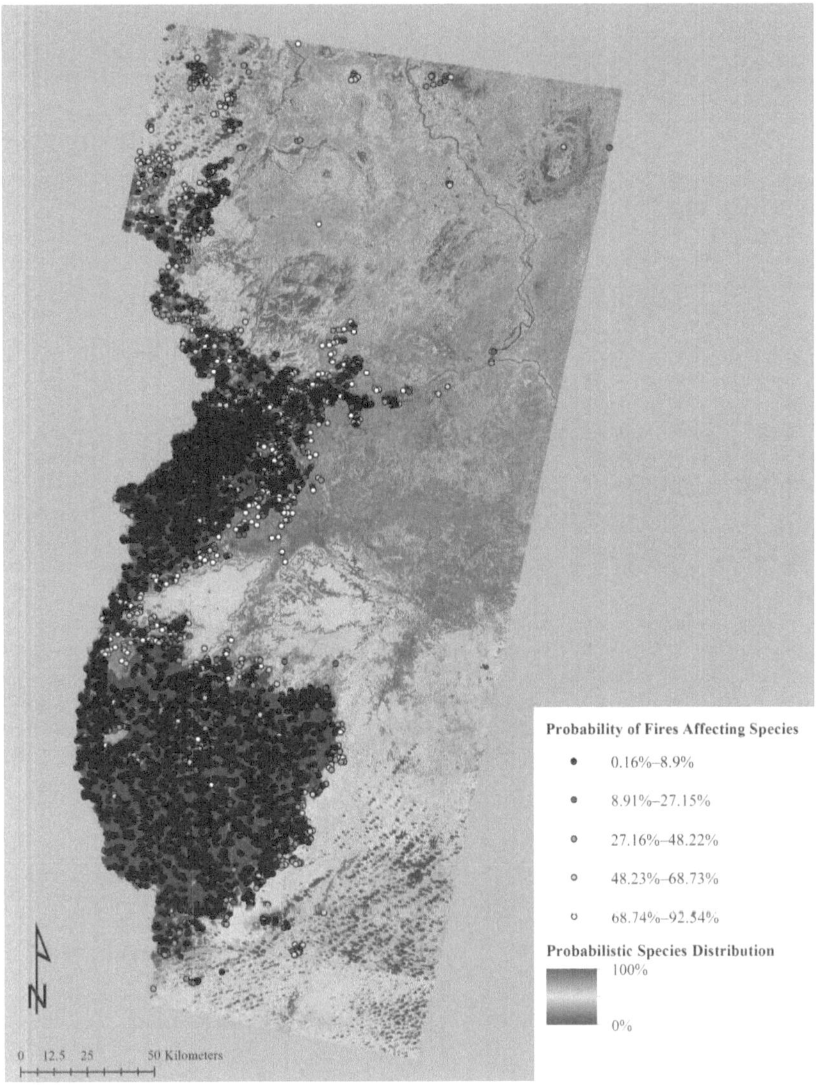


*Figure 5.3b* Maxent models and fire interactions for *M. bidentata*.

area we described here as the "forest edge" or the transition zone between the forest and savannah, which is characterized by indigenous peoples' swidden agriculture plots. Given that indigenous peoples farm and gather on the forest–savannah edge, the location of fires within this region was not surprising, but we note that they also gather from the plant species of interest within this zone, and increased fires here could lead to increased impacts on such plants.

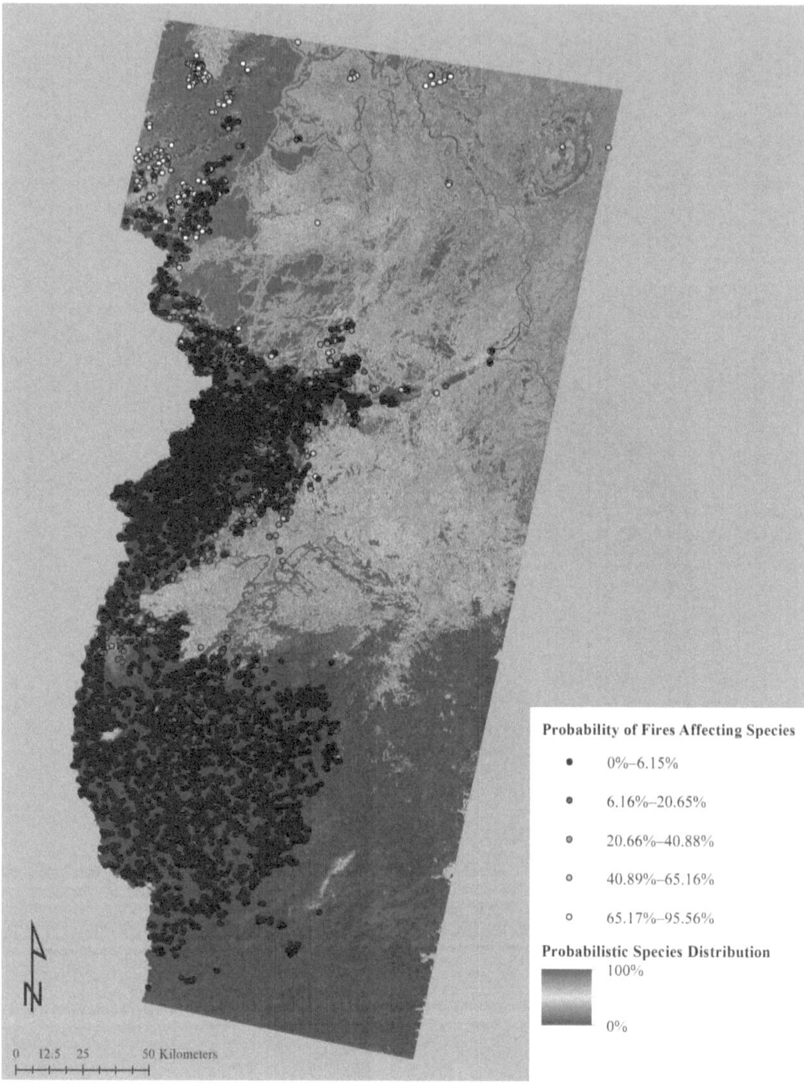


*Figure 5.3c* Maxent models and fire interactions for *C. guianensis*.

## Estimating the Impact of Fires on Species Distribution

Similar to how the probabilistic distribution of the five plant species varied across the landscape, estimates of potential impacts of fires on the distribution of the plants of interest also varied. The mean probability of fires impacting the distribution of the five species suggested that the years when the species would have more impacts from fires did not always correspond to those years that had

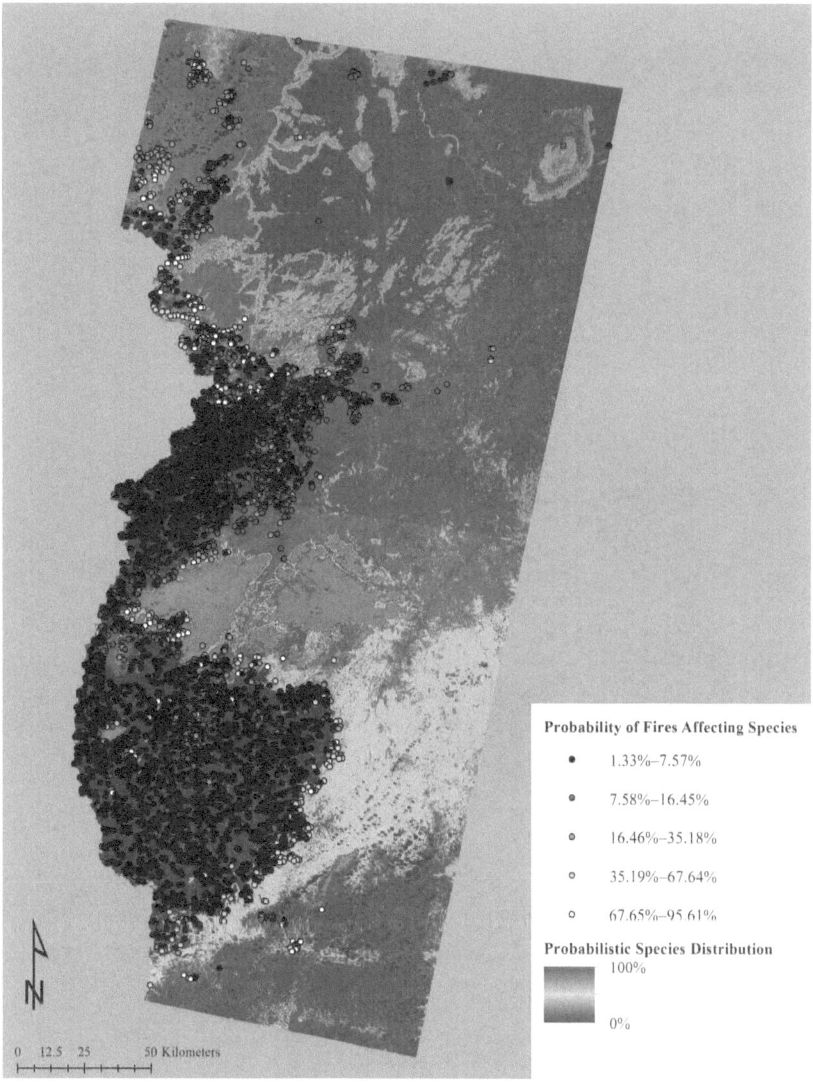


*Figure 5.3d* Maxent models and fire interactions for *H. courbaril*.

the highest number of fires. While the number of fires was highest for 2009 and 2015, the average probability of a species being impacted did not follow this pattern (Figure 5.4; Table 5.5).

The highest potential impact on all species, as measured by the average probability that a species was distributed where the MODIS data detected a fire (see Figure 5.4 and Table 5.5), was in the years 2015, 2008, and 2016, in order

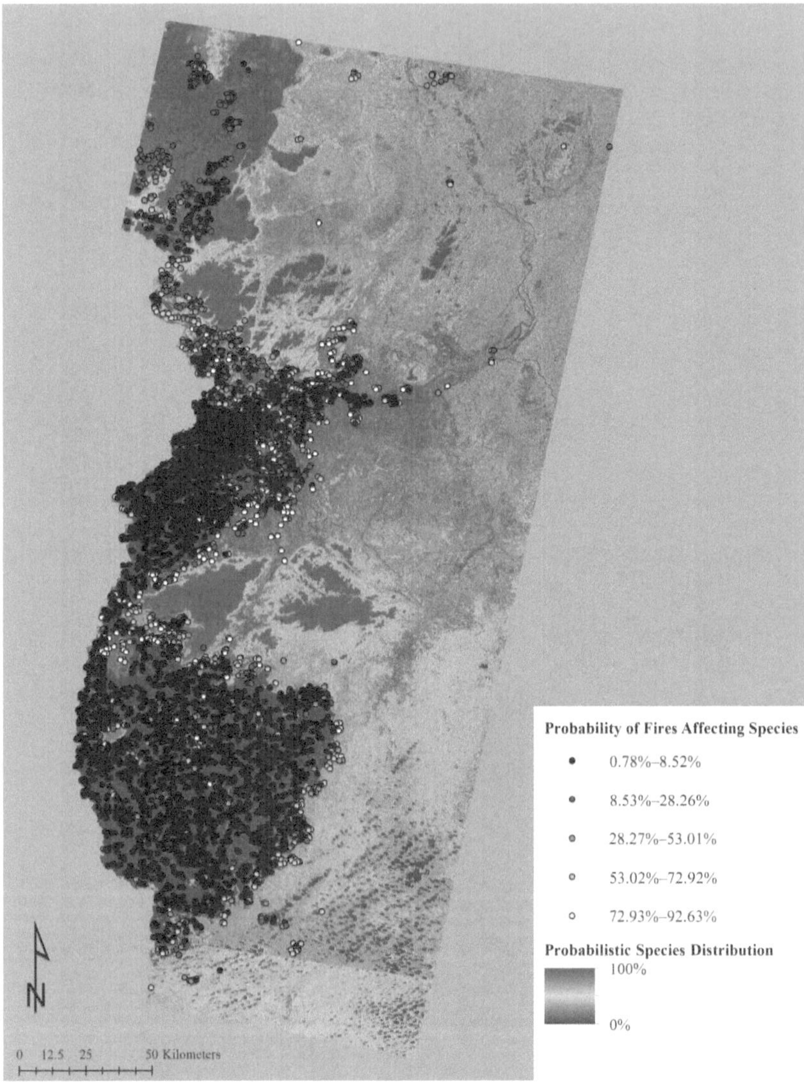


*Figure 5.3e* Maxent models and fire interactions for *A. maripa*.

from lowest to highest probability. Given that the El Niño event covered the years 2009–2010 and 2015–2016, the high number of fires in 2015 and 2016 was expected, as were the higher impacts, but 2008 had the lowest number of fires (Table 5.4) and therefore the high probability of impacts associated with this year was surprising. A sharp increase in the average probability of a species being impacted by fires was noted from the year 2015 to 2016, increasing

*Table 5.4* The ten-year period studied and the number of fires detected by MODIS in each year within the study area

| *Year* | *Number of Fires* |
|---|---|
| 2007 | 665 |
| 2008 | 473 |
| 2009 | 802 |
| 2010 | 367 |
| 2011 | 646 |
| 2012 | 717 |
| 2013 | 663 |
| 2014 | 669 |
| 2015 | 980 |
| 2016 | 452 |

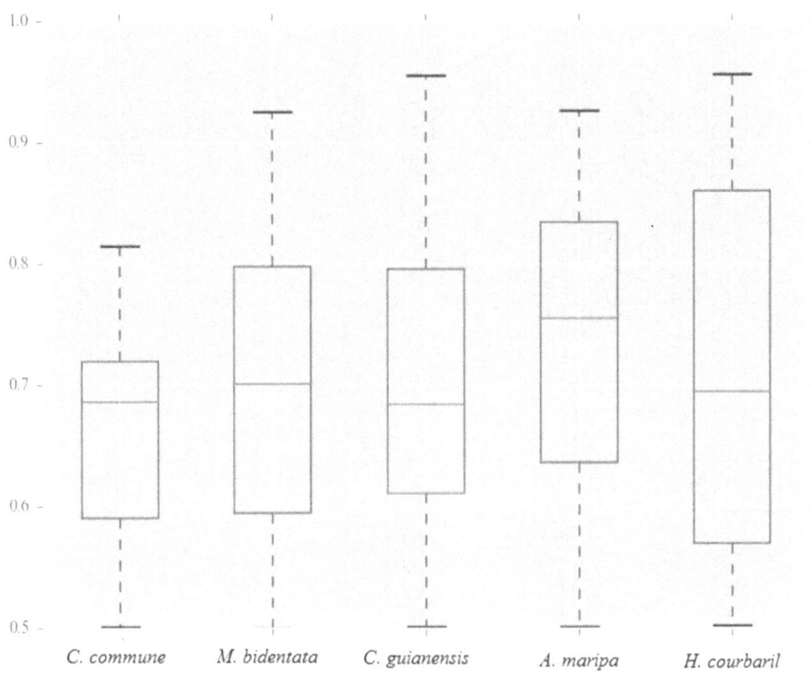


*Figure 5.4a* Fires with probability higher than 0.5 of impacting the plant species of interest.

by a probability of 0.05, 0.06, 0.02, 0.07, and 0.3 for *C. commune*, *M. bidentata*, *C. guianensis*, *H. courbaril*, and *A. maripa*, respectively. There was also an increase in the average probability of impact from 2007 to 2008 (Table 5.5), but this was not as sharp as observed from the 2015 to 2016 period.

When we examined the impacts of fires that occurred in the 2009–2010 El Niño years, we found some variation across species. For *C. commune*,

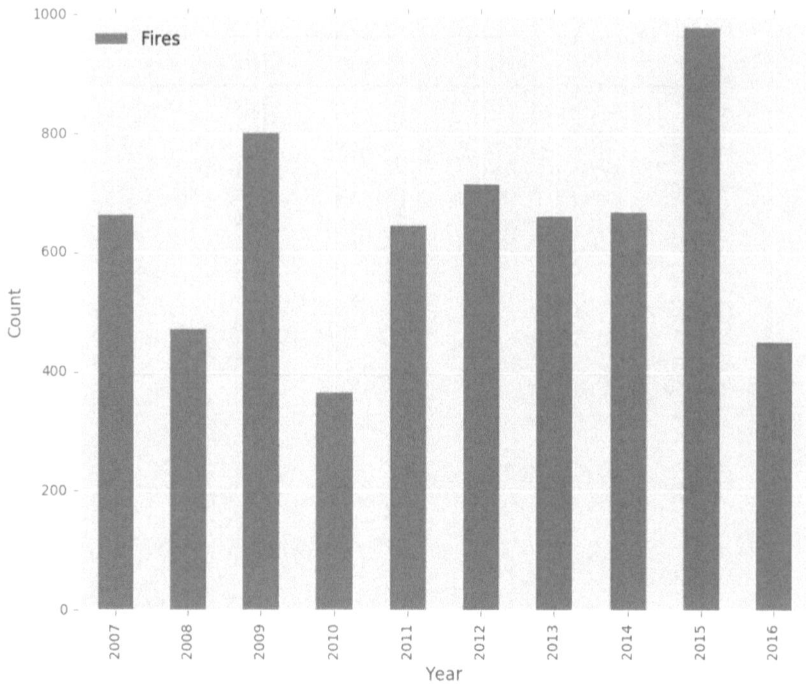


*Figure 5.4b* Distribution of fires by year.

*Table 5.5* The mean probability of a species being impacted by fires in each year

| *Year* | *C. commune* | *M. bidentata* | *C. guianensis* | *A. maripa* | *H. courbaril* |
|---|---|---|---|---|---|
| 2007 | 0.09 | 0.10 | 0.03 | 0.12 | 0.08 |
| 2008 | 0.11 | 0.11 | 0.04 | 0.13 | 0.10 |
| 2009 | 0.08 | 0.09 | 0.02 | 0.12 | 0.09 |
| 2010 | 0.09 | 0.09 | 0.03 | 0.10 | 0.07 |
| 2011 | 0.07 | 0.07 | 0.02 | 0.10 | 0.07 |
| 2012 | 0.09 | 0.09 | 0.04 | 0.11 | 0.08 |
| 2013 | 0.07 | 0.07 | 0.02 | 0.09 | 0.07 |
| 2014 | 0.09 | 0.09 | 0.03 | 0.11 | 0.08 |
| 2015 | 0.11 | 0.11 | 0.04 | 0.13 | 0.09 |
| 2016 | 0.16 | 0.17 | 0.06 | 0.20 | 0.12 |

*C. guianensis*, and *M. bidentata*, the 2010 El Niño year had a greater probability of impact on species distribution than the 2009 El Niño year. The 2010 El Niño year was ranked as the third lowest in terms of potential impact on *A. maripa*, with 2009 ranked the fifth highest for potential impact. In the case of *H. courbaril*, 2009 had the fourth highest potential impact on the species distribution, while 2010 was ranked the year with the third lowest potential impact.

Unlike the 2009–2010 El Niño event, the potential impacts of the 2015–2016 event were the highest recorded in our analysis. The potential impacts of 2015 and 2016, taken by years separately and measured here by the average probability of a species being impacted, were only separated by the year 2008 among years with the highest mean probability of impacting species distributions. The mean probabilities of *C. commune* being impacted in 2015 and 2016 were 0.11 and 0.16 respectively, compared to 0.09 in 2010 and 0.11 in 2008. Overall, the average probability of these plants being impacted ranged from 0.07 in 2011 to 0.16 in 2016. The average probability that *C. guianensis* plants were impacted in 2015 was 0.04 and increased to 0.06 in 2016. In fact, based on the Maxent models, *C. guianensis* had the lowest potential of being impacted by fires across all species. Overall, the average probability of impact associated with *C. guianensis* ranged from 0.02 in 2011 through to 0.06 in 2016, while 2008 and 2015 had a similar probability of 0.04 of being impacted. Similarly, the average probabilities of *M. bidentata* being impacted in 2015 and 2016 were 0.11 and 0.17 respectively, compared to 0.09 in 2010 and 0.11 in 2008. Overall, the average probability of being impacted for *M. bidentata* varied from 0.1 in 2011 to 0.17 in 2016. Both *H. courbaril* and *A. maripa* had the lowest average probability of being impacted by fires in 2013 (0.07 and 0.09 respectively), with the 2016 average probabilities increasing to 0.12 and 0.20 respectively. As noted earlier, 2008 had the second highest impact on most species, and this was also the case for *H. courbaril* and *A. maripa*, which had mean probabilities of being impacted of 0.10 and 0.13 respectively.

When we moved away from the average probability of fires impacting species distributions and considered probabilities ranging from 0.5 to 0.9, a total of 1,494 or 23% of fires met this criterion. The analysis suggested that the potential impacts of these fires contrasted the observation for the average impacts and the years in which these occurred. Over the years, the number of fires that that had the higher probability of impacting the distribution of the five species declined. A total of 418 fires had a probability of impacting species distributions between 0.5 and 0.59, with 376 displaying a probability between 0.6 and 0.69; 353 had a probability between 0.7 and 0.79; 267 had a probability between 0.8 and 0.89; and 80 had a probability greater than 0.9 (Table 5.6). In almost every case, because of the differences in probabilistic species distributions, a single fire had a different probability of impacting two species (Table 5.7). Some of the details on the impacts of fires on species distributions are provided below.

Of the 418 fires that had a probability between 0.5–0.59 of impacting the five species, the El Niño years of 2009, 2016, and 2015 had the highest number of fires, with 42, 57, and 61 respectively. It should be noted, too, that 2007 also had 42 fires with the potential to impact these species. When we examined the potential impacts on species, a total of 127 of these fires had the potential to impact *C. commune*. Similar to the years with the highest number of fires,

*Table 5.6* Fires with probabilities greater than 0.5 of impacting the five target species and their distribution across the study period

| *Years* | *Number of Fires (0.5–0.59)* | *Number of Fires (0.6–0.69)* | *Number of Fires (0.7–0.79)* | *Number of Fires (0.8–0.89)* | *Number of Fires (>0.9)* | *Total* |
|---|---|---|---|---|---|---|
| 2007 | 42 | 38 | 29 | 32 | 10 | 151 |
| 2008 | 36 | 29 | 34 | 25 | 9 | 133 |
| 2009 | 42 | 45 | 27 | 33 | 16 | 163 |
| 2010 | 29 | 21 | 17 | 9 | 2 | 78 |
| 2011 | 33 | 29 | 21 | 20 | 2 | 105 |
| 2012 | 41 | 43 | 37 | 28 | 8 | 157 |
| 2013 | 37 | 24 | 28 | 14 | 4 | 107 |
| 2014 | 40 | 30 | 40 | 22 | 7 | 139 |
| 2015 | 61 | 69 | 64 | 45 | 9 | 248 |
| 2016 | 57 | 48 | 56 | 39 | 13 | 213 |
| Total | 418 | 376 | 353 | 267 | 80 | 1494 |

2009, 2016, and 2015 had 17, 19, and 22 fires respectively that had at least a 50% chance of impacting this species. In the case of *M. bidentata*, 131 fires had the potential of impacting the distribution of this species. Unlike the observation for *C. commune*, the years 2016, 2012, and 2015 had fires with highest potential impact with 16, 18, and 21 respectively. Only 34 or 8% of the 418 fires had a probability greater than 0.5 of impacting the distribution of *C. guianensis*. The highest number of fires that impacted *C. guianensis* occurred in 2007, 2010, 2012, and 2015, with 5, 5, 6, and 7, respectively. A total of 22% of fires had a probability greater than 0.5 of impacting the distribution of *H. courbaril*. Of these fires, the top three years only included the one El Niño of 2016, which observed an equal number of fires with 2011. In a departure from the number of fires observed at this probability for the other species of interest, the highest number of fires impacting *H. courbaril* occurred in 2007 with 13 total. The palm species, *A. maripa*, had a total of 110 fires with a potential probability of 0.5–0.59 of impacting its distribution. Like the general pattern observed for *C. commune*, *A. maripa* saw 2009, 2016, and 2015 as the ones with the highest number of fires with 13, 15, and 16 respectively.

Our analysis of the number of fires with a probability between 0.6 and 0.69 of impacting the distribution of the five species showed that 376 such fires occurred during the study period. Like the observation for the fires that had a probability in the range of 0.5–0.59, the 2009 El Niño year, and the 2015–2016 El Niño years had the highest number of fires with 45, 48, and 69 events respectively. Of these fires, a total of 146 had the potential of impacting *C. commune* distribution, with the years 2016, 2015, and 2012 with the highest number of fires, with 17, 21, and 22, respectively. While the number of fires that could potentially impact *M. bidentata* distribution declined to 114 at this probability, the same years as per *C. commune* had the highest number of fires,

*Table 5.7* The number of fires with a probability greater than 0.5 of impacting the distribution of the five species across the ten-year study period with the number that occurred in each year and the species potentially impacted

| *Probabilities of Impact (Total Number of Fires)* | *Year* | | | | | | | | | | | |
|---|---|---|---|---|---|---|---|---|---|---|---|---|
| | *Species* | *2007* | *2008* | *2009* | *2010* | *2011* | *2012* | *2013* | *2014* | *2015* | *2016* | *Total* |
| Probability = 0.5–0.59 (418) | *C. commune* | 10 | 9 | 17 | 3 | 10 | 11 | 15 | 11 | 22 | 19 | 127 |
| | *H. courbaril* | 13 | 8 | 9 | 6 | 11 | 7 | 7 | 10 | 10 | 11 | 92 |
| | *C. guianensis* | 1 | 5 | 1 | 5 | 1 | 6 | 2 | 2 | 7 | 4 | 34 |
| | *M. bidentata* | 10 | 14 | 11 | 12 | 5 | 18 | 11 | 13 | 21 | 16 | 131 |
| | *A. maripa* | 12 | 12 | 13 | 10 | 8 | 7 | 7 | 10 | 16 | 15 | 110 |
| Probability = 0.6–0.69 (376) | *C. commune* | 16 | 12 | 16 | 12 | 10 | 22 | 8 | 12 | 21 | 17 | 146 |
| | *H. courbaril* | 1 | 3 | 1 | 0 | 2 | 0 | 2 | 2 | 7 | 6 | 24 |
| | *C. guianensis* | 4 | 4 | 4 | 3 | 3 | 7 | 4 | 2 | 10 | 3 | 44 |
| | *M. bidentata* | 11 | 8 | 12 | 7 | 10 | 13 | 7 | 12 | 21 | 13 | 114 |
| | *A. maripa* | 14 | 11 | 20 | 6 | 7 | 13 | 4 | 10 | 24 | 23 | 132 |
| Probability = 0.7–0.79 (353) | *C. commune* | 17 | 19 | 14 | 11 | 8 | 18 | 8 | 17 | 35 | 29 | 176 |
| | *H. courbaril* | 2 | 3 | 2 | 0 | 0 | 2 | 5 | 3 | 7 | 4 | 28 |
| | *C. guianensis* | 0 | 2 | 3 | 1 | 3 | 3 | 5 | 4 | 5 | 5 | 31 |
| | *M. bidentata* | 7 | 11 | 7 | 6 | 9 | 13 | 5 | 11 | 25 | 26 | 120 |
| | *A. maripa* | 10 | 11 | 6 | 6 | 10 | 12 | 10 | 18 | 20 | 19 | 122 |
| Probability = 0.8–0.89 (267) | *C. commune* | 4 | 0 | 0 | 0 | 1 | 2 | 0 | 0 | 1 | 3 | 11 |
| | *H. courbaril* | 4 | 7 | 5 | 1 | 2 | 2 | 1 | 4 | 7 | 5 | 38 |
| | *C. guianensis* | 4 | 2 | 0 | 1 | 2 | 3 | 0 | 1 | 1 | 4 | 18 |
| | *M. bidentata* | 16 | 8 | 17 | 4 | 8 | 11 | 6 | 9 | 12 | 12 | 103 |
| | *A. maripa* | 24 | 16 | 27 | 7 | 16 | 22 | 13 | 16 | 37 | 29 | 207 |
| Probability = > 0.9 (80) | *C. commune* | 0 | 0 | 0 | 0 | 0 | 0 | 0 | 0 | 0 | 0 | 0 |
| | *H. courbaril* | 4 | 5 | 10 | 2 | 2 | 4 | 0 | 3 | 5 | 7 | 42 |
| | *C. guianensis* | 1 | 0 | 1 | 0 | 0 | 3 | 1 | 1 | 2 | 9 | 18 |
| | *M. bidentata* | 5 | 4 | 5 | 0 | 0 | 1 | 3 | 3 | 1 | 6 | 29 |
| | *A. maripa* | 3 | 4 | 4 | 0 | 0 | 0 | 3 | 3 | 2 | 3 | 22 |

albeit with different totals in each year. In 2012 and 2016, 13 fires showed the potential to impact this species, while 2015 had the highest of 21 fires with the potential to impact *M. bidentata* distribution. While at the 0.5–0.59 probability range only 8% of fires showed the potential to impact *C. guianensis* distribution, 12% of fires showed the potential to impact the distribution of this species at the 0.6–0.69 range. Of the 44 fires that showed this potential, ten occurred in 2015, with seven in 2012, and the years 2007, 2008, 2009, and 2013 each recording four fires with this potential level of impact. Slightly more than 6% of fires had the potential of impacting the distribution of *H. courbaril*, with 2008 (three fires), 2016 (six fires), and 2015 (seven fires) the top three years with potential impacts. The palm species, *A. maripa*, saw the second highest number of fires impacting its distribution, with 132 events showing a probability in the range of 0.6–0.69 of impacting this species. The top three years for impacts on *A. maripa* were 2009, 2016, and 2015 with 20, 23, and 24 fires respectively.

The 353 fires that had a probability between 0.7 and 0.79 of impacting the distribution of the five species had the highest occurrence in the years 2014, 2016, and 2015, with 40, 56, and 64 fires respectively. As observed for the previous two probability ranges, the years that had the highest potential impact on species did not always follow this pattern. In the case of *C. commune*, a total of 176 fires had the potential to impact its distribution, with the year 2015 observing the highest number (35), with 2016 (29 fires) and 2008 (19 fires) completing the top three years. The total number of fires that could potentially impact *M. bidentata* was 120 at this probability range, with 2012, 2015, and 2016 with 11, 25, and 26 fires respectively, being the top three years for potential impacts. Only 31 fires showed the potential to impact the distribution of *C. guianensis*, with the years 2013, 2015, and 2016, with three fires each, the years of highest probability of threat to this species distribution. Relative to *C. guianensis*, an even lower number of fires, 28, showed the potential to impact the distribution of *H. courbaril* at the 0.7–0.79 probability range. Like *C. guianensis*, 2016, 2013, and 2015 were the years with the highest potential impacts with four, five, and seven fires respectively. The 122 fires that showed the potential to impact the distribution of *A. maripa* at this probability range had the highest probability of occurrence in the years 2014, 2016 and 2014 with 18, 19 and 20 fires respectively.

A total of 267 fires had a probability range of 0.8–0.89 of impacting the distribution of the five species. Of these fires, three El Niño years, 2009, 2016, and 2015, had the highest number of fires, with 33, 39, and 45 respectively. These fires showed the highest potential for impact on the palm species, *A. maripa*, with 207 or 76% of fires occurring within its range. As per the general observation of when these fires occurred, 2009, 2015, and 2016 were the top three years for potential impact, with 27, 29, and 39 events respectively. For the tree species, *M. bidentata*'s distribution could have potentially been impacted by 103 fires. Unlike the observation for the years with the highest number of fires, the years 2015, 2016, 2007, and 2009 with 12, 12, 16, and 17 fires respectively, were the ones that could potentially impact this species. Thirty-eight fires showed the potential for impacting the distribution of *H. courbaril* at this range of probability, with 2016 and 2009 (five fires each) and 2008 and 2015 (seven fires each) the years with the most events. In the case of *C. guianensis*, 18 fires showed the potential to impact the distribution of this species. The years 2007 and 2016 saw four fires each, while 2012 observed three fires. Unlike the high potential of *C. commune* distribution being impacted at the 0.5–0.79 probability range, this species only saw 11 fires potentially impacting its range at this higher probability. In fact, 2007 had the most fires (4), while 2012 (2) and 2016 (3) accounted for the times with the highest potential impact on this species.

The three years in which the fires with the highest probability of impacting the distribution of the five species were 2007 (10), 2016 (13), and 2009 (16). As a note, in the other El Niño years, 2010 and 2015, the MODIS sensor detected two and nine fires, respectively, that had a probability of greater than 0.9 of impacting the distribution of the five species. With the low number of fires potentially impacting *C. commune* distribution at the 0.8–0.89 probability level, it was not surprising that none of the 80 fires that had a probability greater than 0.9 impacted the distribution of this species. More than 52% of the fires that had a probability greater than 0.9 could have potentially impacted the distribution of *H. courbaril*. The three years associated with El Niño, 2009 (10 fires), 2016 (7 fires), and 2015 (5 fires), were the ones with the highest potential impact. A further 35% of fires had the potential to impact the distribution of *M. bidentata*. The El Niño year, 2016, had six fires with this potential, while 2007 and 2009 recorded five fires each. There were 18 fires with the potential to impact the distribution of *C. guianensis*, with nine occurring in 2016, three in 2012, and two in 2015. A total of 22 fires had the potential to impact *A. maripa*, with the distribution across the years the most uniform observed. The years 2008 and 2009 saw four fires each, while 2007, 2013, 2014, and 2016 all noted three fires with this potential for impacting the distribution of this species.

## Discussion and Conclusions

The MODIS fire product showed that the two El Niño events resulted in an increased number of fires for the Rupununi study area, relative to non-El Niño years (Table 5.4). While investigating the cause and origin of each fire was beyond the scope of this chapter, the end result nonetheless was that each fire had a potential impact on the distribution of one or more species. While we note and emphasize that the Maxent models showed the potential suitability of conditions for the occurrence of the plant species (Phillips et al., 2017) of interest, which we used as a proxy for species presence, our analysis showed that the potential impacts of fires varied by species. The fact that the plant species of interest in our sample are of importance to the livelihoods of the indigenous peoples of the Rupununi (Table 5.2), and by extension Amazonian populations, the methods we explored in this chapter have the potential for being used to study these or similar species in other settings. Our analysis of the impacts of the fire events on the distribution of species brought out some points that are worth noting.

First, our analysis showed that not all fires impact all species in the same way (see Tables 5.5 and 5.7). On average, the probability of fires impacting the distribution of any one of the species was low, at 20% (see Table 5.5). However, even when we used the average probability of a species being impacted by fire, what became apparent was that the identity of the species that was impacted might be most important. In 2016, the second year of the 2015–2016 El Niño event, all species had the highest average probability of being impacted. Of these species, *A. maripa*, a species that is critical for the day-to-day needs of a large proportion of residents within the study area, had the highest probability of being impacted by fires. Without a healthy and thriving population of *A. maripa* palms, the potential for thatching roofs, a reality for most of the Rupununi's indigenous population, will be impaired (see Table 5.2 for details on how this species is used). We also found it interesting that the number of fires with the highest potential for impacts on the five species occurred in El Niño years (Table 5.6; Table 5.7), a direct contrast to average impact when 2008, a non-El Niño year, saw the second highest level of impact.

Second, despite only relying on three environmental variables for developing probabilistic distributions of the five species of interest, the Maxent models showed that the Rupununi had a high suitability for the presence of the species of interest. The probabilistic models showed species distributions, for each species, upwards of 80% which allowed us to demonstrate how the presence of fires may be impacting the species of interest. Based on the models and the MODIS data (Table 5.3), we observed that there was an increase in the number of fires associated with El Niño events and that these can impact the distribution of each of the key species. While our work only considered the point that the fire was detected, based on the MODIS fire product, we acknowledge that each fire will impact an area of the landscape and hence a different level of impact can be potentially determined when the areas are considered. Future work will continue to refine the Maxent models to gain a sense of the distribution of the five plant species and how they may be impacted by the area affected by each of the fires.

Third, beyond understanding the area that was impacted by each fire event, our analysis (Table 5.4) of the number of fires associated with the study area showed a clear increase in the El Niño years. The fact that El Niño has led to an increase in the number of fires is a concern to the distribution of the five plant species of interest and the ecosystem services with which they are associated. In particular, it was of concern to note, that even though there were fewer fires in 2016 than 2015, the 2016 fires had a higher probability of impacting the plant species of interest. While *in situ* data are required to understand exactly how each species was impacted by the 2016 fires, these results may be hinting at the prolonged El Niño leading to more fire encroachment into the forest.

This may be consistent with other recent findings (e.g. Brown & Buis, 2017) that showed that the 2015–2016 El Niño event lead to increased levels of carbon in the atmosphere. While the number of fires in our study did not increase in 2016, their encroachment into the forest will lead to carbon emissions and contribute to the findings of Brown and Buis (2017).

The overarching goal of this chapter was to demonstrate to scholars, practitioners, and members of the nonprofit community, for example, that we can draw on publicly available data and methods to study how natural disasters may impact the distribution of plant species. Our work showed that freely available data, mainly imagery from Landsat, fire data from MODIS, and the secondary products derived from Landsat, could help practitioners to begin gauging the impacts of phenomena such as El Niño on the distribution of plant species that are important to indigenous peoples and the wildlife with which they are associated. In our case, the data on the distribution of plant species were collected *in situ*, and this will perhaps be the only major obstacle for completing similar studies for species of importance in difficult-to-access settings. Once the species presence data are available, however, completing analysis becomes more accessible, especially in settings where GIS software packages are available. While the results of our analysis point towards the gravity changes in El Niño patterns will have for the distribution of species that are important to indigenous people's livelihoods, our approach can be replicated across any other phenomenon of interest. Approaches like ours can be used as a pre-disaster management tool to help managers and others to determine where aid for local people may be required, even under conditions when the natural disaster is not of the same magnitude of those commonly gaining our attention.

## Acknowledgement

Plant species presence data were obtained as a part of the US National Science Foundation BE/CNH Grant 0837531 funded project led by Dr Jose Fragoso.

## References

Abramson, A. 2017. Why it's so hard to predict exactly where wildfires will strike. URL: http://time.com/4977123/wildfire-california-nor-cal-prediction/

Anapol, A. 2017. Oxfam slams US response in Puerto Rico as "slow, inadequate". URL: http://thehill.com/homenews/administration/353563-oxfam-steps-in-to-help-puerto-rico-slamming-us-response-as-slow

Brown, D. 2017. Gov't appeals for international assistance to rebuild hurricane-ravaged Barbuda. URL: https://antiguanewsroom.com/news/govt-appeals-for-international-assistance-to-rebuild-hurricane-ravaged-barbuda/

Brown, D. & Buis, A. 2017. NASA pinpoints cause of earth's recent record carbon dioxide spike. URL: www.nasa.gov/press-release/nasa-pinpoints-cause-of-earth-s-recent-record-carbon-dioxide-spike

Chavez, N. 2017. Mexico earthquake: A rush to save lives amid "new national emergency". URL: www.cnn.com/2017/09/20/americas/mexico-earthquake-rescues/index.html

Coren, M. 2017. An earthquake early warning system helped Mexico City: Trump's budget would kill it in the US. URL: https://qz.com/1082191/an-earthquake-early-warning-system-helped-spare-mexico-city-trumps-budget-would-kill-it-in-the-us/

Cummings, A.R. 2013. For logs, for traditional purposes and for food: Identification of multiple-use plant species of Northern Amazonia and an assessment of factors associated with their distribution (Dissertations e ALL). Paper 17. URL: http://surface.syr.edu/etd/17

Cummings, A.R., Read, J.M. & Fragoso. 2015. Utilizing Amerindian Hunters' Descriptions to Guide the Production of a Vegetation Map. *International Journal of Applied Geospatial Research*, 6(1), 118–142. DOI: 10.4018/ijagr.2015010107

Cummings, A.R. 2016. Mapping hot spots of human-jaguar conflicts and identifying country-level stakeholders for long term conflict resolution in Guyana. Final Report for Panthera.

Cummings, A.R. & Read, J.M. 2016. Drawing on traditional knowledge to identify and describe ecosystem services associated with Northern Amazon's multiple-use plants. *International Journal of Biodiversity Science, Ecosystem Services & Management*, 12, 39–56. DOI:10.1080/21513732.2015.1136841.

Cummings, A.R., Karale, Y., Cummings, G.R., Hamer, E., Moses, P., Norman, Z. & Captain, V. 2017. UAV-derived data for mapping change on a swidden agriculture plot: Preliminary results from a pilot study. *International Journal of Remote Sensing* 38(8–10): 2066–2082.

Denevan, W.M. 1980. Swiddens and cattle versus forest: The imminent demise of the Amazon rain forest reexamined. *Studies in Third World Societies* 13: 25–44.

Denevan, W.M. 1988. Measurement of abandoned terracing from air photos: Colca Valley, Peru. *Conference of Latin Americanist Geographers* 14: 20–30.

Denevan, W.M. 1992. The pristine myth: The landscape of the Americas in 1492. *Annals of the Association of American Geographers* 82(3): 369–385.

Denevan, W.M. 2004. Semi-intensive pre-European cultivation and the origins of anthropogenic dark earth in Amazonia. In Glaser, B. & Woods, W. (Eds.), *Amazonian Dark Earths: Explorations in Space and Time* (pp. 135–143). New York: Springer.

Denevan, W.M. 2006. Pre-European forest cultivation in Amazonia. In Balee, W. & Erickson, C.L. (Eds.), *Time and Complexity in Historical Ecology* (pp. 153–165). New York: Columbia University Press.

Elvidge, C.D., Zhizhin, M., Baugh, K., Hsu, F. & Ghosh, T. 2016. Methods for global survey of natural gas flaring from visible infrared imaging radiometer suite data. *Energies* 9(1).

Forget, P.M. & Hammond, D.S. 2005. Rainforest vertebrates and food plant diversity in the Guiana Shield. In Hammond, D.S. (Ed.), *Tropical Forests of the Guiana Shield* (pp. 233–294). Cambridge: CABI Publishing.

Forte, J. 1996. *Makusipe Komanto Iseru: Sustaining Makushi Way of Life*. Guyana: North Rupununi District Development Board.

Griffiths, T. 2008. Seeing "REDD"? Forests, climate change mitigation and the rights of indigenous peoples and local communities. Forest Peoples Programme. URL: http://unfccc.int/resource/docs/2012/smsn/ngo/242.pdf

Guyana Chronicle. 2015. "El Nino committee" working to combat dry-weather impact on region 9—Rupununi River 13 feet below normal. URL: http://guyanachronicle.com/2015/10/08/el-nino-committee-working-to-combat-dry-weather-impact-on-region-9-rupununi-river-13-feet-below-normal

Hanna, J. 2017. 2 new quakes shake Southern Mexico, already coping with disasters. URL: www.cnn.com/2017/09/23/americas/mexico-oaxaca-earthquake/index.html

Hess, D. & Tasa, D. 2017. *McKnight's Physical Geography: A Landscape Appreciation.* Hoboken, New Jersey: Pearson Education Inc.

Hester, J.L. & Echenique, M. 2017. After hurricane Maria, Puerto Rico's grid needs a complete overhaul. URL: www.wired.com/story/after-hurricane-maria-puerto-ricos-grid-needs-a-complete-overhaul/

Hidore, J.J. 1996. *Global Environmental Change: Its Nature and Impact.* Upper Saddle River: Prentice Hall.

Huffman, M.R. 2013. The many elements of traditional fire knowledge: Synthesis, classification, and aids to cross-cultural problem solving in fire dependent systems around the world. *Ecology & Society* 18(4): 3.

Iwokrama. 2008. Iwokrama plant species list, unpublished data used in Clarke, H.D., Funk, V. & Hollowell, T. 2001. Using checklists and collections data to investigate plant diversity. I: A comparative checklist of the plant diversity of the Iwokrama forest, Guyana. *Sida Botanical Miscellany* 21.

Kauffman, J.B., Uhl, C. & Cummings, D.L. 1988. Fire in the Venezuelan Amazon 1: Fuel biomass and fire chemistry in the evergreen rainforest of Venezuela. *Oikos* 53: 167–175.

Lehmann, J., Kern, D.C., German, L., McCann, J.M., Martines, G.C. & Moreira, A. 2003. Soil fertility and production potential. In Lehmann, J., Kern, D.C., Glaser, B. & Woods, W.I. (Eds.), *Amazonian Dark Earths: Origin, Properties, Management* (pp. 105–124). Dordrecht, The Netherlands: Kluwer.

Liu, Z., Yang, J. & Dwomoh, F. 2016. Mapping recent burned patches in Siberian larch forest using Landsat and MODIS data. *European Journal of Remote Sensing* 49: 861–887.

Lopez, G. 2017. The research on race that could explain Trump's slow response to Puerto Rico. URL: www.vox.com/identities/2017/10/3/16390230/puerto-rico-trump-racism

Lu, D. & Alcantara, C. 2017. Most of Puerto Rico has been in the dark for 23 days, 8 hours and 19 minutes. URL: www.washingtonpost.com/graphics/2017/national/puerto-rico-hurricane-recovery/?utm_term=.1bfd1f14bb3f

Luzar, J.B., Silvius, K.M., Overman, H., Giery, S.T., Read, J.M. & Fragoso, J.M.V. 2011. Large-scale environmental monitoring by indigenous peoples. *BioScience* 61: 771–781.

Major, J., diTommaso, A., Lehmann, J. & Falção, N.P.S. 2005. Weed dynamics on Amazonian dark earth and adjacent soils of Brazil. *Agriculture, Ecosystems and Environment* 111: 1–12.

Malhi, Y., Roberts, J.T., Betts, R.A., Killeen, T.J., Li, W. & Nobre, C.A. 2008. Climate change, deforestation, and the fate of the amazon. *Science* 319(5860): 169–172. doi:10.1126/science.1146961

Matricardi, E.A.T., Skole, D.L., Pedlowski, M.A., Chomentowski, W. & Fernandes, L.C. 2010. Assessment of tropical forest degradation by selective logging and fire using Landsat imagery. *Remote Sensing of Environment* 114(5): 1117–1129.

McPhate, M. 2017. California today: Mexico has a quake warning system. Where is California's? URL: www.nytimes.com/2017/09/21/us/california-today-mexico-has-a-quake-warning-system-where-is-californias.html

Mistry, J., Bilbao, B.A. & Berardi, A. 2016. Community owned solutions for fire management in tropical ecosystems: Case studies from indigenous communities of South America. *Philosophical Transactions* B 371(1696).

Morton, D.C., DeFries, R.S., Nagol, J., Souza, C.M., Kasischke, E.S., Hurtt, G.C. & Dubayah, R. 2011. Mapping canopy damage from understory fires in Amazon forests using annual time series of Landsat and MODIS data. *Remote Sensing of Environment* 115(7): 1706–1720.

Mufson, S. 2017. Hurricane Maria has dealt a heavy blow to Puerto Rico's bankrupt utility and fragile electric grid. URL: www.washingtonpost.com/news/energy-environment/wp/2017/09/20/puerto-ricos-power-company-was-already-bankrupt-then-hurricane-maria-hit/?utm_term=.d01653aea81d

Plew, M.G. 2005. The archaeology of Iwokrama and the North Rupununi. Proceedings of the Academy of Natural Sciences of Philadelphia 154: 7–28.

Phillips, S.J., Anderson, R.P., Dudík, M., Schapire, R.E. & Blair, M.E. 2017. Opening the black box: An open-source release of Maxent. *Ecography* 40: 887–893.

Phillips, S.J., Anderson, R.P. & Schapire, R.E. 2006. Maximum entropy modeling of species geographic distributions. *Ecological Modelling* 190: 231–259.

Phillips, S.J. & Dudik, M. 2008. Modeling of species distributions with Maxent: New extensions and a comprehensive evaluation. *Ecography* 31: 161–175.

Polak, A.M. 1992. *Major timber trees of Guyana: A field guide, Tropenbos series 2.* Wageningen, The Netherlands: The Tropenbos Foundation.

Posey, D.A. 1982. The keepers of the forest. *Garden* 6: 18–24.

Posey, D.A. 1985. Indigenous management of tropical forest ecosystems: The case of the Kayapó Indians of the Brazilian Amazon. *Agroforestry Systems* 3(2): 139–158.

Raish, C., González-Cabán, A. & Condie, C.J. 2005. The importance of traditional fire use and management practices for contemporary land managers in the American Southwest. *Environmental Hazards* 6: 115–122.

Raphael, T.J. 2017. For first time in 300 years, there's not a single living person on the island of Barbuda. URL: www.usatoday.com/story/news/world/2017/09/14/barbuda-hurricane-irama-devastation/665950001/

Read, J.M., Fragoso, J.M.V., Silvius, K.M., Luzar, J., Overman, H., Cummings, A., Giery, S.T. & de Oliveira, F. 2010. Space, place, and hunting patterns among indigenous peoples of the Guyanese Rupununi region. *Journal of Latin American Geography* 9(5): 213–243.

Roosmalen, M. 1985. *Fruits of the Guianan flora.* Institute of Systematic Botany. Utrecht, The Netherlands: Utrecht University.

Roy, D.P. & Kumar, S.S. 2017. Multi-year MODIS active fire type classification over the Brazilian tropical moist forest biome. *International Journal of Digital Earth* 10(1): 54–84.

Semple, K., Villegas, P. & Malkin, E. 2017. Mexico earthquake kills hundreds, trapping many under rubble. URL: www.nytimes.com/2017/09/19/world/americas/mexico-earthquake.html

Sivasailam, A. & Cummings, A.R. 2016. Does the location of Amerindian communities provide signals about the spatial distribution of tree and palm species? In Griffith, D., Chun, Y. & Dean, D. (Eds.), *Advances in Geocomputation.* New York: Springer.

Stabroeknews. 2017. Hurricane-hit Guyanese return. URL: www.stabroeknews.com/2017/news/stories/10/10/hurricane-hit-guyanese-return/

Sutherland, G. 2009. El Nino bakes South Rupununi. URL: www.stabroeknews.com/2009/news/stories/09/02/el-nino-bakes-south-rupununi/

Sutherland, G. 2016. Rupununi farmers in battle to save crops from unrelenting El Nino. URL: www.stabroeknews.com/2016/news/stories/02/14/rupununi-farmers-battle-save-crops-unrelenting-el-nino/

Uhl, C., Kauffman J. B. & Cummings, D.L. 1988. Fire in the Venezuelan Amazon 2: environmental conditions necessary for forest fires in the evergreen rainforest of Venezuela. *Oikos* 53:176-184.

Uhl, C. 1987. Factors controlling succession following slash and burn agriculture in Amazonia. *Journal of Ecology* 75: 377–407.

Uhl, C., Clark, H., Clark, K. & Maquirino, P. 1982. Successional patterns associated with slash and burn agriculture in the Upper Rio Negro region of the Amazon Basin. *Biotropica* 14: 249–254.

Uhl, C. & Kauffman, J.B. 1990. Deforestation, fire susceptibility, and potential tree responses to fire in the Eastern Amazon. *Ecology* 71: 437–449.

van Andel, T. 2000. *Non-timber forest products of the North-West District of Guyana Part II*. Georgetown, Guyana: Tropenbos-Guyana Series 8b.

Walker, A. 2017. Mexico's earthquake early warning system gave some over a minute's notice. URL: https://la.curbed.com/2017/9/8/16276982/mexico-earthquake-early-warning-system

Welch, J.R., Brondízio, E.S., Hetrick, S.S. & Coimbra Jr., C.E.A. 2013. Indigenous burning as conservation practice: Neotropical savanna recovery amid agribusiness deforestation in central Brazil. *PLoS One* 8(12).

Williams, G.W. 2000. Introduction to aboriginal fire use in North America. *Fire Management Today* 60(3): 8–12.

# 6 Understanding Threats to Crowdsourced Geographic Data Quality Through a Study of OpenStreetMap Contributor Bans

*Sterling Quinn and Floyd Bull*

## Introduction and Related Work

OpenStreetMap (OSM) is fundamentally a GIS database into which any logged-in user with an Internet connection can contribute information about the world. OSM data is freely available under an Open Database License (ODBL) for people to download, restyle, and use in their own maps. Now over a decade old, OSM has grown to the point where many governments and businesses are considering it a potentially valuable source of geographic data that can supplement their everyday mapping services and perhaps reduce bottom-line costs of data acquisition.

OSM is often described as being similar to Wikipedia, although one main difference is that OSM does not allow anonymous edits; in other words, all contributors to OSM must create a user account. Once logged in, contributors typically draw points, lines, or areas representing real-world features, then apply one or more "tags" describing the features. Although anyone can tag any entity with any tag (even made-up ones), in practice most contributors stick to a community-defined set of tags explained on the OSM wiki page. Adhering to standard tags allows the entities to be recognized and drawn into OSM maps like the ones on the openstreetmap.org home page.

In some parts of the world, principally urban areas in Western Europe, OSM has amassed road data rivaling that of government sources (Haklay 2010; Graser et al. 2014). In other cases, where governments have not collected or shared geographic databases, OSM may be the most complete, or the only, source available for vector basemap data.

The same crowdsourcing approach that invites local expert knowledge into OSM also enables non-locals, non-experts, or both to introduce error. OSM is thus susceptible to data damage, which could occur accidentally or on purpose. Although OSM technicians can revert edits, this takes time, effort, and technical expertise. Errors also reduce the credibility and utility of the data and harm the long-term viability of the project.

Johnson and Sieber (2013) examined the adoption of Volunteered Geographic Information (VGI) such as OSM by governments and found that many officials struggled to view it as a serious source of data, due to the involvement of hobbyists and people untrained in cartographic data production. Quinn and MacEachren (2018) mention anecdotes from geospatial professionals in government and private industry who hesitated to use OSM data because they themselves had noticed errors in their map areas of interest. All the same, some institutions such as Portland Tri-Met in the United States have adopted OSM as their principal source of data while paying employees to ensure that the data in the local area of interest is maintained at high quality (McHugh 2014). This is the approach taken by the cloud-based mapping services company Mapbox, which employs dozens of people spread around the world to manually update OSM data as well as develop tools to automatically detect anomalies in edits submitted to OSM (Barth 2015). TeleNav is another example of a large location services company that has built products around OSM while investing heavily in OSM quality monitoring and repair (Van Exel 2014; Illisei and Van Exel 2016).

Despite the number of resources some organizations have invested towards maintaining OSM data quality, the threats to OSM data integrity and usefulness are myriad. They range from inexperienced newbies accidentally dragging street corners across the screen, to angry contributors repeatedly undoing each other's work, to sophisticated vandals repeatedly creating new accounts to evade administrators (Neis et al. 2012; Ballatore 2014). These types of issues are not specific to OSM and occur in Wikipedia as well as various other VGI-based map projects. For instance, Google Map Maker saw users fabricating places in an attempt to influence the game Pokémon GO (Tuoi Tre News 2016). Volunteer contributors to Google Maps have sketched rude shapes on the landscape (Hern 2015), and a synagogue in Hungary was defaced in Wikimapia with anti-Semitic place description referencing the Holocaust (Bittner 2017b).[1]

In this chapter, we investigate threats to VGI quality by studying the reasons that OSM administrators block users from contributing to the project. OSM is governed by a number of volunteer committees that oversee the project's technical implementation, data integrity, publicity, and so forth. The committee in charge of data quality is called the Data Working Group (DWG). The DWG has the power to block user accounts from contributing edits for a given amount of time depending on the severity and pervasiveness of the infraction.[2]

The DWG publishes information about user bans in publicly available web pages. These ban descriptions constitute a rich source of qualitative information about carto-vandalism, as well as the myriad errors committed by well-meaning contributors. Neis et al. (2012) studied the ban descriptions to learn more about vandalism incidents, with the end of developing automated tools to detect malicious edits. Their study involved about 200 bans; now there are over 1,000. Quinn and Tucker (2017) used the ban history to identify cases where geopolitical disputes influenced the production of OSM. We are unaware of any other attempts to systematically leverage these ban descriptions to learn more about problematic edits in OSM, especially those that lie outside the realms of geopolitical disputes or traditional notions of vandalism. In this study, we scrutinize the user ban descriptions to better understand how people damage OSM data, as well as derive ideas about how harmful edits can be avoided or preempted.

## Methods

The DWG places descriptions of OSM user bans in individual web pages (one for each ban) that use the address format www.openstreetmap.org/user_blocks/<ID> where ID is the identification number of the ban. The page includes the name of the user being banned, the reason for the ban, the duration of the ban, the time of the ban's implementation, and the user name of the DWG member applying the ban. We created a table of this information by retrieving each page in sequential fashion and extracting the key information using Python code and the Beautiful Soup HTML parsing library. This "scraping" of the ban descriptions was performed with a time delay on each request so as not to overburden OSM servers (although the risk for disruption was already low due to the rudimentary format of the page and the relatively small number of bans).

Using these methods, we collected information on 1,218 bans spanning from October 12, 2009 to March 20, 2017. Because bans are sometimes issued to the same users repeatedly or to groups of users all at once, we faced the decision of whether to omit repetitious bans. Because each ban represents work that needs to be performed by the DWG, such as blocking the user and reverting problematic edits, we chose to leave most of the bans in the database and count them individually.

In several extreme situations, we made exceptions. In one case, someone created 108 accounts at once for the purpose of mass importing data. These were all banned on the same day, and we treated the incident as a single ban in our analysis. We also eliminated 69 bans for conducting mechanical edits during a one-time event where these were not allowed,[3] 40 bans because they did not contain enough information in the description, and 8 bans that were instigated by the DWG for test purposes. These omissions left us with 994 bans that we were further able to analyze.

Although the vast majority of the ban descriptions were originally written in English, a few were in German, French, and other languages. In order to study all the bans, we machine-translated non-English ban descriptions into English using the Google Translate online service. Although the translations sometimes resulted in awkward wording, the reason for the ban was still discernable in virtually all cases.

With the ban information extracted into tabular form, we each independently read through a subset of the ban descriptions. Then we consulted together to enumerate the most common themes we had seen. This enabled us to derive a set of ban categories.

With categories determined, we each independently went through the entire list of ban descriptions and assigned every ban into one of the categories in our set. After this, we went through a reconciling process to review all bans where we had disagreed on the category. Eventually we arrived at a final consensus on the category of each.

The above process of assigning a single category to each ban has several notable advantages and disadvantages. One advantage is that it allowed us to calculate an intuitive percentage of how much each ban type contributed to the whole. This method also allowed us to focus on the main reason for each ban. That being said, there were many situations where a ban could have reasonably fit into two or more categories. An alternate approach wherein each ban could be placed in multiple categories might help acknowledge the complexity of the ban process. In this approach, category weights would still need to be debated. There is also a risk that generously applying multiple categories to the bans might lead to an overestimation of the influence of each category.

## Results

We identified 12 categories of bans, which helped us to derive four broader themes of problems, which we call "Nefariousness", "Obstinance", "Ignorance", and "Mechanical Problems". Table 6.1 describes how each ban category fit into these broader themes.

## Nefariousness

Sometimes people edit OpenStreetMap for self-serving purposes that run contrary to the overall ethos of the community, whether to sell a product, make a political statement, or get a thrill from introducing artistic embellishments or inaccuracies into the data. In enumerating motivations to contribute to VGI projects, Coleman et al. (2009) included negative motivations alongside their

*Table 6.1* Themes observed in the bans

| *Broader Themes* | *Percentage of Bans* | *Ban Categories (In Order of Prevalence)* |
|---|---|---|
| Nefariousness | 31 | Vandalism<br>Politically motivated edits<br>Sock puppetry<br>Spam |
| Obstinance | 26 | Failure to cooperate with the OSM community<br>Deleting other people's work<br>Edit wars |
| Ignorance | 23 | Misunderstanding of OSM practices or software<br>Copyright violations<br>Erroneous edits |
| Mechanical Problems | 20 | Data imports conducted incorrectly<br>Bots unintentionally corrupting data |

longer list of constructive motivations. These negative motivations were largely derived from literature on Wikipedia, and include mischief, agenda, and malice. These situations fall under the umbrella of what we term "nefarious" edits, in that the contributors demonstrate no interest in the overall goals of the project. Many of these bans were committed by one-time editors or very new accounts.

Nefarious edits were the most common cause of the bans we observed. Below we describe the categories of nefariousness that we identified.

### *Vandalism*

In the OSM literature, the term "vandalism" has been invoked to describe all kinds of undesirable behaviors such as deleting data, spamming people, disputing on wiki pages, and committing copyright violations (Neis et al. 2012; Ballatore 2014). We took a somewhat narrower view and considered vandalism as any action that intentionally harmed the accuracy or credibility of the data. In some cases, the vandalism was malicious in nature; in other cases it was playful (although the DWG members did not see anything funny about it). Malicious vandalism included deliberately inserting false names or geometries into the database in an attempt to damage the project. Playful vandalism involved tracing messages or user names on the landscape, drawing fictitious features, or adding supposedly humorous names and labels such as "Swamp girl lives here" or "Trail of Zombies".

A website called OpenGeoFiction.net (Figure 6.1) has been established for people who want to use the OSM technology to create fictitious worlds in an environment that doesn't interfere with the real map. Wikimapia has a similar polygon art exhibition area in a remote part of the South Pacific Ocean. Such digital canvases can be compared to urban walls dedicated specifically to graffiti or street art in order to discourage vandalism on other buildings; however, they may not offer the same thrill or excitement associated with corrupting the utility of real data used by everyone.

With some bans, the question of whether the damage was intentional or not was impossible to discern. When the problematic edits added no information that benefited the map and were repeated despite a previous ban, we considered these cases as vandalism.

### *Politically Motivated Edits*

Given that OSM is open to edits from people around the world, it is unsurprising that occasional disagreements arise over territorial sovereignty, boundary locations, and place names. OSM nominally follows an "on the ground" policy wherein contributors are urged to map things as they would appear to someone visiting the physical location.[4] Although the DWG has approved or enforced exceptions in a few cases, contributors can be banned for "going rogue" and applying their own preferred names and boundaries, especially if the change is inflammatory or occurs on a repeated basis.

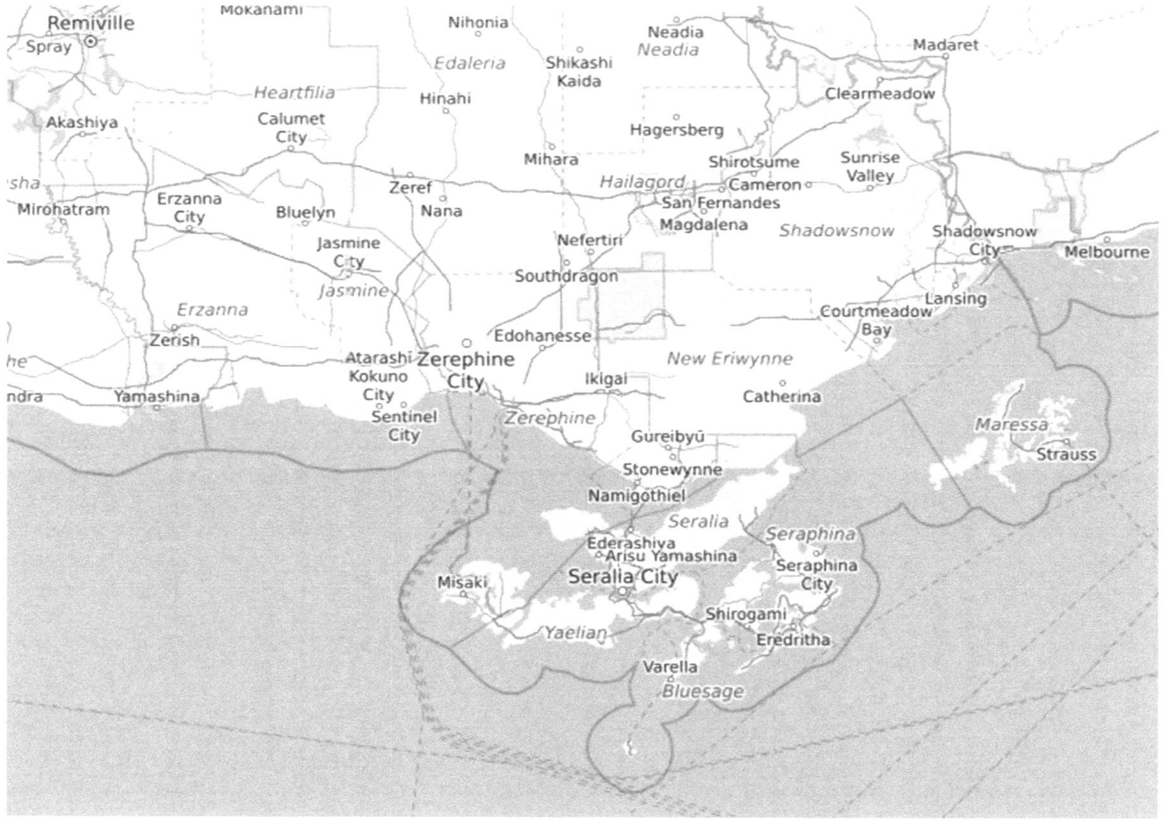


*Figure 6.1* A fantasy landscape built with OSM tools on the OpenGeoFiction website.

Most of the politically motivated edits we observed in the ban descriptions occurred in Eastern Europe, where a relatively active OSM community is mapping regions of high irredentist or separatist sentiment. These include regions in Georgia and Azerbaijan. The Crimea saw editors changing the languages of place names *en masse* between Russian and Ukrainian. Other hotbeds included the South China Sea, Morocco, Sardinia, and Kosovo. Quinn and Tucker (2017) offer some maps and theoretical analysis of these incidents.

### *Sock Puppetry*

Sometimes contributors attempt to circumvent a ban by creating a new user account and continuing their prohibited activity. This pattern of behavior is referred to across the Internet as "sock puppetry". We observed dozens of bans for sock puppetry, but sometimes these were issued to repeat offenders. In many situations the DWG swiftly detected the offending account because the geographic location and nature of the edits matched some other recent ban. For example, this situation where we refer to the banned contributors as User A and User B:

> Dear User B, yesterday I asked User A on behalf of the Austrian community to stop his mass editing of data in Austria and discuss with them before he continues. Shortly after, your account has been created, and continues where User A left off. What I said to User A applies to you as well.[5]

### *Spam*

In a handful of cases, people used the OSM tagging or messaging frameworks as a place to advertise a service or spread hyperlinks to product websites. Sometimes this was done as a search engine optimization strategy.

Although there is not any rule against adding one's own place of business to OSM, the insertions must match current conditions "on the ground". The use of overtly enterprising language in tags is frowned upon. As one member of the DWG informed a banned contributor:

> OpenStreetMap is not a business directory. If you have a bricks-and-mortar business to add, please do so (provided that it is visible from the street and therefore verifiable by other mappers). Please do not include guff like "many customers have found out just how easy it can be to make sure that they are getting a simple and easy". That's not a descriptive address or other details; it's just spam.[6]

## Obstinance

The crowdsourced nature of OSM creates frequent situations where contributors modify each other's work. Furthermore, a person's contributions must live alongside other people's edits in a map that would ideally appear seamless to the reader. In some categories of bans we observed a theme of obstinance, wherein a contributor was attempting to enrich OSM solely through his or her own view of how the map should be constructed. With these types of bans, attempts at correction or collaboration were met with indifference, stubbornness, or hostility. Such behavior might not cause overt breakage of the data, but could lead to a dataset that falls short of its potential level of quality. We describe these categories of obstinance below.

### *Failure to Cooperate With the OSM Community*

OSM has a strong user community built through wiki pages, message boards, a comment system for each edit, and a private messaging system. Contributors working on the same part of the map often attempt to contact each other through these channels. When the behavior of a single contributor runs contrary to the norms or practices established by local groups of mappers, and he or she ignores good-faith inquiries, the community can request help from the DWG to temporarily or permanently block the contributor.

Errant behaviors in this category include not replying to fellow users when messaged about problematic edits, making high-impact edits affecting others' work without submitting any comment about why, and refusing to conform to community-agreed standards published on the OSM wiki pages, even after much experience editing OSM.

This category also included any bans related to name-calling, personal insults, intimidation, and slanderous edits towards groups or individuals, and profanity directed at other contributors.

### *Deleting Other People's Work*

Some contributors delete OSM data that still exists on the landscape, often without any notification or justification. In some situations, the contributor disagrees with the way that the features were originally mapped. In other cases, the contributor believes the features are sensitive and must not be mapped (as in the case of an Israeli contributor who deleted military installations).[7]

Sometimes the contributor offers no explanation at all, and these cases are difficult to categorize. The act may constitute a form of deliberate vandalism, an honest accident, or a failure to understand OSM norms or work with the community. For this reason, we put "deleting data" into its own category.

### *Edit Wars*

Edit wars occur in crowdsourced projects when two or more people disagree about a contribution and repeatedly undo each other's work. These types of conflicts are not unique to OSM; edit wars are a fact of daily life in Wikipedia and their role in the lifespan of an article is portrayed vividly by Viégas et al. (2004).

Given this, it was somewhat surprising to us that (non-political) edit warring was one of the least common reasons for observing a ban in OSM. Wroclawski (2014), a member of the DWG, believes that the frequency of edit wars in OSM is much lower than Wikipedia precisely because the "on the ground" principle allows most disputes to work their way to a verifiable resolution.

The cases that did occur tended to involve disagreements about which name to put on a feature or how to tag a particular item. Often these disputes were highly local in nature, but one longtime user instigated enough edit wars over how to map turn restrictions that the case went all the way to the OpenStreetMap Foundation (OSMF) board and resulted in an indefinite ban.[8]

Although there may be some overlap of this category with politically motivated edits, we observed that many politically motivated edits are of a one-time "hit and run" nature and don't involve animosity developing between individual contributors.

## Ignorance

Hundreds of bans involved what appeared to be well-meaning behavior by people who were unaware that they were doing anything wrong. Reasons include a misunderstanding of OSM standards, software, or scope; unintentional misrepresentation of features on the map; and failure to comply with OSM's data copyright policy. In these cases, the DWG often applies a temporary ban that is lifted as soon as the contributor reads the ban notification text. This kind of ban does not constitute a punitive measure; rather, it serves as a teaching instrument while instituting an emergency moratorium on the problematic edits.

### *Misunderstanding of OSM*

We observed many bans wherein people seemed to be unaware that their edits would be visible to others or even permanently recorded in a database. This includes sketches or other markings made for practice, as well as data of a personal nature.

In other cases, contributors appeared to misunderstand basic tagging norms and unwittingly corrupted the data. Or they did not understand how to properly align imagery to trace.

Finally, some misunderstandings were facilitated by software. For example, the popular mobile app MAPS.ME allows users to add items to OSM and has increased contributions by new users; however, the design of the app has led many users to believe they are adding personal notes rather than information that will be publicly visible.[9] So many contributors uploaded personal information to OSM via MAPS.ME that at one point the DWG composed its own gentle instructions about how to create a personal bookmark in MAPS.ME, which it then pasted into multiple ban descriptions.[10]

### *Copyright Infringement*

Contributors to OSM are not allowed to copy names or entities from any source not compatible with OSM's own license. This includes copyrighted paper maps and some widely available online maps like Google Maps. Users who don't know about this policy or choose to ignore it can face a ban if the infraction is detected. The widespread addition of street names in difficult-to-reach areas or places where public data doesn't exist is one red flag that sometimes indicates copying, and can lead to a ban.[11]

Tracing imagery from Google Maps is also considered an infraction. In fact, contributors who are unaware of OSM policies will sometimes mention directly in a changeset comment that they took information from Google or other proprietary sources, thereby alerting other community members of a copyright problem.[12] Cases where contributors mention that they traced Google Maps can be difficult to sort out because there are many kinds of satellite images available and allowed for tracing in the OSM editors, yet sometimes new contributors are in the habit of referring to any satellite image as "Google Maps", no matter the source.

### *Erroneous Edits*

Some contributions appear to involve realistic data, but inexplicably do not match items on the ground. In other cases, contributors accidentally move features or introduce some tag that does not apply. We used this category of "Erroneous edits" for bans involving incorrect data that did not seem to be put there out of a sense of maliciousness or playfulness (as is the case with vandalism).

Although the category of erroneous edits contained the smallest number of bans under the theme of "Ignorance", it should be remembered that these kinds of errors are sometimes difficult to detect. Subtle mistakes in data may not be as glaring as other types of problems in OSM. They often require an interaction with some other contributor who has local knowledge, which may be rare in rural areas or other undermapped places.

## Mechanical Problems

OSM offers an application programming interface (API) that allows the mass uploading and editing of data through code. Executing an automated edit is a complex task that requires adherence to OSM community standards, knowledge of correct OSM tagging practices and ontologies, and proper testing and execution of code.

### *Data Imports Conducted Incorrectly*

In certain cases, OSM allows contributors to import publicly available geographic datasets whose licenses are compatible with the OSM license. Such imports have been used to bring massive amounts of buildings (Hoff 2014) or streets (Zielstra et al. 2013) into the map that would otherwise be time-consuming or difficult to comprehensively collect if mapped by individuals. At the same time, some have criticized imports for stifling the growth of active mapping communities (McConchie 2015).

Regardless of how one feels about imports in OSM, the process of importing data is fraught with technical and procedural peril. Prospective importers are asked to familiarize themselves with OSM, gain the buy-in of the existing OSM community in the area of import, ensure that the imported data license is compatible with OSM's, document all import activities, get approval for the import, create a special account for the import activities, apply appropriate tags to the data, and post a report when done.[13] Additionally, certain types of data have been prohibited from imports, such as parcel boundaries, terrain, and some types of land ownership data.[14] In cases of bad imports, OSM administrators must often go to great efforts to revert the changes.

The OSM user ban archives are replete with instances where the importer was either not aware of one or more of the above guidelines, chose to ignore them, or was not able to implement them successfully. Some of the ban descriptions vividly portray the technical challenges and community frustrations introduced by these edits. For example:

> You seem to be importing CORINE landuse data in a rather crass violation of all our import guidelines. You haven't talked to the communities affected—the Italians seem to be pretty unhappy for one!—and you are importing without regard to already existing data, just slapping your polygons on top of what is already there.
>
> Please stop this immediately. The data you have already imported will likely have to be reverted. You are not helping OpenStreetMap with this, you are actually annoyig [sic] the very people on whose hard mapping work OSM's success is based.[15]

### *Bots Unintentionally Corrupting Data*

OSM users can write short pieces of code, or scripts, that make mass edits with the goal of fixing small errors and cleaning up the project to conform to community-established norms. Such programs are called "bots", and they are also commonplace in other crowdsourced projects such as Wikipedia. For example, some bots are designed to detect and fix obvious typos in tags.

As with data imports, bot activity in OSM can go awry. Contributors are supposed to test their bots on small amounts of data, but some bots are unleashed without testing and can get out of hand, either writing incorrect data, modifying a wider scope of data than intended (or approved), or getting into edit wars with themselves or other bots and users.[16] Although bots can be used to commit deliberate vandalism, we observed that most incidents were perpetrated by well-meaning users.

Because bots are often deployed on large areas, including the entire world in some cases, their scope of affected data can be much larger than with imports. Mistakes are a source of immediate alarm and consternation to the OSM community, such as in this ban message from the DWG:

> Please, stop!
>
> You are carrying out a series of mechanical edits without giving any thought to the data that you are actually changing.
>
> Several hours, several changesets and many thousands of object edits ago I suggested on www.openstreetmap.org/changeset/35588464 that you really shouldn't be changing shops that you have not surveyed.[17]

## Discussion

The public record of OSM bans confirms that many things can and do go wrong when assembling a crowdsourced database. These issues cover a broad spectrum. Some problems are technical in nature, while others involve human factors such as relationships between contributors and the psychology behind individual edits.

Would-be users of OSM data are right to be concerned about issues such as vandalism and data corruption. The record of bans shows that these can happen at any moment. It is also disturbing that nefarious intentions were the most common theme we saw behind the bans.

However, the record also reveals a vigilant community that is quick to report errors and mishaps, as well as a responsive DWG with some power to quell damaging edits. As OSM adoption increases in the corporate sector, we anticipate further proliferation of quality assurance (QA) tools that will quickly detect egregious errors and the contributors that introduce them. A prime example is the OSM Changeset Analyzer (OSMcha) utility developed by Mapbox, which scans incoming OSM changesets in near real time for geometric abnormalities and problematic attribute changes (Ganesh 2017).[18] This tool looks for profanity in a list of "suspicious words", while also checking for copyright violations by detecting the names of other map data providers in the "source" tag.[19]

Currently OSMcha only raises warnings and does not automatically revert contributors' work. As OSM grows in volume, there may be a temptation to introduce utilities for automatic reversion of problematic edits; however, these could actually have an effect of stifling the very community they are meant to assist. Halfaker et al. (2013) demonstrate that heavy-handed quality control algorithms seem to be driving away desirable contributors from Wikipedia. New users often encounter harsh messages and no personal engagement, then flee the project. Although these algorithms have prevented some damage to articles, the project as a whole is suffering a decline in the size of its active community. OSM may want to avoid this road.

## Potential Interventions

We believe that studying OSM bans is a helpful exercise for identifying interventions that could reduce the rate of problematic contributions and improve the quality of OSM data. For example, to preempt the insertion of personal information into OSM, the OSMF could request that OSM editing apps display a message warning "Your changes will be viewable by everyone" prior to a contributor's first edit with the tool. Actions like this that cause a contributor to think twice before uploading are already starting to appear in OSM tools. For example, the iD editor (commonly used by new OSM contributors) allows people to check a box when they save their edits, indicating they would like someone else to review the changes. This adds a tag to the uploaded features that a review is requested. The system still relies on volunteers to find and check the changesets and modify the tag.

To prevent against politically motivated edits, the DWG could investigate the feasibility of locking access to sensitive items (like borders), in the same fashion that Wikipedia locks articles to stop edit wars. Such suggestions have already proved controversial in the OSM community, as they are perceived to reduce the openness of the project.[20] In several cases, the DWG has monitored and reverted the changes of anyone who modified particular controversial features (such as the name of Jerusalem or the sovereignty of the Crimea). This instituted a de facto locking system that, in at least the case of Jerusalem, grew lax over time (Bittner 2017a).

Finally, to reduce issues with mechanical edits, OSM might investigate some gatekeeping measures at the software level, perhaps requiring API users to supply a unique token or passcode at the time that imports or bots are implemented. This authorization might be issued by the DWG or other similar committee after the would-be contributor presented sufficient evidence of OSM community buy-in and knowledge of import procedures. Such an approach could have challenges with scalability as the project grows; and, like other restrictive measures, it may be viewed as damaging to the open feel of the project.

Ultimately, as OSM grows and the stakes increase for those who build their operations on top of it, the OSM community will need to struggle with the question of how much power contributors are allowed to wield. Interventions and restrictions that seemed unthinkable in years past may be met with different reactions over time.

## Human Factors in the DWG

DWG members must strike a careful balance of firmness against egregious offenders and kindness towards well-meaning mappers who are making mistakes. Although the characteristics of many banned OSM contributors are still somewhat mysterious, the personalities of the DWG members are on full display throughout the ban descriptions.

In some situations, DWG members played the role of mediators, attempting to pacify warring mappers with all the diplomacy of an elementary school playground supervisor:

> Hello User A, I see that you have added a number of things to OSM that do not correspond to available aerial imagery. . . . User B was right in removing these, and it was not ok of you to delete User B's work in retaliation.[21]

The cultural context, native language, and gender of DWG members may play a role in how contribution problems are addressed and how the offending parties interpret their ban descriptions. Some explanations were verbose, others were short and terse, a few were almost apologetic, and some were written in broken English. DWG members occasionally mentioned that they had machine-translated ban descriptions in order to reach contributors who did not appear to speak English. When reading any particular ban description, it's interesting to consider how the wording might be rendered by different members of the DWG. Perhaps some styles and practices of communication are more effective at deterring repeat behavior than others.

Our research does not examine whether the DWG and OSMF possess sufficient technical hardware, staff, and skills to handle future expansion of the contributor community or a broad-scale coordinated attack on the data or account infrastructures. The DWG has the power to revert edits, it is true, but comments in the ban descriptions allude that this is a time and work-intensive process. OSM has deployed some automated protections to mitigate damage. For example, there are limits on the number of features allowed in a changeset, or the number of communications that can be sent with the OSM messaging framework at one time. The closest event we can see to an organized threat was the situation where 108 users were created (and banned) in a single day for the same action, but this was an outlier. In a handful of other situations, small teams of editors working for businesses or school classes received bans because of faulty OSM editing practices such as entering personal data. OSM appears to be a small enough project for a volunteer-based DWG to handle at this stage, but the scope, politics, and dynamics of OSM administration could rapidly change as more organizations develop business models that rely on OSM.

## Limitations and Possibilities for Further Work

This study examined the utility of the OSM ban archives for learning more about vulnerabilities in OSM and the common problems introduced by contributors. As such, it did not examine minor issues or situations where a ban would be considered an overreaction. An active and communicative OSM community may be the best defense against petty vandalism or uninformed contributors. The correction of small errors among community members is important because the DWG cannot feasibly handle each case and because seemingly innocuous errors can erode the credibility of the data.

Due to our desire to gain some holistic understanding of the dataset, we have not been able to pursue deeper questions such as which types of bans follow other bans and how often contributors commit repeat offenses. It would be interesting to know, for example, which categories of bans tend to result in sock puppetry, where contributors are most determined to work around the ban.

The influence of time, when analyzed with the bans, could reveal much more about contributor personas and habits. For example, which types of infractions are committed by more seasoned contributors, versus newer ones? And what do people tend to do after the bans? Do they leave the project, repeat the infractions, or "learn" from their errors and continue as productive contributors to the project?

Tallying the tags and features most commonly involved in the bans could inform strategies for monitoring future data contributions and detecting the most frequent problems. The offending changesets are often easy to identify because they are either referenced directly in the ban description or they are timestamped just prior to the ban, yet such research is time consuming for a large number of bans.

Returning to the human factors in the DWG, it would be useful to learn if bans discriminate against any particular class or group of contributors. Are some kinds of serious problems resulting in light treatment, while other, less damaging offenses are resulting in full bans? How have enforcement trends changed over time?

We encourage these continued explorations of the bans as OSM continues to mature and evolve into new phases (especially as the number of for-hire contributors grows), and we hope that our work will inspire others to use the ban archives as a resource for OSM studies. We propose that elements of OSM's social history as recorded in the bans can be informative for people studying other crowdsourced data repositories such as Wikipedia or Wikimapia. We recommend the use of OSM ban descriptions for informing policies and practices around the creation and use of OSM and other crowdsourced data.

## Notes

1. http://wikimapia.org/#lang=en&lat=47.496035&lon=19.060609&z=18&m=b&show=/object/history/show/?object_type=&id=19829&rev=20&lng=en.
2. See the OpenStreetMap Ban Policy at https://wiki.osmfoundation.org/wiki/Ban_Policy.
3. In 2012, OSM changed licenses and its administrators needed to make a series of complicated edits to remove existing data contributed by those who did not accept the new license. During this time, known as the OSM Redaction Period, mechanical edits such as data imports and bot activity were not allowed.
4. See the policy document here: https://wiki.osmfoundation.org/w/images/d/d8/DisputedTerritoriesInformation.pdf.
5. www.openstreetmap.org/user_blocks/9.
6. www.openstreetmap.org/user_blocks/865.
7. https://forum.openstreetmap.org/viewtopic.php?id=3820.

8. www.openstreetmap.org/user_blocks/348.
9. See this discussion on the OSM forum, for example. https://forum.openstreetmap.org/viewtopic.php?id=58889.
10. For an example of the DWG response, see www.openstreetmap.org/user_blocks/1086
11. See for example www.openstreetmap.org/user_blocks/628.
12. See for example www.openstreetmap.org/user_blocks/1165.
13. See the OSM import guidelines at https://wiki.openstreetmap.org/wiki/Import/Guidelines.
14. Some of these discouraged datasets are mentioned at https://wiki.openstreetmap.org/wiki/Import/Past_Problems.
15. www.openstreetmap.org/user_blocks/33.
16. See www.openstreetmap.org/user_blocks/45: "Your robot appears to be warring with itself".
17. www.openstreetmap.org/user_blocks/855.
18. https://osmcha.mapbox.com/.
19. The full list of flagged "suspect" words is stored in the OSMcha GitHub page at https://github.com/willemarcel/osmcha/blob/master/osmcha/suspect_words.yaml.
20. See the discussion at https://help.openstreetmap.org/questions/7841/is-it-possible-to-lockprotect-some-content-nodes-ways-relations. This thread includes commentary by a prominent member of the DWG, Frederik Ramm, opposing the idea of locking features.
21. www.openstreetmap.org/user_blocks/1178.

## References

Ballatore, A. (2014). Defacing the map: Cartographic vandalism in the digital commons. *The Cartographic Journal*. Retrieved from www.maneyonline.com/doi/abs/10.1179/1743277414Y.0000000085

Barth, A. (2015). The paid mappers are coming. *State of the Map US 2015*. Retrieved from http://stateofthemap.us/the-paid-mappers-are-coming/

Bittner, C. (2017a). OpenStreetMap in Israel and Palestine—'Game changer' or reproducer of contested cartographies? *Political Geography*, *57*, 34–48. https://doi.org/10.1016/j.polgeo.2016.11.010

Bittner, C. (2017b). Social structures of Wikimapia. Presented at the American Association of Geographers Annual Meeting, Boston, MA.

Coleman, D. J., Georgiadou, Y., & Labonte, J. (2009). Volunteered geographic information: The nature and motivation of producers. *International Journal of Spatial Data Infrastructures Research*, *4*(1), 332–358.

Ganesh, A. (2017). Validating OpenStreetMap. Presented at the State of the Map 2017, Fukushima, Japan. Retrieved from https://2017.stateofthemap.org/2017/validating-openstreetmap/

Graser, A., Straub, M., & Dragaschnig, M. (2014). Towards an open source analysis toolbox for street network comparison: Indicators, tools and results of a comparison of OSM and the official Austrian reference graph. *Transactions in GIS*, *18*(4), 510–526.

Haklay, M. (2010). How good is volunteered geographical information? A comparative study of OpenStreetMap and ordnance survey datasets. *Environment and Planning. B, Planning & Design*, *37*(4), 682.

Halfaker, A., Geiger, R. S., Morgan, J. T., & Riedl, J. (2013). The rise and decline of an open collaboration system: How Wikipedia's reaction to popularity is causing its decline. *American Behavioral Scientist*, *57*(5), 664–688. https://doi.org/10.1177/0002764212469365

Hern, A. (2015, April 24). Google Maps hides an image of the Android robot urinating on Apple. *The Guardian*. Retrieved from www.theguardian.com/technology/2015/apr/24/google-maps-hides-an-image-of-the-android-robot-pissing-on-apple

Hoff, H. (2014). Dutch address and building import. Presented at the State of the Map 2014, Buenos Aires, Argentina. Retrieved from http://vimeo.com/album/3134207/video/115363425

Illisei, A., & Van Exel, M. (2016). OpenStreetView. Presented at the State of the Map US 2016, Seattle, Washington, DC. Retrieved from https://2016.stateofthemap.us/openstreetview/

Johnson, P. A., & Sieber, R. E. (2013). Situating the adoption of VGI by government. In D. Sui, S. Elwood, & M. Goodchild (Eds.), *Crowdsourcing geographic knowledge* (pp. 65–81). The Netherlands: Springer. Retrieved from http://link.springer.com/chapter/10.1007/978-94-007-4587-2_5

McConchie, A. (2015). Tracing patterns of growth and maintenance in OpenStreetMap. In *State of the map US 2015*. New York. Retrieved from http://stateofthemap.us/tracing-patterns-of-growth-and-maintenance-in-openstreetmap

McHugh, B. (2014). Government as a contributing member of the OpenStreetMap (OSM) community. In *FOSS4G 2014*. Portland, OR. Retrieved from https://vimeo.com/album/3606079/video/106226528

Neis, P., Goetz, M., & Zipf, A. (2012). Towards automatic vandalism detection in OpenStreetMap. *ISPRS International Journal of Geo-Information*, *1*(3), 315–332. https://doi.org/10.3390/ijgi1030315

Quinn, S. D., & MacEachren, A. M. (2018). A geovisual analytics exploration of the OpenStreetMap crowd. *Cartography and Geographic Information Science*, *45*(2), 140–155. https://doi.org/10.1080/15230406.2016.1276479

Quinn, S. D., & Tucker, D. A. (2017). How geopolitical conflict shapes the mass-produced online map. *First Monday*, *22*(11). Retrieved from http://firstmonday.org/ojs/index.php/fm/article/view/7922

Tuoi Tre News. (2016, August 11). Vietnamese Pokémon GO addicts abuse Google map maker, ruining national map. Retrieved from https://tuoitrenews.vn/society/36444/vietnamese-pokemon-go-addicts-abuse-google-map-maker-ruining-national-map

Van Exel, M. (2014). OpenStreetMap and TeleNav; Past, present and future. In *State of the map 2014*. Buenos Aires, Argentina. Retrieved from https://vimeo.com/album/3134207/video/112305387

Viégas, F. B., Wattenberg, M., & Dave, K. (2004). Studying cooperation and conflict between authors with history flow visualizations. In *Proceedings of the SIGCHI conference on human factors in computing systems* (pp. 575–582). New York: ACM. https://doi.org/10.1145/985692.985765

Wroclawski, S. (2014, January 17). Edit wars in OpenStreetMap. Retrieved June 26, 2018, from https://blog.emacsen.net/blog/2014/01/17/edit-wars-in-openstreetmap/

Zielstra, D., Hochmair, H. H., & Neis, P. (2013). Assessing the effect of data imports on the completeness of OpenStreetMap—A United States case study. *Transactions in GIS*, *17*(3), 315–334. https://doi.org/10.1111/tgis.12037

# Section III

# Applied Research Using GIS

# 7 More Than Meets the Eye

## The Methodological and Epistemological Hazards of GIS Map Use in the Public Sphere

*Nathan F. Alleman and L. Neal Holly*

### Introduction

Developing compelling policy recommendations is often as much a matter of data representation as the data itself. However, just like collection and analysis stages, representation may also be laced with meaning-making expectations and imbued with assumptions of which groups ought to have access to the tools of policy formation. This chapter explores the implications and challenges of one particular data representation approach: Geographic Information Systems (GIS) mapping. GIS is "a computer system capable of capturing, storing, analyzing, and displaying geographically referenced information; that is, data identified according to location. Practitioners also define a GIS as including the procedures, operating personnel, and spatial data that go into the system" (USGS Website, 2007, para 2).

Based on a federal College Access Challenge Grant and administrated by the State Council of Higher Education for Virginia (SCHEV), the larger study from which this analysis emerged examined college access provider organizations in the Commonwealth of Virginia. College access providers are nonprofit groups that promote college-going among K–12 students, often focusing on traditionally underrepresented groups and targeting resources needed for a successful transition to postsecondary education. In that study, we sought to identify the type and distribution of college access provider organizations as well as the resources and activities they offered to students in their service areas. Although prior studies (most significantly Gandara & Bial, 2001; Gullatt & Jan, 2003: Perna, 2002; Perna & Swail, 2001) have offered valuable nationally generalized descriptions, analyses, and typologies of such programs, this was the first study to pursue a comprehensive, state-level analysis upon which policy recommendations can be built. GIS mapping offered an easily accessible method for showcasing areas of college access need and success that correlate with past related policy initiatives and show areas of need for future policy action.

Virginia is a state of 132 K–12 school divisions, each facing unique demographic and achievement obstacles using a unique set of resources. The challenge of this study was to translate large amounts of school demographic and achievement data, along with college access provider data, into a format that was both accessible and descriptive. Adding to this challenge, the mandate for this study included a directive that findings be distributed to a wide range of constituents, including educators at all educational levels, college access organization administrators, and policymakers, which included state and local public officials.

The variety of constituents targeted by this study emerged as a complicating issue as we considered using GIS mapping to represent our data. Data consumers often lend greater legitimacy to maps and other visual data representations as self-evident data points. Consumers are also less apt to recognize the socially constructed nature of mapping and may fail to subject it to the same critique as other policy data (Monmonier, 1991). Furthermore, the visual simplicity and approachability of many maps belie the often-complex processes of data collection and interpretation from which the maps emerged. Mapping, according to some critics (Taylor, 1990), thus represents a new sort of scientific empiricism: a complex and biased argument cloaked in the apparent conceptual clarity of a visual fact. As noted by Schuurman (2000), GIS is not the first type of mapping to receive this critique. However, the application of GIS to a wide variety of fields and disciplines, such as the health sciences, education, and ecological research, that are often linked to policy decision-making and questions about who has access to this powerful technology have renewed concerns about responsible use.

This chapter explores and analyzes GIS mapping from the perspective of educational researchers employing GIS as a tool to further policy development at the state level. Yet, embedded in GIS use were issues concerning the hidden power of the researchers, the logistical manipulation of data, and the representational outcomes of the process. Some elements of this conversation reflect aspects of an ongoing dialogue and controversy in the cartography and geography fields (Schuurman, 2000; Sieber, 2006), and other elements represent broader data representation issues that arose in the context of our study. This ongoing conversation, in the context of educational research, presses practitioners and researchers to reflect on the hazards and opportunities of graphically representing data generally, and use of GIS mapping specifically.

## GIS Mapping: Opportunities and Complications

We came to use GIS mapping through a process of exploration and modification. Early in the project we recognized that displaying the distribution of access providers visually would simplify our efforts to convey complex state-level data. After exploring several less technologically sophisticated systems (such as the use of paper maps and online Google Maps), we connected with a faculty member at our institution's geography department, who was at that time creating GIS-based maps of community colleges and local demographics for a colleague. Our initial meetings with the faculty member challenged our neophyte understanding of the GIS mapping process, and we became increasingly aware of the amount of time necessary to prepare our data to be compatible with the GIS software. Complications quickly multiplied. Although our initial hope had been to connect our findings to individual high schools, the smallest available geographic unit of analysis was an existing division-level GIS dataset. Although the research team provided the data, the geographer and his assistant advised our process, including best approaches to representing data, processes for converting data to mesh with the GIS software, and the layout of the mapping products (see Appendix: College access provider distribution map (color coded 1–13 by density) with regional demarcations).

Visually representing data through GIS mapping is an issue that has received increased scrutiny and attention over the past two decades, largely dividing technicians, who view GIS capabilities as a credible and descriptive tool, from geography theorists, who tend to critique GIS mapping as a new tool of positivism and therefore imbued with false assumptions of value-neutrality and subject–object disconnection (Aitken & Michel, 1995; Pickles, 1995; Schuurman, 2000). Geographers have noted the particular power of maps generally as a persuasive and seemingly irrefutable self-evident fact (Monmonier, 1991). According to Obermeyer (1998), the issue at stake contains important practical policy implications:

> The use of geographic information systems can make it increasingly difficult for average citizens to participate in ongoing policy debates. This difficulty arises because using GIS simplifies the performance of spatial analysis and the preparation of excellent graphics (maps being the most obvious example), which lend an aura of persuasiveness to the reports on policy that public and private institutions prepare. No matter how sound (or unsound) the underlying ideas, the GIS can make a report seem more authentic and authoritative than it otherwise might seem.
>
> (p. 2)

These critical and theoretical perspectives on mapping are often grouped under the moniker GIS Society, or "GISoc". Many GISoc theorists conceive of mapping as a socially constructed phenomenon that is subject to the same bias, access and exclusion issues, and majority group dominance that has plagued other forms of inquiry and expression historically (Sheppard, 1995). Given this critique, the question arises: can GIS mapping be wrested from the exclusive control of academic, governmental, and private sector interests and used to empower and equip these same individuals and groups who are frequently excluded from policy decision-making?

To some scholars, the answer is a qualified "yes" (Ghose, 2001; MacEachren, 2000). Under the banner of Public Participation GIS, or "PPGIS", researchers and activists create user-friendly tools, hold seminars, and engage in community organizing that promotes access to GIS tools as a means of local participation in public policy and decision-making. Those engaged in PPGIS have found, however, that although mapping can be an avenue for indigenous and underrepresented groups to advance their interests, circumstances such as limited access to databases, limited technical expertise, group turnover, and unforeseen or undesirable responses to mapping sometimes frustrate such efforts (Sieber, 2006).

Access to mapping is complicated by the tools and knowledge needed to harness them, ranging from the simple to the sophisticated. Popular free internet programs, such as Google Earth, are based on the GIS platform and are designed for users to work on small projects using the provided, but limited, maps. Professional GIS programs, such as ArcGIS, cost thousands of dollars for a license and require specific training to use. Not only do GIS professionals need to understand what types of maps and data are already available for use (for instance, school division maps in Virginia were already available and did not need to be developed for the project), but users also need advanced knowledge in the use of databases and data entry software in order to construct new maps and layers and integrate data from secondary sources.

Researchers note that the increasing use of GIS mapping for education, health-care, and public policy argument-making represents a potent resource for delivering compelling data that must be used conscientiously and judiciously (Haque, 2001; Kwaku Kyem, 2004). However, as interest in GIS mapping has increased, it has increased attention from diverse disciplines, fields, and interest groups. These newly involved parties, often not privy to insider conversations about mapping access, ethics, and representation, are discovering the opportunities and hazards of this work on their own. Like many researchers, we initially engaged in mapping strictly as a representational tool, working cooperatively but dependently with a professional geographer. In retrospect, we now understand that through the process of map development, we occupied the positions of power majority (to the school divisions and access provider organizations we sought to describe) and advocating minority (to SCHEV and other governmental agencies we sought to convince) simultaneously. Finding a balance between these positions of power was an unforeseen challenge that led to an ongoing conversation about the influence of mapping and its impact on our overall study.

## Mapping Processes and Challenges

In this chapter, we explore three methodological and epistemological challenge areas: *logistical issues* (the basic mapping challenges we initially faced that led to GIS map use); *representational issues* (the difficulties we experienced as we compiled and interpreted complex data from which the maps were derived); and *interpretational issues* (our political and symbolic concerns about the ways constituents might misapply or misconstrue the maps). More than an ancillary aspect of the study, mapping methodology was intertwined with the logistical and representational challenges of this project in general. Consequently, the methodology of map designing will be treated as both process and result in our analysis.

### *Logistical Issues*

Although college access organizations are a familiar research topic (Gandara & Bial, 2001; Gullatt & Jan, 2003; Perna, 2002; Perna & Swail, 2001; Tierney & Jun, 2001), our novel state-level analysis approach meant we could not benefit from existing models to help us design a data-gathering process, or to anticipate constituent and political obstacles during the research and reporting stages. Our research team identified college access provider organizations in Virginia through state and nonprofit databases, as well as a snowball technique through an online survey. From this initiative, we identified 480 access provider instances[1] spread over 132 school divisions.

The two central logistical challenges posed by GIS mapping dealt with managing the strategic advantages and disadvantages of this process. The first logistical challenge we faced was determining the unit of analysis. Although the access provider data we had gathered would serve as the basis for the maps, conceptualizing the unit of analysis was problematic. The access providers' administrative locations and mailing addresses often did not correspond with the site of services. For parents, students, and educators, the distribution of service sites was the issue of interest. Developing maps based on provider mailing addresses or home offices would be technically accurate, but functionally of little use. Thus, the schools themselves as the site of most service interventions (providers typically bring services to those served), and not the access provider's office locations, became our mapping focal point. However, this decision led a subsequent logistical challenge.

The second logistical challenge arose from the databases used to construct provider maps. Generally, the geographic and demographic data available is constrained by the scope of the most basic unit of analysis. In our case, describing the distribution of providers at the school level would have yielded the most precise maps, but this approach faced two impediments: first, because of the sheer volume of data, we would be confined to a set of regional maps and would not be able to display a state-level map with the detail desired. Second, and even more important, at that time, no school-level GIS maps existed that would allow us to identify the geographic boundaries of each unit. Although several national mapping initiatives are under way, high schools in Virginia, as in most states, operate on a feeder system from elementary schools to middle schools, and on to high schools. As a result, although paper maps may exist in division offices, there were no state-level digital maps of the boundaries of individual schools. The smallest unit of analysis available was the school division, or clusters of school districts, most often defined by county or city borders.

### *Representational Issues*

These logistical issues are easily overlooked as the trifling obstacles that are part of any research project. However, limitations inherent to translating social data into geographic data forced us to conform our ideas of data representation to those best suited for the maps. In essence, map-making shifted from a resource to a process driver, determining our unit of analysis and forcing us to reconfigure data to match the input needs of the software. Despite these encumbrances, our increased investment in the mapping process revealed three additional representational issues that helpfully challenged us to consider the most useful form and delivery of data to constituents.

The school boundary problem created our first representational issue. Identifying access providers by school district reduced the descriptive accuracy of our findings, since the number of schools contained in one division varies by local population, history, and other factors. For example, both Fairfax County and Alexandria City Public Schools had eight college access providers (nonprofit organizations, public agencies, or higher education institutions) operating within their divisions. However, Alexandria City included one public high school while Fairfax County Schools included 26 public high schools. On a provider distribution density map, the two divisions appear to be equally serviced, yet students in Alexandria City had access to the full complement of access services described by the provider count, while students in Fairfax County may not, since that same number of providers is unequally distributed among a large number of schools. To parents or students, the map misleadingly appears to indicate equal services among these two school districts, as it would to a local philanthropic organization interested in supporting or initiating an access provider organization. Thus, although to say both districts have eight providers is correct, the availability of access services or the urgency for the development of new services has been inaccurately represented. And although the original study included figures that described and illustrated these differences, the translation to and accessibility of mapping may reduce the likelihood that study consumers will invest the time necessary to understand these crucial nuances by reading the complete study.

A second representational issue dealt with the varied types of access organizations that constituted the provider count for any given school division. Our total count included all public and private not-for-profit college access providers whose primary purpose fit the following definition, developed from our data collection and analysis: any organization through which an individual gains the knowledge, skills, or support necessary for college aspiration, qualification, application, and enrollment (based on Cabrera & La Nasa, 2001). To qualify as an access provider in Virginia, an organization must have staff physically working within the Commonwealth and, thus, within a school division. However, the services, resources, and organizational missions of these varied groups, in aggregate, resulted in combinations that may or may not meet the needs of local constituents. For example, both Henrico County Schools and Prince Edward County Schools had five "college access providers" working in their respective districts. Four of the providers in Henrico County were traditional community-based private organizations working within the schools, and the fifth was a community college-based Career Coach operating in a similar manner. By contrast, Prince Edward County Schools had one traditional access provider organization, a Career Coach location, a federally funded GEAR UP location, and two colleges or universities (one public, one private) which were also included in the access provider count. Thus, the density and distribution map fails to capture the important distinction between types of provider organizations, with significant implications for the types of services that may be available.

In our data analysis process, we were challenged by a state policymaker who, upon reading a draft of our study, asked what the provider count really indicated to readers of the study. To accurately represent the type of organizations, we constructed a table with nine categories of providers (including private, locally based organizations, state-funded initiatives, federally funded initiatives, and the aforementioned degree-granting two- or four-year colleges and universities) listed by school division. One might imagine that adding additional map layers illustrating population and provider type could easily alleviate these representational challenges. Yet, adding these layers resulted in maps that were too crowded and difficult for constituents to understand, highlighting the tension between representation and accessibility.

Thus, although revealing the layers of variation that were part of the provider count became an interpretational issue, it was first a representational one: despite the fact that the table clarified the nature of the accumulated count by school division, we found no way to reflect that detail through GIS maps.[2] In summary, although the mapping project faced a variety of representational issues, perhaps the most important was the combined effect of the dissimilar school division sizes and the disparate types and missions of the access provider organizations. The maps, though visually impressive, cloak the complexity of these two factors in the deceptively simple and self-explanatory guise of a single access provider count data point.

### *Interpretational Issues*

The representational issues establish the context for and content of issues of sense-making among constituents of this study, raising several questions about the role of the authors in developing and disseminating the findings of the report. First, we questioned what sense various constituents and stakeholders would make of the provider density maps, and our responsibility in that meaning-making process. At the state level, we were subtly encouraged not to report our findings in a way that cast the ongoing college access initiatives of the Commonwealth in a particularly negative light. In this regard, the map data cut both ways, reflecting the increased resources SCHEV and other agencies had targeted towards particular regions, but also (in conjunction with demographic and achievement data) highlighting areas of acute need with little or no state response. We were deliberate in our efforts to link the maps to data and discussions of the complexity of the access provider environment. However, we quickly realized that despite our role as authors and designers of the study, once this product entered the public arena, we were no longer in control of the interpretation process or product.

Realizing our limited control over constituent interpretations and use of the maps raised a second set of questions, which were complicated by a growing level of interest by SCHEV, legislators, and other stakeholders as they learned that these maps were under development. At the state and local level, we were concerned that provider distribution data would be interpreted apart from important demographic, population density, and achievement data. We wondered: would state legislators, each of whom also received a SCHEV-designed and -distributed four-color brochure prominently featuring the density map, use it alternatively as evidence of a rampant problem or as the absence of a college access problem in their district or in the state in general? Would college access providers interpret the maps (and hence, our study) as championing their work and as evidence for additional support, or as misconstruing and underrepresenting the effect size of their efforts? Would local school officials receive this data as indicative of significant needs and seek out cooperative relationships with access providers, or view it as an unwelcome public indictment of their schools? Although we share the concerns of writers critical of GIS mapping for its empiricist roots and apparent value-neutrality (Lake, 1993), the above questions also highlight that meaning emerges through discursive communities and the interchange of language within them (Gergen, 1992), beyond the control of those who originate the subject matter. As a result, our role in setting the agenda through the map creation was only one element in the continuous meaning-construction of a variety of overlapping political, social, and educational communities. These communities are neither (or not simply) hapless victims of map data, nor are they immune to the possibly disruptive or persuasive influence that the maps may levy. Nevertheless, we also acknowledged our responsibility to be actively engaged in this public conversation, and to hear the interpretations and concerns of state and local constituents through a forthcoming assessment of our initial study.

## Conclusions

GIS mapping is yet another juncture in the ongoing struggle between modern and post-modern perspectives of research interpretation, pitting advances of empirical science against critiques of sweeping narratives and frameworks that mask and disregard the voices of those not part of the dominant milieu. Like other contested ground (gender, the media, public policy, etc.), the fight did not originate with this topic, and though GIS mapping may provide an arena where these ongoing feuds can find new expression, neither will it see its conclusion. However, similar to the history of feminist critiques of the natural sciences (Harding, 1996; Keller, 1982), as criticisms of power use and resource access were gradually acknowledged by the established order, one positive outcome has been an increasing openness, dialogue, and tendency towards scholarly self-policing. Despite occasional blazes of vitriol on both sides, ground gained as the legitimacy of criticisms are gradually acknowledged leads to a movement towards a self-policing and critiquing community of scholars and practitioners. The emergence of PPGIS is an example of just such an intra-field adjustment. This peer group is, at its best, aware of the tendencies of the discipline to exclude the perspectives of individuals and groups and is willing to engage in a lively dialogue about power, privilege, access, and voice. Nevertheless, the broad application and increasing accessibility of GIS in recent years has resulted in a range of constituents attracted to the representational and analytic opportunities it affords, with little to no appreciation for or interest in the epistemological issues and conversations related to its use. In other words, the opportunities for intentional and unintentional abuse grow when such tools are used apart from the influence of peer review and professional interaction.

The proliferation of GIS mapping as a promoted commodity adds an additional layer to concerns about ethical use and social responsibility. As we developed our project, our partner geographer was aiding in the creation of a campus-based, grant-funded, multi-million-dollar GIS laboratory aimed at developing its own geographic projects as well as promoting inter- and multidisciplinary partnership projects across the institution. At no point did this professional geographer engage with us in a conversation about the implications of mapping apart from base data accuracy. Whether it was his responsibility to do so is part of the question we broach here. The simple allure and self-evidence of mapping, particularly in projects designed for consumption by the uninformed patron, indicates that GIS and next-generation mapping software will continue to grow in popularity. Whether the burden of responsibility for fair representation rests with the researcher, the geographer, the policymaker, or the consumer is a vital question and worthy of further conversation.

As we invested in the mapping process and committed time and resources to this representational form, the demands of the mapping process increasingly shaped how we formatted data to comply with the GIS software. The format of the data, in turn, impacted how we interacted with the data, how we thought about the data, how we talked about the data, and ultimately the sense we made of the data. Gradually, mapping changed from a logistical and representational tool to an interpretational agent. As mapping novices, we realized that not only could the mapping product impact unreflective audiences in potentially subversive ways, but also how the demands of mapping could impact our sense-making in the process of data analysis in ways that might not be just, equitable, or even ethical to groups or individuals represented by the data.

Certainly, our research team is neither the first nor the last to discuss the challenges of data representation and interpretation. Other researchers have encountered similar challenges through traditional visual methods (Cooper et al., 2003; Crowe, 2006; Weaver & Converse, 2008). However, we intend this chapter to introduce some of the challenges, issues, and obstacles unique and related to GIS map use in general, and mapping access provider organizations in particular. At the state level, a full assessment of access provider resources is a laudable goal, especially given the calls for increased numbers of college graduates. However, conveying needs and resources must be done with care. The debate over racial and ethnic categorization by governmental and educational entities highlights both the frequently spurious process of category development and the far-reaching implications of those metrics (Omi, 1997). Similarly, mapping in this context is a relatively simple process with extensive social and political consequences.

Thus, we suggest three specific areas for ongoing map-related conversations related specifically to college access, and generally to the study of higher education. First, stakeholders interested in college access as a state policy issue need to engage in a dialogue about how to count and categorize college access providers and ways to transmit that data to interested parties, including legislators, educators, private citizens, and the access providers themselves. We hope that the work emanating from our original study is contributing to this goal. Second, educational researchers must engage in a dialogue regarding the hazards and benefits of using GIS mapping as a tool for representing geographically based data, including sensitive demographic, achievement, and resource information. We found both positive and negative research experiences associated with the GIS mapping and interpretation processes. Finally, researchers, practitioners, and policymakers using these tools have a duty to participate in the ongoing dialogue about the responsibilities of scholars using GIS mapping, and to reflect on the expedience and accessibility of the medium when delivering data into the public policy arena.

## Notes

1. The term "instances" is used since many providers operate as semi-autonomous branches of or as members within a larger organizational network. Since the number of networks is less important than the specific locations they serve, we elected to base our count on areas served by distinct entities of service to increase descriptive power.
2. Although constructing web-based interactive maps may have provided more options for representation, this approach would also have limited opportunities for display and presentation. Ultimately, SCHEV elected to use the data from this study and construct those very maps as a tool for parents, educators, and policymakers. The maps are available through their website: www.SCHEV.edu.

## References

Aitken, S. C., & Michel, S. M. (1995). Who contrives the "real" in GIS? Geographic information, planning and critical theory. *Cartography and Geographic Information Systems, 22*(1), 17–29.

Cabrera, A. F., & La Nasa, S. M. (2001). On the path to college: Three critical tasks facing America's disadvantaged. *Research in Higher Education, 42*, 119–149.

Cooper, R. J., Schriger, D. L., Wallace, R. C., Mikulich, V. J., & Wilkes, M. S. (2003). The quantity and quality of scientific graphs in pharmaceutical advertisements. *Journal of General Internal Medicine, 18*(4), 294–297.

Crowe, A. R. (2006). Technology, citizenship, and the social studies classroom: Education for democracy in a technological age. *International Journal of Social Education, 21*(1), 111–121.

Gandara, P. C., & Bial, D. (2001). *Paving the way to postsecondary education: K-12 intervention programs for underrepresented youth.* Washington, DC: U.S. Department of Education, National Center for Education Statistics.

Gergen, K. J. (1992). Organizational theory in the postmodern era. In M. Reed & M. Hughes (Eds.). *Rethinking organization: New directions in organizational theory and analysis.* London: Sage.

Ghose, R. (2001). Use of information technology for community empowerment: Transforming geographic information systems into community information systems. *Transactions in GIS, 5*(2), 141–163.

Gullatt, Y., & Jan, W. (2003). *How do pre-collegiate academic outreach programs impact college-going among underrepresented students?* Boston: Pathways to College Network Clearinghouse.

Haque, A. (2001). GIS, public service, and the issue of democratic governance. *Public Administrative Review, 61*(3), 259–265.

Harding, S. (1996). Feminism, science, and the anti-enlightenment critiques. In Ann Garry & Marilyn Pearsall (Eds.). *Women, knowledge and reality: Explorations in feminist philosophy.* London: Routledge.

Keller, E. F. (1982). Feminism and science. *Feminist Theory, 7*(3), 589–602.

Kwaku Kyem, P. (2004). Of intractable conflicts and participatory GIS systems: The search for consensus amidst competing claims and institutional demands. *Annuls of the Association of American Geographers, 94*(1), 37–57.

Lake, R.W. (1993). Planning and applied geography: Positivism, ethics, and geographic information systems. *Progress in Human Geography* 17, 404–413.

MacEachren, A. M. (2000). Cartography and GIS: Facilitating collaboration. *Progress in Human Geography, 24*(3), 445–456.

Monmonier, M. (1991). *How to lie with maps.* Chicago: The University of Chicago Press.

Obermeyer, N. J. (1998). The evolution of public participation GIS. *Cartography and Geographic Information Systems, 25*(2), 65–66.

Omi, M. (1997). Racial identity and the state: The dilemmas of classification. *Law and Inequality, 7*(19).

Perna, L. W. (2002). Precollege outreach programs: Characteristics of programs serving historically underrepresented groups of students. *Journal of College Student Development, 43*(1), 64–83.

Perna, L. W., & Swail, W. S. (2001). Pre-college outreach and early intervention. *Thought and Action: The NEA Higher Education Journal, 27*, 99–110.

Pickles, J. (1995). Representations in an electronic age: Geography, GIS, and democracy. In J. Pickles (Ed.). *Ground truth.* New York: Guilford Press.

Schuurman, N. (2000). Trouble in the heartland: GIS and its critics in the 1990s. *Progress in Human Geography, 24*(4), 569–590. DOI:10.1191/030913200100189111

Sheppard, E. (1995). GIS and society: Toward a research agenda. *Cartography and Geographic Information Systems, 22*(1), 5–16.

Sieber, R. (2006). Public participation geographic information systems: A literature review and framework. *Annuals of the Association of American Cartographers, 96*(3), 491–507.

Taylor, P. J. (1990). GKS. *Political Geography Quarterly*, *9*, 211–212.

Tierney, W. G., & Jun, A. (2001, March–April). A university helps prepare low income youths for college: Tracking school success. *The Journal of Higher Education*, *72*(2), 205–225.

United States Geological Survey. (2007, February). *Geographic information systems*. Retrieved from http://egsc.usgs.gov/isb/pubs/gis_poster/

Weaver, C. L., & Converse, D. (2008). Picture this: Strategies for communicating data to decision makers. *NASJE News Quarterly*, *23*(4). Retrieved from http://nasje.org/news/newsletter0804/02-resources01.php

# Appendix

The map below is a density map of the number of college access provider organizations by county and by region (numbers 1-9).

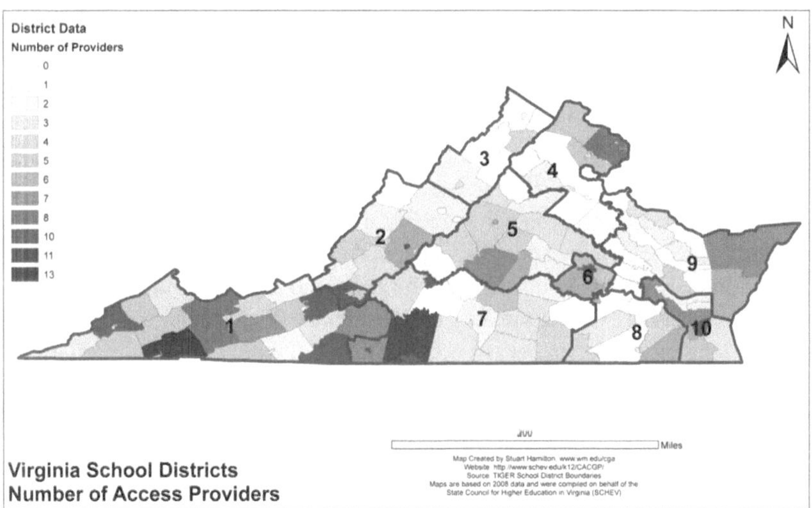

# 8 Protecting Surface Water Drinking Supplies in WV With Zones of Critical Concern

*Michael P. Strager*

## Introduction

In January 2014, Charleston, West Virginia made the national news for all the wrong reasons. A leak from a chemical tank located along the bank of the Elk River, which is less than half a mile upstream of Charleston, spilled a chemical called Methylcyclohexanemethanol (MCHM) in the river. Over 10,000 gallons of the chemical, which is used to clean coal before it is used in coal-fired power plants, made its way to the surface water intake and circulated throughout the city and extending to a nine-county area. This made all water contact from the faucet unavailable for consumption or even washing for 300,000 people. Reports of rashes and hospital visits were frequent throughout the area. Businesses had to close, and residents scrambled to purchase water or wait in lines at water buffalo stations. The social and economic impact of this event has had a wide-ranging impact on the area. Many people were forced to move out and have yet to return due to a perceived existing threat to their health and well-being.

The state legislature in West Virginia moved quickly to tighten regulations regarding above-ground storage tanks near rivers and streams in order to prevent future spills across the state. Senate Bill 373 was enacted in June of 2014, six months after the spill. The bill and subsequent additions required a registration period of all above-ground storage tanks, and NPDES general permit holders with above-ground storage tanks within a newly defined zone of critical concern were required to apply for a permit and perform engineering-level inspections. All tanks needed to be registered, and tank owners must submit spill prevention plans by qualified inspectors or engineers. Costs for registration and spill response plans typically averaged $3,500 per tank in the zone of critical concern. Companies scrambled to move their tanks and to determine whether or not they were in the ZCC.

To aid in modeling and mapping, West Virginia University was contracted by the West Virginia Bureau of Public Health to assist in the delineation of the ZCCs statewide. For each of the surface water intakes (n = 175), a five-hour time of travel was determined above the intake. For each of the mainstem river segments, a 1,000-foot buffer had to be created, and a 500-foot buffer for each tributary. If the intake was in a reservoir, the reservoir would be buffered 1,000 feet and all tributaries to the reservoir buffered 500 feet.

## Approach

(*The following section references the work in Strager 2012.*)

A spatial modeling approach using hydrological data was needed to create a time of travel estimate for all streams five hours upstream of the surface water intakes. Runoff is a function of climate, morphology, land cover, watershed state properties (soil, storage, topography), antecedent moisture, and land use. Ideally, these all would be considered to estimate the real-time stream flow condition and water volume calculations to perform the modeling. After an extensive literature search, it was determined that surprisingly few time of travel modeling approaches have been developed in the spatial modeling area. The choice was made to integrate an equation and study by Jobson (1996), which predicted the travel time and longitudinal dispersion of rivers and streams in the United States. In this report, data were analyzed for over 980 subreaches, or about 90 different rivers, in the United States representing a wide range of river sizes, slopes, and geomorphic types. The authors found that four variables were available in sufficient quantities for a regression analysis. The variables included the drainage area ($D_a$), the reach slope (S), the mean annual river discharge ($Q_a$), and the discharge at the section at time of the measurement (Q). The report defines peak velocity as:

$$V'_p = V_p D_a / Q$$

and the dimensionless drainage area as:

$$D'_a = D_a 1.25 * \text{sqrt}\left(g\right) / Q_a$$

where g is the acceleration of gravity. The dimensionless relative discharge is defined as:

$$Q'_a = Q / Q_a$$

The equations are homogeneous, so any consistent system of units can $m/s^2$ be used in the dimensionless groups. The regression equation that follows has a constant term that has specific units, meters per second. The most convenient set of units for use with the equation are: velocity in meters per second, discharge in cubic meters per second, drainage area in square meters, acceleration of gravity in and slope in meters per meter.

The equation derived in the report and the equation used in this study for peak velocity in meters per second was the following:

$$V_p = 0.094 + 0.0143 * \left(D'_a\right) 0.919 * \left(Q'_a\right) - 0.469 * S\ 0.159 * Q / D_a$$

The standard error estimates of the constant and slope are 0.026 m/s and 0.0003, respectively. This prediction equation had an $R^2$ of 0.70 and an RMS error of 0.157 m/s.

Once a velocity grid was calculated as described above, it was used as an inverse weight grid in the flowlength ArcGIS (ESRI, 2010) command. The flowlength command calculates a stream length in meters. If velocity is in meters per second, the inverse velocity as a weight grid will return seconds in the output grid. This calculation of seconds tracks how long water takes to move from every cell in the state where a stream is located to where it leaves the state. The higher values will exist in the headwater sections of a watershed. By querying the grid, it is possible to add the appropriate travel time to the cell value to find the time it takes water to reach the site. For each intake cell location, a value of 18,000 (18,000 seconds for 5 hours) was added to determine the extent to reach the intake. To use this methodology, GIS data layers had to be calculated for drainage area, stream slope, annual average flow, and bank-full flow for all of West Virginia. The sections below describe how each of these grids was created.

### *Drainage Area*

Obtaining a drainage area calculation for every stream cell in the state required a hydrologically correct DEM. The process of creating a hydrologically correct DEM is discussed by Jenson and Domingue (1988). Essentially, from the DEM the flow direction and flow accumulation values for each stream cell are derived. The output of the flow direction request is an integer grid, the values of which range from 1 to 255. The values for each direction from the center are:

| | | |
|---|---|---|
| 32 | 64 | 128 |
| 16 | X | 1 |
| 8 | 4 | 2 |

For example, if the direction of steepest drop were to the left of the current processing cell, its flow direction would be coded as 16. If a cell is lower than its eight neighbors, that cell is given the value of its lowest neighbor and flow is defined towards this cell (ESRI, 2010).

The accumulated flow is based upon the number of cells flowing into each cell in the output grid. The current processing cell is not considered in this accumulation. Output cells with a high flow accumulation are areas of concentrated flow and may be used to identify stream channels. Output cells with a flow accumulation of zero are local topographic highs and may be used to identify ridges. The equation to calculate drainage area from a 20-meter cell sized flow accumulation grid was: (cell value of flow accumulation grid + 1) * 400 = drainage area in meters squared.

### *Stream Slope*

Stream slope was calculated for each stream reach in the state. A stream reach is not necessarily an entire stream, only the section of a stream between junctions.

The GIS command streamlink was first used to find all unique streams between stream intersections or junctions. For each of these reaches, the length was calculated from the flowlength GIS command. Having the original DEM allowed us to find the maximum and minimum values for each of the stream reaches. The difference in the maximum and minimum elevations for the stream reach divided by the total reach length gave us our stream reach slope in meters per meter.

### *Annual Average Flow*

Annual average flow for each stream cell location was found based on a relationship between drainage area and gauged stream flow. For 88 gauging stations in West Virginia, covering many different rainfall, geological, and elevation regions, we assembled a table of drainage areas for the gauges versus the historic annual stream flow for the gauge. After fitting a linear regression line for this dataset, we found the following equation for annual stream flow, setting the y intercept to zero.

Annual stream flow in cfs = 2.05 * drainage area in square miles

This equation had a corrected $R^2$ of .9729. The XY plot and equation are shown in Figure 8.1.

Since drainage area is already calculated for each stream cell location, this equation incorporated the drainage area grid to compute a separate grid layer of annual stream flow. This would be another input for the velocity calculation.

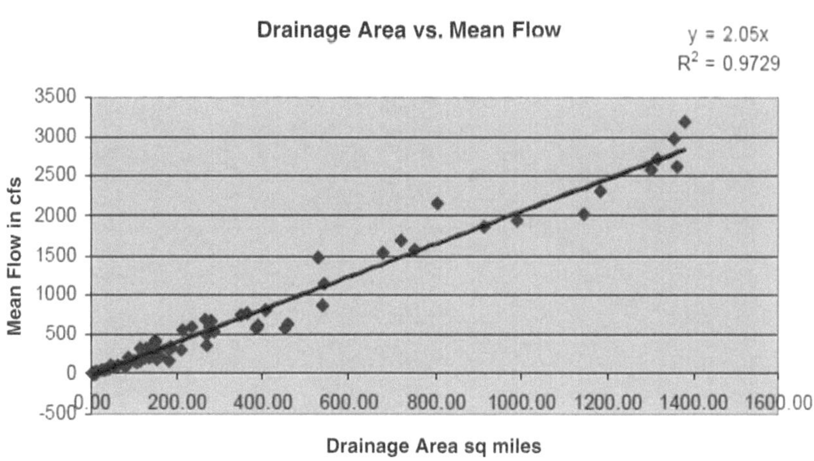


*Figure 8.1* Annual stream flow from gauged stations and drainage area at the gauges.

***Bank-Full Flow***

The last input for the velocity equation was the bank-full flow measure. Just as with annual average flow, this required a modeled value for every raster stream cell in West Virginia. Using the same approach to regressing drainage area to gauged stream flow as performed to find an annual average flow equation, this equation was used to find bank-full flow. Bank-full flow as defined by the Bureau of Public Health is 90% of the annual high flow. To find 90% of high flow for each gauging station, all historic daily stream flow data was downloaded for each of the 88 gauging stations. This data was sorted lowest to highest and then numbered lowest to highest after removing repeating values. The value of flow at 90% of the data became the bank-full flow value for that gauge. These values were then regressed against drainage area at the gauge. The linear regression equation for bank-full stream flow, setting the y intercept to zero, is listed below.

Bank-full stream flow in cfs = 4.357 * drainage area in square miles

This equation had a corrected $R^2$ of .9265. The XY plot and equation are shown in Figure 8.2.

This equation could be applied to the drainage area grid to calculate the bank-full flow for any stream cell in the state. It was the final input needed in the velocity calculation.

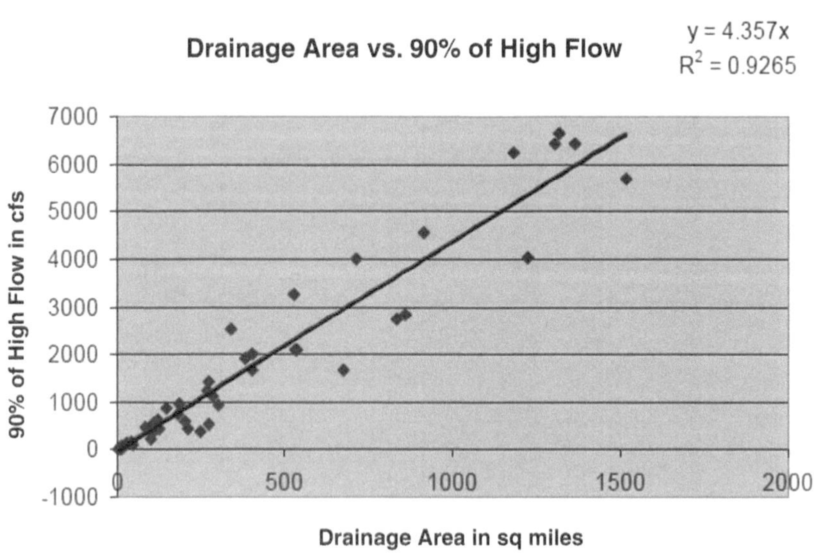


*Figure 8.2* Bank-full stream flow from gauged stations and drainage area at the gauges.

## Results

In Figure 8.3, the raster stream network can be seen, which follows the stream centerline path of water in the Elk River. For the specific location where the surface water intake is shown, the time of travel value can be queried. This value means that water at that cell takes 119,369 seconds to leave the state at Huntington, West Virginia. All drainage leaving the state is time 0, and values larger than zero represent the time for water to reach those outlets.

At the intake location, 180,000 seconds, which represents five hours, can be added to the site to find the total upstream extent. This is shown in Figure 8.4.

By querying for the time of travel in this extent, all the raster cells can be selected and then converted to vector for accurate buffers. Using an attribute for mainstem versus tributary, the segments of streams can be buffered at either 1,000 feet or 500 feet accordingly. Figure 8.5 shows the five-hour extent and the buffers for mainstem and tributaries. This process was completed for all 175 intakes throughout West Virginia.

An analysis of land use and cover as well as potential sources of pollution were inventoried for the areas within the ZCC. Features of interest included the national pollution discharge elimination system sites (NPDES), landfills, superfund sites (CERCLIS), hazardous and solid waste sites (RCRIS), toxic release inventory sites, coal dams, abandoned mine lands, animal feed lots, major highways, and railroads. The degree of potential threat for the surface water intake can be analyzed with the ZCC and these potential sources of pollution using straightforward GIS overlays and summaries. In addition to these potential sources, the goal of the approach was to focus on the above-ground

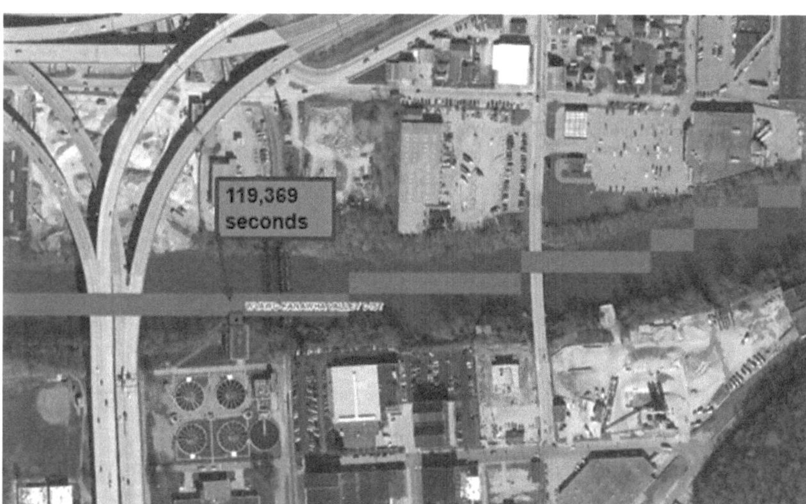


*Figure 8.3* Example of time of travel calculation at surface water intake.

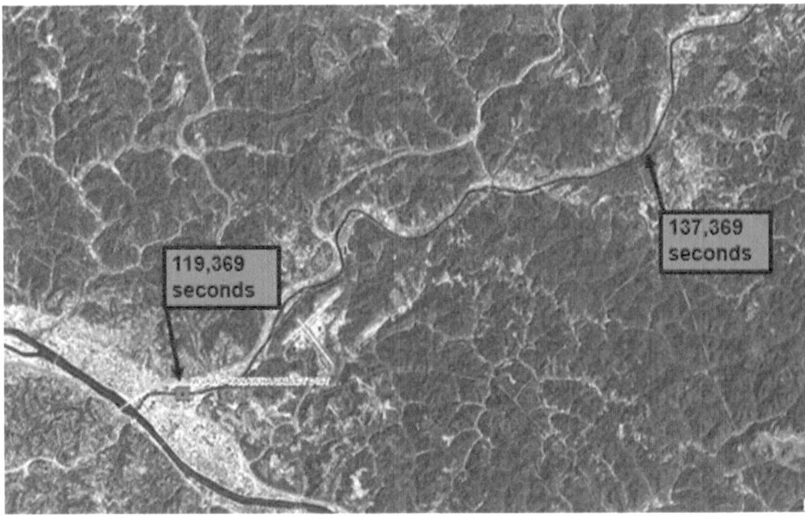


*Figure 8.4* 180,000 seconds or five-hour travel time upstream of intake.

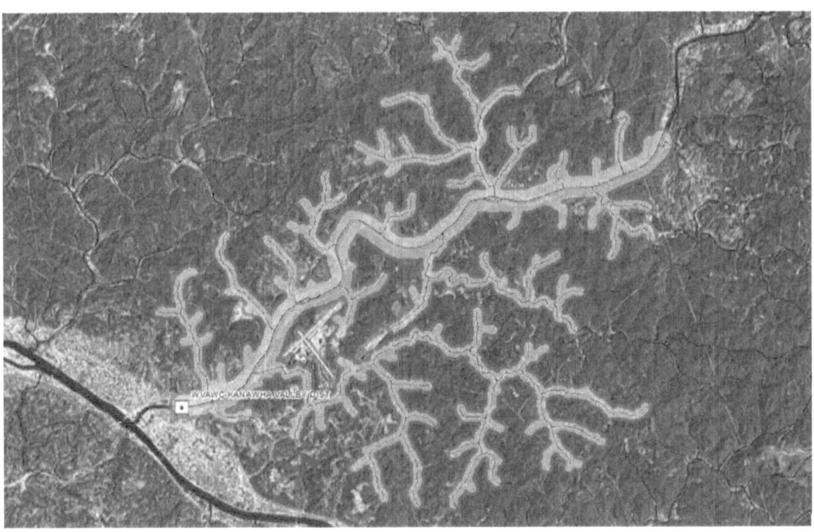

*Figure 8.5* Example of a ZCC of five-hour time of travel with mainstem and tributary buffers.

storage tanks (ASTs). The number, capacity, and ages of the tanks are summarized in Figures 8.6 and 8.7. This information has proven to be extremely valuable for identifying the potential problem tanks and vulnerable systems that have these ASTs present in their ZCC.

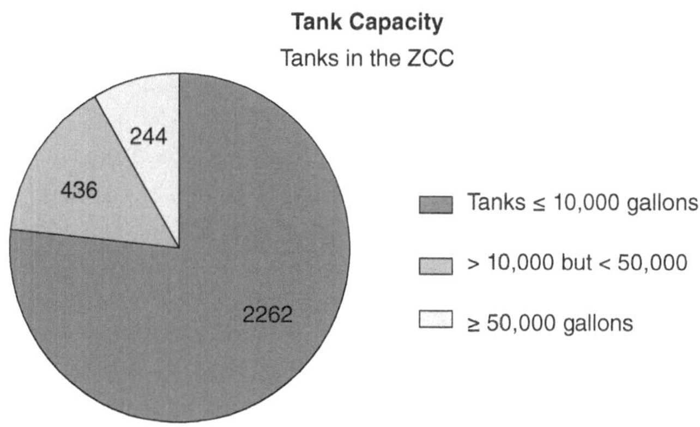


*Figure 8.6* Tank capacity in the ZCC statewide.

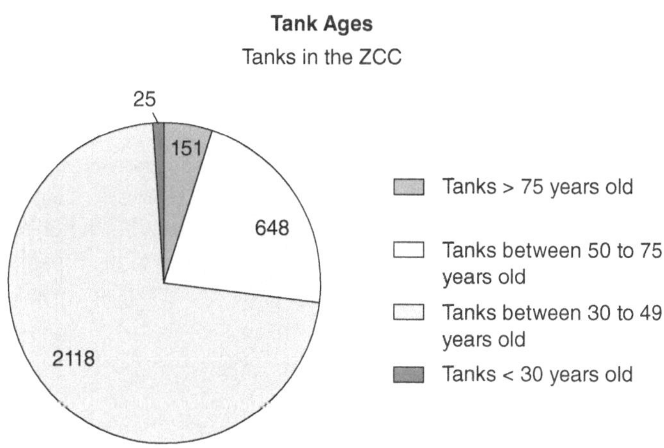


*Figure 8.7* Tank ages in the ZCC statewide.

## Discussion and Conclusions

The need to have tanks registered and inspected has meant additional cost and inconvenience for owners in the ZCCs. In 2016, the AST industry challenged the ZCC approach and implementation. The West Virginia Environmental Quality Board heard the case and decided to uphold the science, approach, and implementation of the AST Act for West Virginia, which uses the ZCCs. It was acknowledged that the best available science and approach at the time was implemented to protect the surface water intakes at the statewide West Virginia scale. The process does have its faults, mainly in the calculation of 2D distance from the mapped river shoreline 1,000 feet back, but also in the assumption that average annual flow is sufficient. Arguments could be made that both a high flow and low flow ZCC could be used or models built to better understand the complexities and intricacies of site-specific topography and watershed hydrology across different parts of the state. In addition, since the drainage area and slope calculations are important variables in the time of travel equation, a more accurate and timely elevation dataset such as those available from LiDAR would improve these values. The elevation data used in the study was from 2003 and was a statewide 3-meter resolution. This was considerably better than the next best alternative, which was the statewide 1:24,000 10-meter data from the mid-1970s assembled from the US Geological Survey. Within just West Virginia, LiDAR was flown for about 40% of the state in 2010 and has a 1-meter spatial resolution. This data could be integrated once it available statewide. Other limitations include the hydrology layer, mapped at 1:4,800 scale from the 2003 State Address Mapping Board hypsography. It is possible that many of the streams are intermittent or too small in size to be effective conduits for water flow during a chemical spill. The Jobson (1996) equation notes the importance of more local chemical spill and plume dispersion studies to capture the impacts of chemicals that are more or less soluble or that suspend in different parts of the water column. This can be expensive and time-consuming work but would be a critical component to understanding the potential downstream dispersion differences across the state and also to better understanding the chemical response options.

Even with these limitations and cautions with the approach implemented, it should be understood that the purpose of the ZCC was to conservatively protect surface water intakes as a pre-spill planning tool that is not contingent upon instantaneous flow or seasonal conditions. The use of the five-hour travel time distance further reinforces the protective nature of this approach.

## References

Environmental Systems Research Institute (ESRI)., 2010. ArcInfo ArcMap. Redlands, CA.

Jenson, S.K., Domingue, J.O., 1988. Extracting topographic structure from digital elevation data for geographic information system analysis. *Photogrammetric Engineering and Remote Sensing* 54 (11), 1593–1600.

Jobson, H.E., 1996. Prediction of travel time and longitudinal dispersion in rivers and streams: U.S. geological survey water-resources investigations report 96–4013, p. 69; https://pubs.usgs.gov/of/1996/4013.

Strager, M.P., 2012. Tools for watershed planning—development of a statewide source water protection system (SWPS). *Water Resources Management and Modeling.*

# Section IV

# Practitioner Use of GIS in Public and Nonprofit Organizations

# 9 Uses of Geospatial Information Systems (GIS) for Public Higher Education Institutions

*Nicolas A. Valcik and Daniel Servian*

## Introduction

College and university administrators face difficult and complex issues unique to higher education institutions. Problems at public institutions can be further compounded by local, state, and federal rules and regulations, which overlay more restrictions on what institutions can and cannot do to resolve certain problems. For example, complex issues can arise from right-of-way and storm water management to hazardous material (HAZMAT) locations to jurisdictional purview for university law enforcement officials. To resolve difficult and complex problems, administration needs to be innovative and must be willing to use new technology, which can provide additional information for administrative decision-making processes.

The examples throughout this chapter will tie in academic innovations utilizing GIS to provide spatial data that can potentially be useful in resolving complex issues for upper-level administrators. This chapter will discuss how GIS can be leveraged to quickly analyze how students and employees of a large public university intersect with additional large regional employers, insufficient transportation networks, and topography that can potentially strain existing infrastructure. Unlike an academic or classroom setting, a practitioner can face potential consequences if an administrator makes an error in the decision-making process. To illustrate situations in which GIS can be used administratively at universities and colleges in the decision-making process, several different examples encountered at West Virginia University will be highlighted.

## Prior Research

Dr. John Snow is credited with not only the start of the field of epidemiology but also the beginning of using maps for operational action. In 1854, Dr. Snow began mapping cholera outbreaks related to water pumps in London to determine the source of the outbreaks and thus identify the source of the illness (UCLA, 2014). What might appear to be a simple exercise was actually considered cutting-edge data usage, with epidemiology intersecting with geographic data. As Figures 9.1, 9.2, and 9.3 show, the data by itself is limited until it is layered with the geographic data (Kukaswadia, 2013).

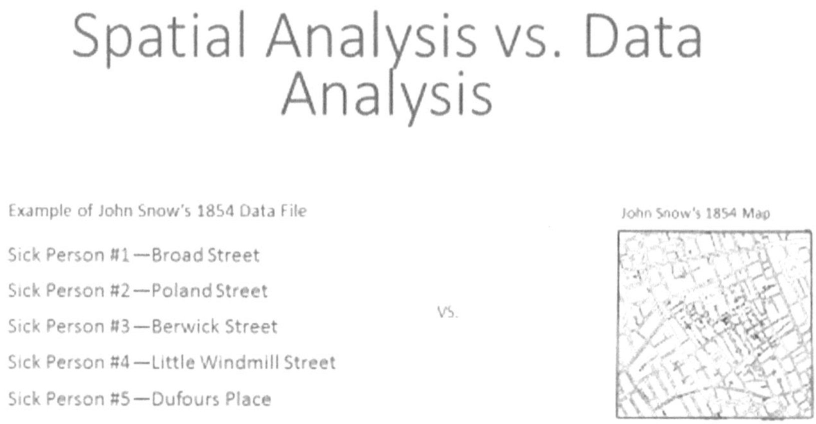


*Figure 9.1* List of infected persons vs. infected persons pinpointed on a map.

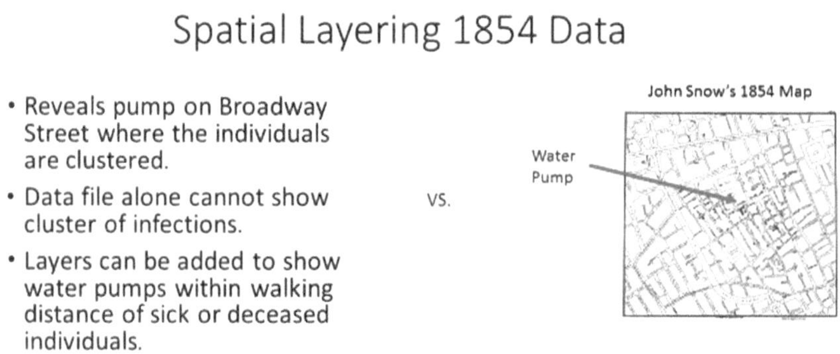


*Figure 9.2* Water pump location.

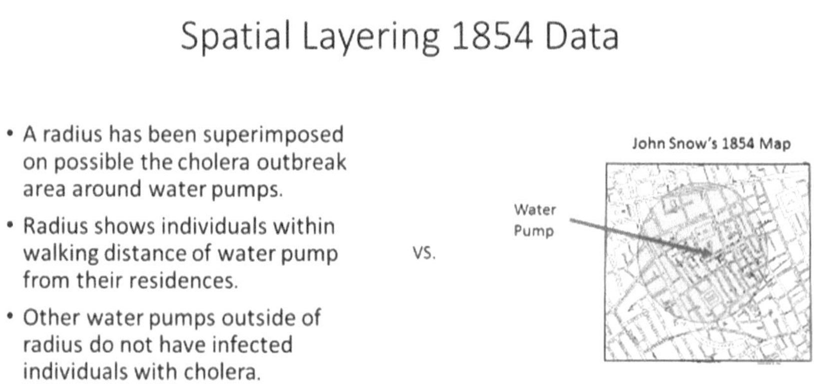


*Figure 9.3* As can be seen in Figures 9.1, 9.2, and 9.3, the data allows decision-making to be made operationally since the data is triangulated with more than one data source.

## GIS as a Tool for Administration

What is GIS, and why should higher education institutions use it as opposed to using Computer Aided Drafting (CAD) software? CAD is still an industry standard for architects and draftsmen for facility construction (United States Department of Agriculture Natural Resources Conservation Service, 2006). CAD is heavily used in public organizations, which in some cases have been using it since its inception in the 1970s. Using this resource has required organizations to train personnel, obtain hardware, and pay for software to keep up with current CAD capabilities and retain viability for universities and colleges. Frequently, CAD users are located in the facility management departments at colleges and universities in which facility information resides. However, for administrative purposes, CAD is very limited in both capability and interoperability for providing information to different administrative departments within a college or university. While CAD has been used extensively by architects and drafters, it has not been used by staff or faculty in administration or social science disciplines. This is because in addition to requiring specialized training, CAD is unable to utilize large informational databases on the same level as GIS, which can analyze and layer information.

In contrast to CAD's existing capabilities, GIS has evolved over the years. GIS not only ties in large amounts of data to very specific locations but also can capture anything from floor plans to three-dimensional renderings to coordinate geometry. The expansion of GIS technology provides researchers, practitioners, and students a tool with which to investigate a wide array of research initiatives. CAD systems, however, have not evolved to intuitively accommodate those types of research or practitioner-based initiatives. Administrators need to use the right tool for the right job, and for many, administrative GIS is a superior tool for the decision-making process.

Additionally, GIS has the capability utilize a wide array of coordinate systems, elevation models, satellite imagery, aerial photography, and seamless integration with server databases (i.e. Microsoft SQL Server, Oracle etc.). GIS has effectively created a new generation of geographers and geoscientists with a reputation for being able to perform research with high-tech tools (Golledge, 2001). Gone are the days of geographers making maps with pen and paper (Titus, 2001). The perception of geographers and geoscientists using laptops and laser scanners is becoming more commonplace within the academic community. With the advent of GIS, universities and colleges now have newly created GIS academic programs that are enrolling students at the undergraduate, professional, and graduate level. With these types of degree offerings come the opportunity to integrate GIS with new administrative procedures and research in addition to the many education applications in higher education (Pilesjö and Mårtensson, 2009; Space Daily, 2012).

The effective use of GIS by administration in higher education can assist in resolving and researching a number of issues faced by almost every campus throughout its lifecycle. The Harvard Planning and Project Management at Harvard University for example, maintains the university's GIS capability, which is used to create maps and analyses. The GIS group provides standard and custom maps, geographic data, and tools that enable staff to develop their own maps, geographic analyses, data development, and 3D modeling (Harvard University, 2015).

While GIS has been used for epidemiology and in the social sciences, GIS usage for administrative purposes in higher education has been very limited (2018). The administrative use of GIS is growing with institutions that have a robust GIS academic program (e.g. the University of Texas at Dallas, West Virginia University, Penn State University, Stanford University, and Central Washington University). With the support of academic units in the form of software licensing, expertise, and student workers, there have been more higher education institutions using GIS for a variety of purposes over the past few years. The University of Arizona has been using GIS for a number of years and has implemented an enterprise GIS component for planning throughout their campus (McCormick, 2003).

Ohio State University has been using GIS for admissions and recruiting efforts since the late 1990s (Mora, 2003). The university is also using GIS to map down enrolled students and combine that data with United States Census data to obtain additional information on enrolled students (Granados, 2003). Binghamton University has been using GIS to analyze patterns of alumni giving to the university, and the University of Wisconsin system has utilized GIS to analyze survey data and to plan how surveys are administered (Blough, 2003; Jardine, 2003). Western Kentucky University, which currently uses GIS for planning and construction for the university, is an example of GIS becoming more commonly used (Western Kentucky University, 2014). The University of Texas at Dallas used GIS in conjunction with the Logistical Tracking System (LTS) not only to construct floor plans but also to track inventory and HAZMAT throughout the university (Valcik, 2007, 2010). Prior research on proximity analysis is very limited in terms of university administration decision-making processes that use GIS.

## Background on Using GIS at West Virginia University

GIS has a substantial presence at West Virginia University, with an active academic program that offers a bachelor's degree, master's degree, and PhD in GIS (West Virginia University—Geography Program, 2014). The agriculture, geography, geology, and medical departments at West Virginia University currently utilize GIS software for both research and academic purposes. Additionally, the State of West Virginia's GIS Technical Center (WV GIS Tech Center) is located at West Virginia University. The WV GIS Tech Center was created in 1993 by Executive Order 4–93 and was established at West Virginia University in 1998. The department's current objectives are as follows:

- Reduce the duplication of data development efforts among organizations
- Catalog and distribute GIS spatial data and information free-of-charge through the Internet

- Coordinate acquisition of new data additions to the West Virginia Spatial Data Infrastructure
- Assist with strategic planning, development and implementation of statewide mapping guidelines
- Provide advisory services and training programs in the field of geographic information science
- Conduct research and provide education towards improvement of geographic information technologies

(West Virginia GIS Technical Center, 2015)

Until recently, West Virginia University traditionally outsourced administrative GIS work for facility information and land inventory. The university has since invested time and resources in looking at the utilization of GIS for planning purposes at the institution. Over the past several years, West Virginia University's Facilities Planning and Scheduling department has been utilizing GIS. The major utilization of GIS has been for the organization and management of the university's deeded and leased properties. In addition to managing the university's land holdings, GIS has been utilized as a tool for many different types of projects. West Virginia University also uses GIS for projects such as statistical spatial analysis of recruitment, storm water management, and space allocation analysis, and to create web-based map apps for internal departmental usage.

## Unique West Virginia University Campus Characteristics

West Virginia University is the flagship higher education campus in the State of West Virginia. The university has an agriculture research and academic program along with health sciences, which has led to it to have a presence in every county in the State of West Virginia. These extensive land holdings either are property for agriculture purposes or provide health services mission. In addition to having property for education and outreach, West Virginia University owns many tracts of land and minerals, which serve a dual role as an outdoor laboratory and valuable natural resources, such as timber and coal. The campus itself has anywhere from three to six campus segments, depending on who defines what a "campus" comprises for each segment of the university. Currently, there is the original downtown campus, the Evansdale campus, and the health sciences campus. There are also three other segments of the campus: the law school (often lumped into the Evansdale campus), the athletic complex (basketball coliseum, soccer fields, etc., which are lumped into Evansdale), and the administrative areas, which are located off Waterfront Place, one mile from the downtown campus. To link the three campuses together, in the 1970s West Virginia University developed the Personal Rapid Transportation (PRT) thanks to a federal grant; this moves students, employees, and citizens throughout the three locations (West Virginia University—Personal Rapid Transportation, 2014). The PRT transports students throughout the three regions of the university's main campus via a pseudo train system, without the use of personal vehicles or bus lines (West Virginia University GIS Technical Center, 2015). However, the student population has necessitated bus transportation to be added.

The PRT was specifically designed and constructed for students, faculty, and staff to travel between the three regional areas' housing university facilities. It is currently being upgraded, as it was originally designed as a unique transportation system that only served the campus's three main segments along the initial track. However, the campus has now expanded beyond its original boundaries, with the administrative areas located a mile away from the downtown campus. Due to the costs associated with expansion and the limited amount of right of way that can be acquired, it is unlikely that the PRT will ever be expanded. This is in spite of the substantial growth of the population of Morgantown and the fact that traffic patterns have become even more congested since the PRT was initially developed and constructed. In addition to the PRT, a series of buses supplement the transportation needs, which still rely on the same traditional roads surrounding the campuses.

## Tightly Congested Areas

Parking and traffic congestion are important issues that many university and college administrators face and can have both consequences and benefits that hinge on the decision-making process. This section will describe how GIS can be used by administrators to understand and resolve a very difficult administrative issue frequently tied to stakeholder agendas and political machinations.

West Virginia University is not the only university or college to have issues with traffic congestion and parking. Regardless of its student population size, most if not all institutes of higher learning will have issues with adequate parking. Along with insufficient parking facilities, many institutions can affect surrounding communities with increased traffic congestion. For traffic patterns and parking, larger universities should be regarded as cities when infrastructure is discussed. A large university or college is similar to a city in terms of how the organization can address issues of adding or altering existing infrastructure and overlapping infrastructure that consists of independent infrastructure networks. The overlapping, independent infrastructure network that exists in Morgantown, West Virginia will be highlighted in this section. For a large campus, West Virginia University has a very complicated situation due to the three campuses that make up its main campus, located in a three-mile mountainous area with rivers. The natural features limit where buildings and roadways can be built, which is compounded by the jurisdictional control of city, county, and state agencies. The various agencies can control different segments of the streets surrounding West Virginia University with regard to right of way and ownership. Questions in the past over ownership, such as whether or not a street is controlled by the city, the county, the state, or the university, have led to problems with maintenance and even with snow removal. Natural geographic features also dictate how wide the roadways can be constructed and prevent any type of traditional grid traffic pattern from being established. Additionally, the university is land-locked, with the central (main) campus co-located next to the City of Morgantown's downtown area (Map 9.1).

West Virginia University has a fall 2016 enrollment of 28,488 students for the main campus and health sciences center. Traffic flow between the main campus's three regions and throughout Morgantown is a concern for the university. There are variables affecting traffic flow that GIS, and thus this study, cannot forecast or control, such as road conditions. These variables are caused primarily by weather and can only be fixed by the public agency overseeing those specific routes. When the university offers classes during the school year, traffic is frequently gridlocked in the City of Morgantown. The key question becomes: "Is there a way for administrators at West Virginia University to reduce the amount of traffic throughout the City of Morgantown?"

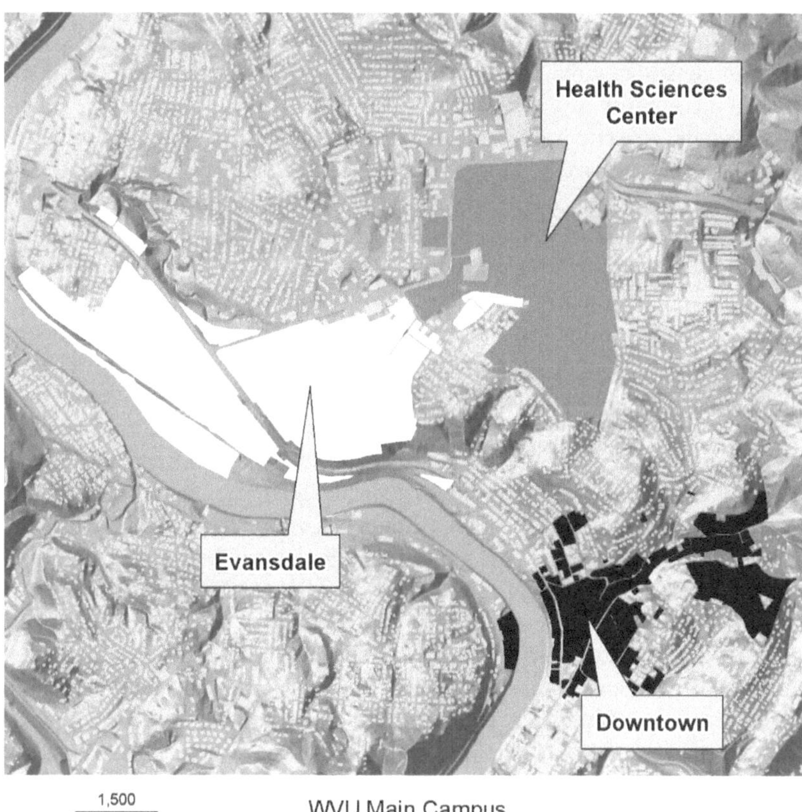


*Map 9.1* WVU Campus Areas in Morgantown.

## Proximity Analysis of University Students and Staff

There are many purposes for geocoding the addresses of staff, faculty, and student populations in relation to where the university is located. West Virginia University's core area has three regions, consisting of the main campus in addition to several other buildings scattered throughout the City of Morgantown. This geographical core area forms a triangle with a perimeter of six miles and is primarily located alongside the Monongahela River. Various non-university-owned properties are scattered within the six-mile triangle, ranging from the downtown business district to other businesses as well as private residential homes and apartments.

With 28,488 students (Fall 2016) on the main campus as well as employees, and in conjunction with surrounding businesses, the infrastructure surrounding the various university properties are frequently above peak load capacity (West Virginia University—Office of Institutional Research, 2015). A 2012 report conducted for the Morgantown Monongalia Metropolitan Planning Organization analyzed Morgantown's transportation networks Level of Service (LOS), which is a measure of corridor operations. The report concluded, through a capacity deficiency analysis, that 11 roads or corridors are at an unacceptable LOS and constitute a major safety concern. Roadway capacity is often compared to the number of vehicles that travel the corridor. However, the maximum roadway capacity is often greater than the number acceptable to travelers in a community the size of Morgantown. The difference between the acceptable number of vehicles and the capacity is important because as more vehicles try to travel through an intersection, the greater the level of delay resulting for all travelers through the intersection. The report found that the volumes of vehicles on the roadway facilities are an integral component in evaluating the existing transportation conditions. The report also found that between June 2008 and December 2011, 4,060 vehicle accidents occurred, which translated to 3–4 accidents per day (Burgess and Niple, 2012).

The university characteristics of needing more infrastructure for students, faculty, and staff lend itself to housing, parking, and traffic improvement needed due to the growth in the university and the surrounding city. This indicates that careful planning is essential when assessing future infrastructure for the institution as well as for the City of Morgantown. The need for planning is complicated by the issue of repairing or even possibly expanding roadways within and around this core area. Completion of primary roadway construction and expansions typically occur during certain times of the year due to weather and traffic congestion. When the students and faculty are on summer break, the traffic congestion throughout the City of Morgantown lessens considerably, allowing for such work. Planning certain activities, such as road construction, requires university administrators and city planners to understand which areas of the city and university will most likely be vacated during the summer months in order to hold traffic congestion down to a minimum. Over the past few years, planning between the university, the state, the county, and the City of Morgantown has improved. As with any planning process, there are always improvements between the governmental entities that are being sought.

## Building Upon Previous Methodology

In addition to facility planning, proximity analysis can also be undertaken to analyze student retention; based on the geocoded address students provide, analysis can determine if location has an impact upon academic performance when compared to distance from students' local residences to their academic locations. According to Bolstad, the proximity function is among the most powerful and common spatial analysis tools (Bolstad, 2016). A proximity analysis utilizes a buffer around a specific area or feature of a specified distance and finds and calculates what falls within this buffer. This methodology builds on a similar methodology used by the University of Texas at Dallas, which developed a shapefile in 2010 to map student and employees in relation to the campus (Valcik, 2013). Unlike the University of Texas at Dallas, however, the core area of West Virginia University is not in one area, and therefore analysis is not contained within a centralized and circular buffer. To provide a more accurate analysis of the West Virginia University core area, a new buffer shape was required to capture the campus's triangular core shape (Figure 9.4; Figure 9.5).

As can be seen in Figure 9.4 and Figure 9.5, the university has several buildings and properties spread out across the triangular radius. There are some shortcomings using this methodology at both the University of Texas at Dallas and West Virginia University in the form of obtaining accurate addresses from student and employees. Accurate and precise student addressing information in particular proved to be difficult to obtain. With the advent of the Internet and cell phone technology, students do not have to report a local mailing address to the university. Thus, the business processes for most universities have moved away from utilizing a student's physical mailing address.

When West Virginia University first attempted to map down student addresses, several student addresses, indicated by the substantial distances in relation to the campus, could not possibly commute on a daily basis. This distance was not in adherence to Tobler's first law of geography, which states: This distance was not in adherence to Tobler's first law of geography, where Tobler indicates that everything is related to everything else location wise, but the closer the items are that are being examined, they are more related than distant items being examined (Tobler, 1970). In simpler terms, a student who lists their address in southern West Virginia is more likely to have that address as their permanent address, since it would be a four-hour commute one way to West Virginia University, which is not feasible.

In addition, West Virginia University's student housing complexes did not show the appropriate number of students living in those residences. Therefore, a file had to be "compiled" from not only what the students reported as their local address but also the university's own student housing information. Many

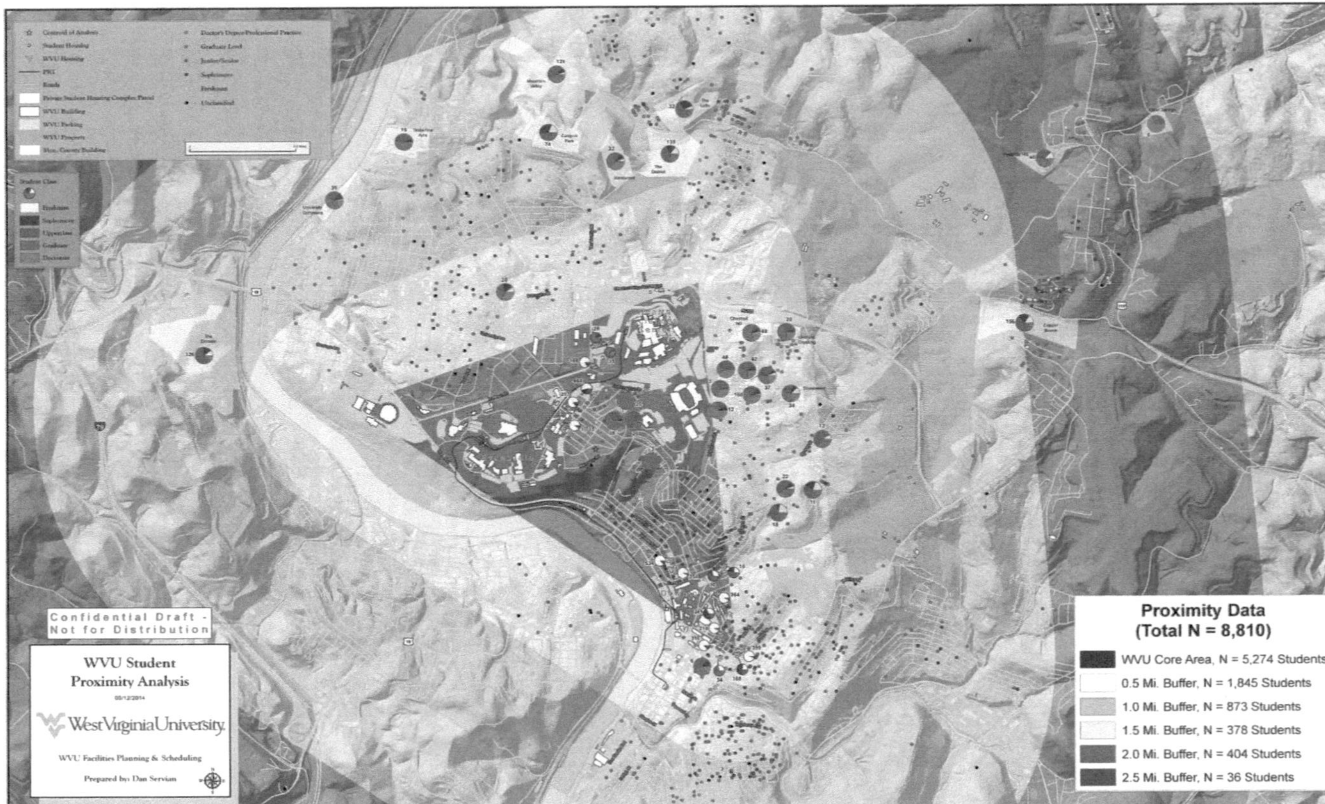
Confidential Draft - Not for Distribution
WVU Student
Proximity Analysis
West Virginia University
WVU Facilities Planning & Scheduling
Prepared by: Dan Servian
Proximity Data
(Total N = 8,810)
WVU Core Area, N = 5,274 Students
0.5 Mi. Buffer, N = 1,845 Students
1.0 Mi. Buffer, N = 873 Students
1.5 Mi. Buffer, N = 378 Students
2.0 Mi. Buffer, N = 404 Students
2.5 Mi. Buffer, N = 36 Students

*Figure 9.4* West Virginia University student proximity analysis.

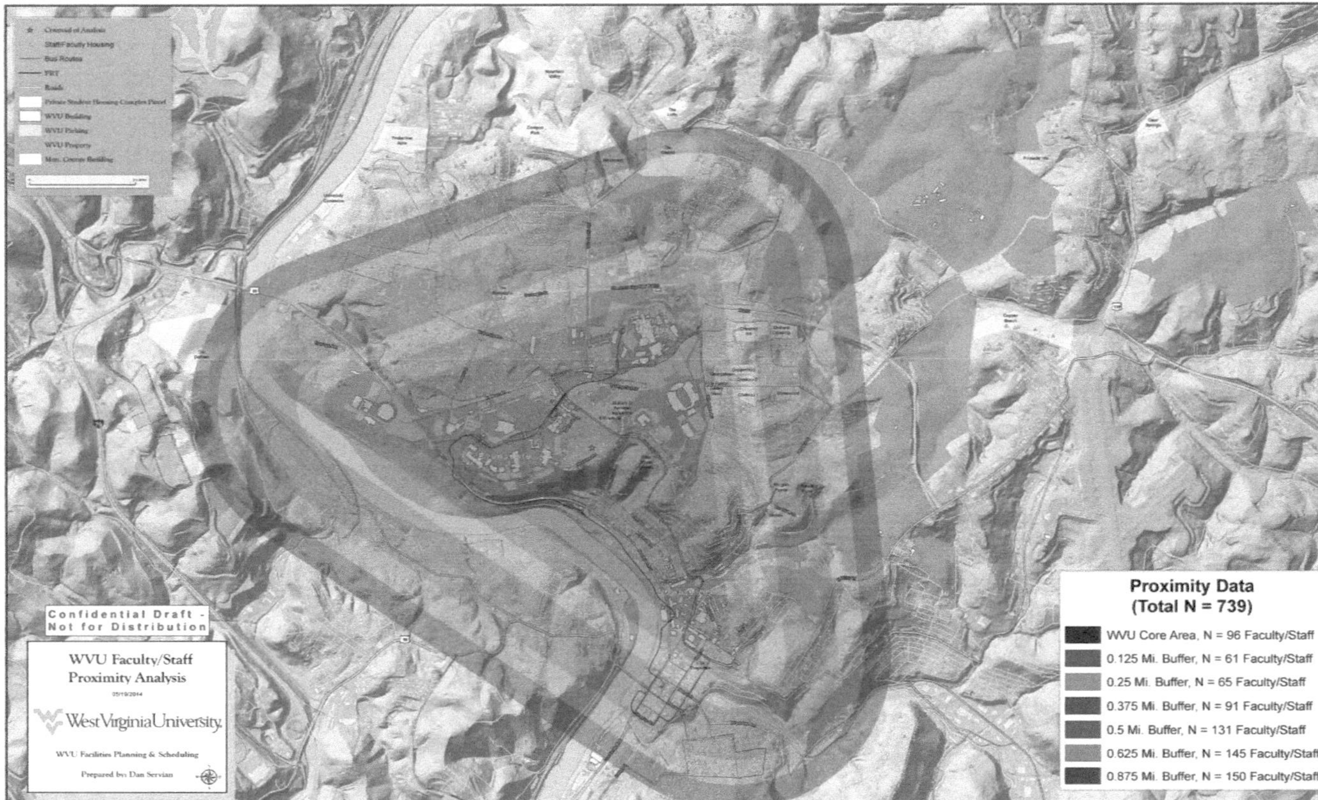
Proximity Data
(Total N = 739)
WVU Core Area, N = 96 Faculty/Staff
0.125 Mi. Buffer, N = 61 Faculty/Staff
0.25 Mi. Buffer, N = 65 Faculty/Staff
0.375 Mi. Buffer, N = 91 Faculty/Staff
0.5 Mi. Buffer, N = 131 Faculty/Staff
0.625 Mi. Buffer, N = 145 Faculty/Staff
0.875 Mi. Buffer, N = 150 Faculty/Staff
Confidential Draft - Not for Distribution
WVU Faculty/Staff
Proximity Analysis
WestVirginiaUniversity
WVU Facilities Planning & Scheduling
Prepared by: Dan Servian

*Figure 9.5* West Virginia University faculty/staff proximity analysis.

of the addresses provided by students appeared to be permanent addresses, most likely their parents' address. When mapping addresses in GIS, there is no method by which students (or employees) can be mapped to a specific location if they have a post office box or rural route, so those data points were excluded.

At the University of Texas at Dallas in particular, a file was constructed that had two different sources for information when inaccurate addresses were discovered. The University of Texas at Dallas discovered the issue when almost no students listed the dorm as their local residence (The University of Texas at Dallas—Office of Strategic Planning and Analysis, 2013). The University of Texas at Dallas's student housing information was obtained from the student information system as well as the department responsible for student housing. While the information analyzed may not be completely accurate, the information is accurate enough to use for planning purposes.

Even with the limitations of the data, the mapped information revealed the neighborhoods within and surrounding the City of Morgantown that held clusters of students who appeared to be leasing or renting houses. This information points to the possibility that property values could be depreciating in certain areas of the city. Information from the appraisal and taxing authority must be obtained to verify that hypothesis. As of 2014, that information was not available in electronic format in Monongalia County. If the information becomes available, that data mapped to where students live can also lead to analysis of whether more affordable student housing is potentially needed in the future for university students.

On the employee and faculty map, a proximity analysis shows where employees live in relation to the campus area. Government employees and elected officials routinely ask how many employees (as well as students) live within a certain radius of the campus. With this type of map, responses to those questions are possible with a fair amount of certainty. Employee maps for West Virginia University used a different methodology than the University of Texas at Dallas because not all employees were located in one state. Zip codes were required as neighboring states' address shapefiles were not available to West Virginia University and thus the distribution of where the university's employees lived could not be observed (Figure 9.6). As with the previous analysis, this analysis was potentially limited by an employee listing the correct zip code or updating the zip code when needed.

Figure 9.6 shows that the majority of West Virginia University's employees live in three different states: West Virginia, Pennsylvania, and Maryland. By analyzing the map, government and university administrators can make assumptions about the possible route (interstates or local roads) employees take to the university. Using this map for inclement weather also makes it possible for administrators to see the impact of a decision such as whether to close the university.

Unlike the University of Texas at Dallas, which is in a dense metro area and has a more centralized employee population, West Virginia University's employees live across a wider regional area and face potentially different

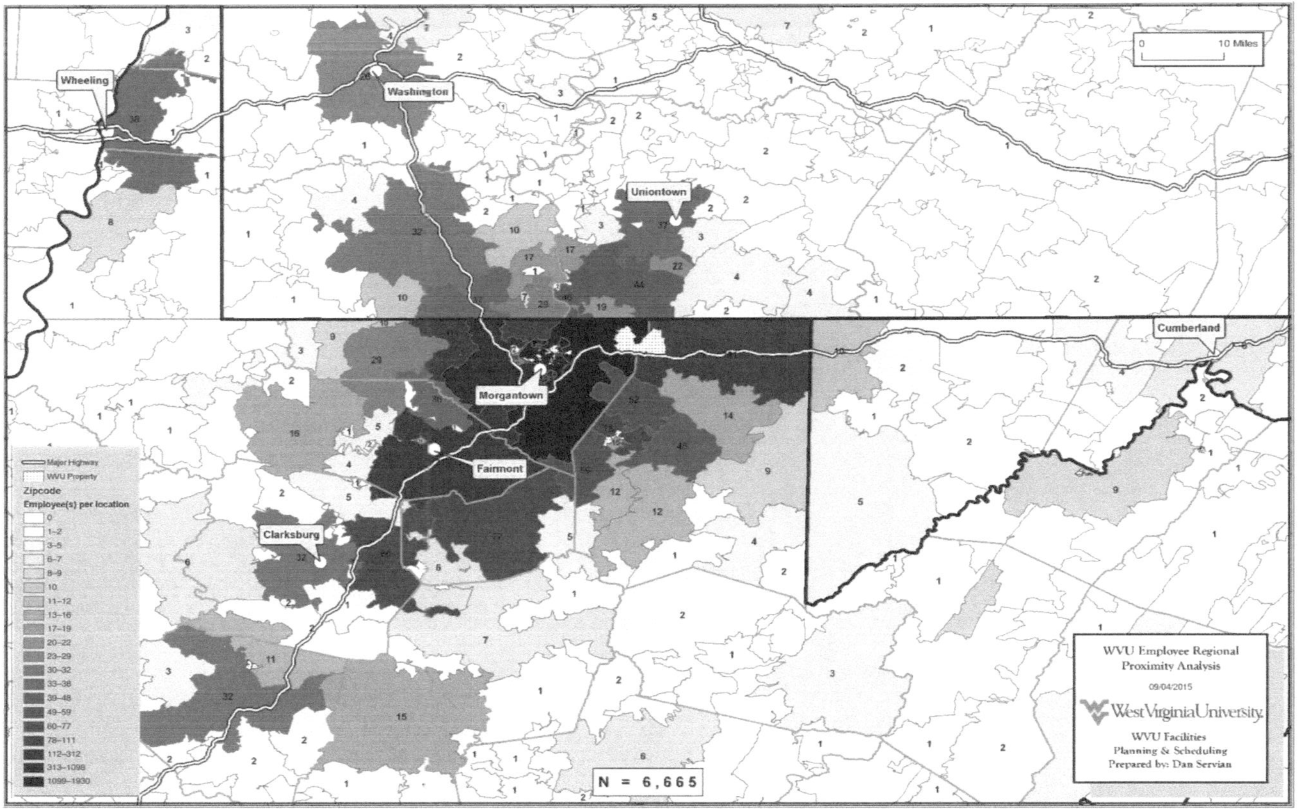


*Figure 9.6* West Virginia University faculty/staff regional proximity analysis.

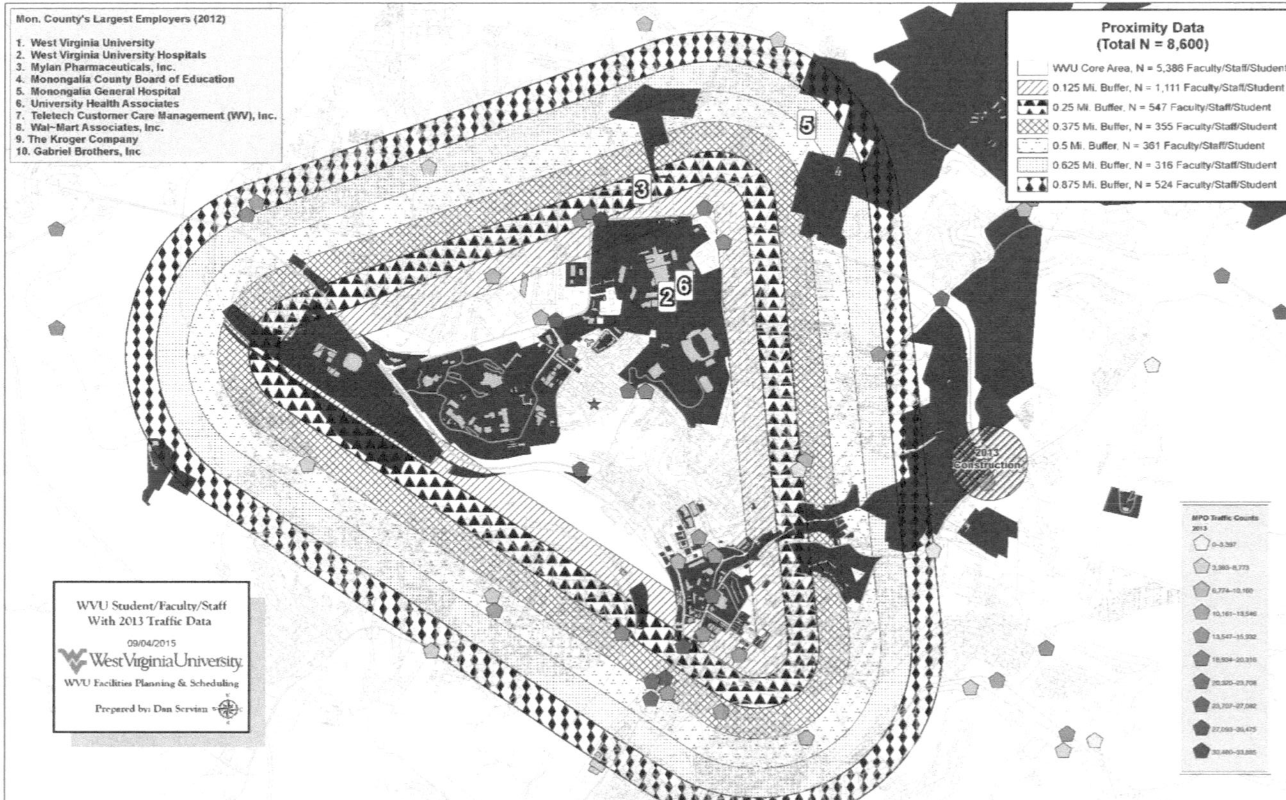


*Figure 9.7* WVU student/faculty/staff regional proximity analysis with traffic data.

roadway conditions. Similar to the student map, analysis of property values from the employee map is possible if data is available from the appraisal and taxing authorities. The analysis can potentially reveal if affordable housing is an issue for university employees. This issue in particular not only affects existing employees but can also influence the university's efforts when attempting to recruit and hire employees and faculty members. Potential salary offers may need to adjust to the real estate realities of the City of Morgantown compared to other areas of the country.

As can been seen from Figure 9.4 and Figure 9.5, the residential data provides information about which students and employees may potentially be using different roadways to access the campuses, as well as when. West Virginia University is located in hilly terrain, with a river running next to the grounds the institution currently owns. This dictates where roadways are located and even how some of these roadways can potentially expand to accommodate the traffic congestion. Additionally, the proximity maps have bus and PRT routes superimposed to show where mass transit possibilities exist.

The bus lines in particular are useful for university administrators. Administrators can review the information to see if an appropriate level of service is available to populations of students and employees. This information is important since the university pays a subsidy to the bus lines. If the bus lines are nowhere near population centers of those employed by or studying at the university, the subsidy is not warranted for a particular bus line or route.

When administrators and city officials review the information with traffic counts included in the analysis, it may be revealed that the university is not the only contributing factor to traffic congestion. As can be seen in Figure 9.7, traffic congestion also occurs around West Virginia University Hospital and Mylan Pharmaceuticals, Inc. as well as Monongalia General Hospital. These three entities are large employers within the city; employees work in shifts, and there are also a large number of visitors to the hospitals. This influx of people as shifts come into and leave the area contributes to traffic congestion. This information can provide both university officials and city planners with a way to create a strategy to alleviate traffic congestion during certain times by seeing if one or more of those employers can (or are willing to) adjust shift times. By staggering shift times, traffic may not be as congested as heavily throughout different parts of the city.

## WVU Proximity Analysis Methodology

Collection of institutional data, consisting of both student and faculty/staff data, is extracted from West Virginia University's Student and Human Resource systems. Extraction of the data from the system results in a file, which is then joined into ArcGIS. To protect individuals' personal information, the creation of a unique identifier is paramount before any analysis of students and staff. The unique identification number takes the place of the contact's name, address, and any other sensitive personal information. Before creating this unique ID, the joining of additional information is necessary for this analysis. The additional data columns for the student dataset included college major and school, student ranking (freshman, sophomore, etc.), and mailing address. The faculty and staff database includes position title, classified/unclassified, and mailing address. Both databases have the ability to join many different databases, allowing for multiple distribution topics.

Unlike the University of Texas at Dallas, the typical circular buffer cannot represent West Virginia University's core region. Construction of West Virginia University's core region is a triangular buffer that best reflects the parameters of the three main campuses. Since a typical buffer analysis is circular in nature, radiating from a centroid or point shapefile, use of the triangle shapefile calculates the employees inside the buffers. The position of the triangle buffer is the centroid of West Virginia University's core region, located at the calculated centroid of all West Virginia University buildings. The defined core buffer extents capture the majority of the university's main campus buildings. There are two different calculations (0.125 miles and 0.5 miles) to calculate the buffer linear distance, with each buffer distance also having multiple buffers rings calculated. Including West Virginia University's core area, there were seven buffer rings calculated for the 0.125 mi. buffer and six buffer rings calculated for the 0.5 mi. buffer.

Each of the individual buffer rings sum the spatially related geocoded point files as well as any manually placed data points. This calculation uses the first geocoding address layer in the database. The students, faculty, and staff that did not geocode were examined and when possible manually mapped. Because of the address schema and design of the buildings, West Virginia University's housing did not geocode; thus, creation of a separate file was required for each of West Virginia University's housing units. Each of the manually generated points relating to the university's housing displayed an aggregation of that building's total residents. However, the spatial data utilized for geocoding was 11 years old, which created issues since not all of the new housing complexes and individual homes were geocoded on the existing file. Manual mapping of new properties onto the spatial data was conducted whenever possible.

Once the data had been geocoded and the symbology tool built into ArcMap had been applied, the data could be used to show the distribution of students' class rankings or the distribution of West Virginia University's faculty and staff positions, among many other variables. Adding layers such as mass transit routes, traffic counts, or the location of large businesses adds to the analysis.

The second distribution analysis is a choropleth map conducted on West Virginia University's faculty and staff. This project made use of the prior faculty and staff proximity analysis database, but mapped the data regionally, via zip code, versus the local view of the geocoded proximity analysis. Similar to the methods described above, to view the distribution, each zip code must sum the number of faculty and staff that reside in an individual zip code. This action creates a new database that should only contain the zip code and total number of corresponding faculty and staff. To create the choropleth database, a summary table is created from the faculty and staff attribute table summing the total occurrences of each zip code. This choropleth database is then uploaded into ArcMap and joined to the US Census TIGER zip code file via the zip code, which is used as the key to link the databases. Once the join is complete, symbology is used to display each zip code's quantity of West Virginia University's faculty and staff.

## GIS Used for Tracking Student Movements Between Campuses

At West Virginia University, scheduling courses can be a challenge given classes take place at all three campuses that make up the university's main campus. In an attempt to streamline where courses are offered (which campus) and reduce travel time between campuses, a file has been compiled on when and where students take classes, their majors, and their classifications (i.e. freshmen, sophomores, juniors, seniors, graduate, or professional). After compiling the file, it is necessary to join the student information with facilities information for a certain block of time during a particular day. Patterns are created by tying all students to facilities and time blocks, which (when animated) can provide a daily view on when and where students transition between the campuses. This also shows the potential usage of the bus lines along those routes as well as the PRT. This can be seen in Figures 9.8–9.12, which exhibit screenshots of an animation analysis.

What Figures 9.8–9.12 show us is the formation of a cluster of seven out of ten randomly chosen students. As seen in Figure 9.8, four students are scheduled at the downtown campus. Figures 9.9 and 9.10 show the accumulation of an additional student, bringing the total to five students scheduled to be downtown. The student majoring in Industrial Engineering (J) has moved from the Evansdale campus to the downtown campus, presumably via the PRT. What cannot be seen in this particular GIS map is the topography the student had to cross between classes, which was a low to high elevation point. In Figure 9.11, the student coded as D, Chemical Engineering, has moved from the location they were at in Figures 9.9–9.11 to a new location south of their previous position. Additionally, Figure 9.11 shows the addition of students E and C, while student G has moved to the Evansdale campus (not shown). Finally, Figure 9.12 shows that certain students have left the downtown campus; other students have transitioned to other locations, but the cluster begins to dissipate.

By reviewing this type of information, university administrators can see what buildings different majors access and look at which classes could potentially be offered at an alternate location. The information essentially illustrates which majors cluster into certain buildings. If university administrators can schedule classes for majors to be on one campus, this reduces traffic congestion throughout the City of Morgantown between the three campuses and results in students having better schedules.

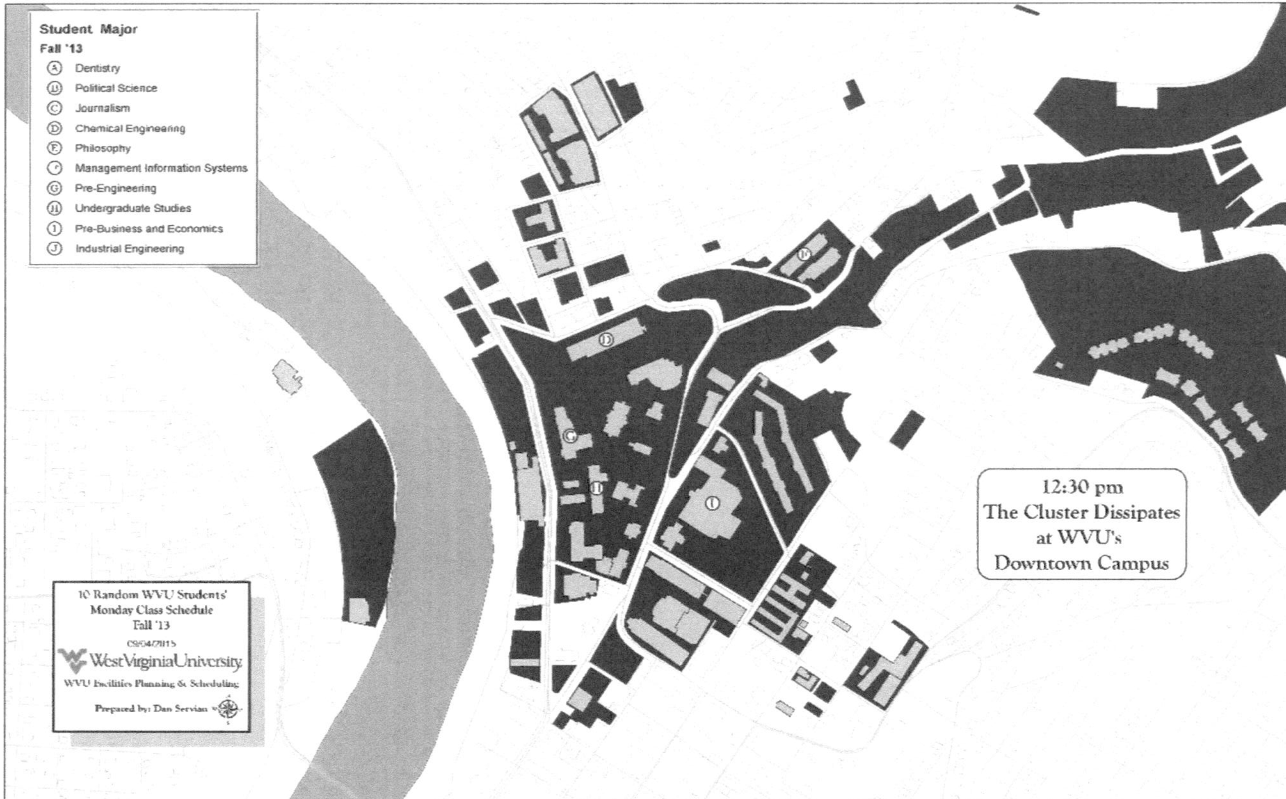


*Figure 9.8* Ten random West Virginia University student class schedules.

Note: Fall 2013, Monday—12:30 p.m.

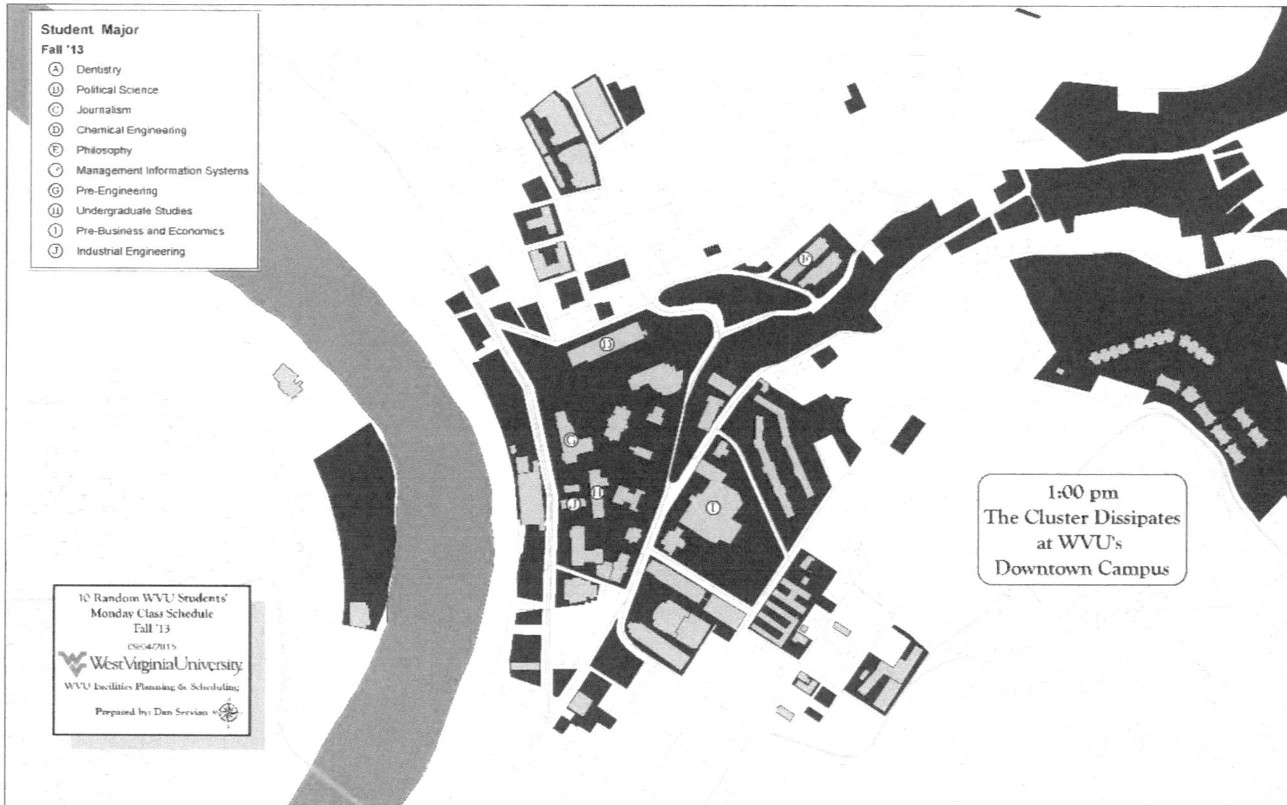


*Figure 9.9* Time lapse for Fall 2013, Monday—1:00 p.m.

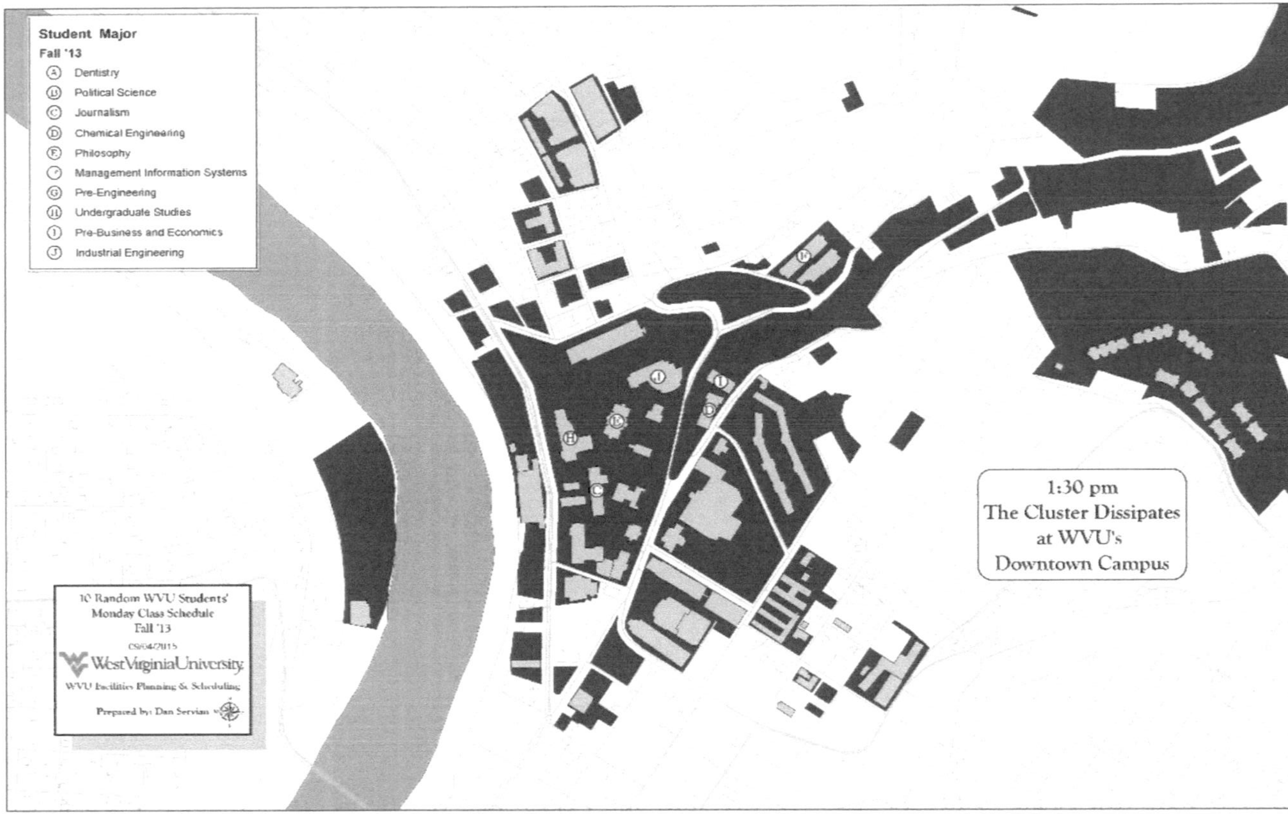


*Figure 9.10* Time lapse for Fall 2013, Monday—1:30 p.m.

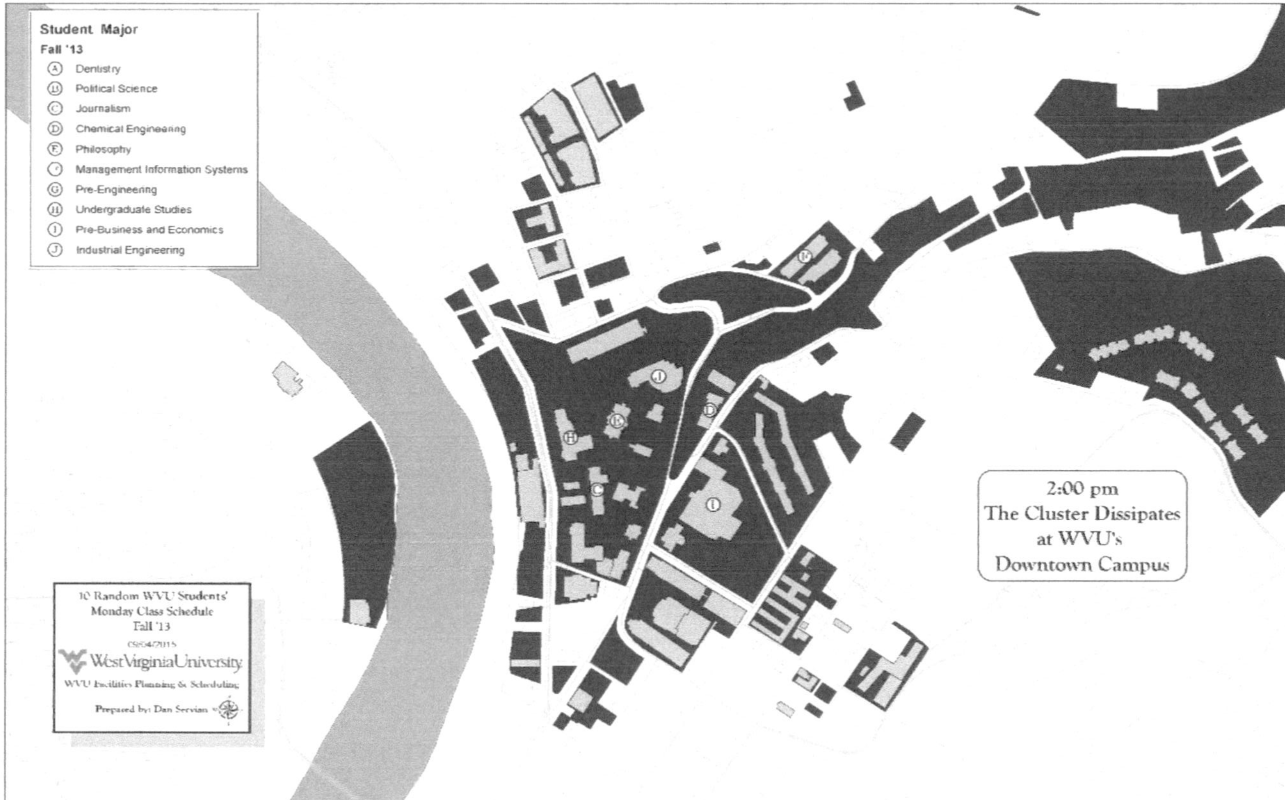


*Figure 9.11* Time lapse for Fall 2013, Monday—2:00 p.m.

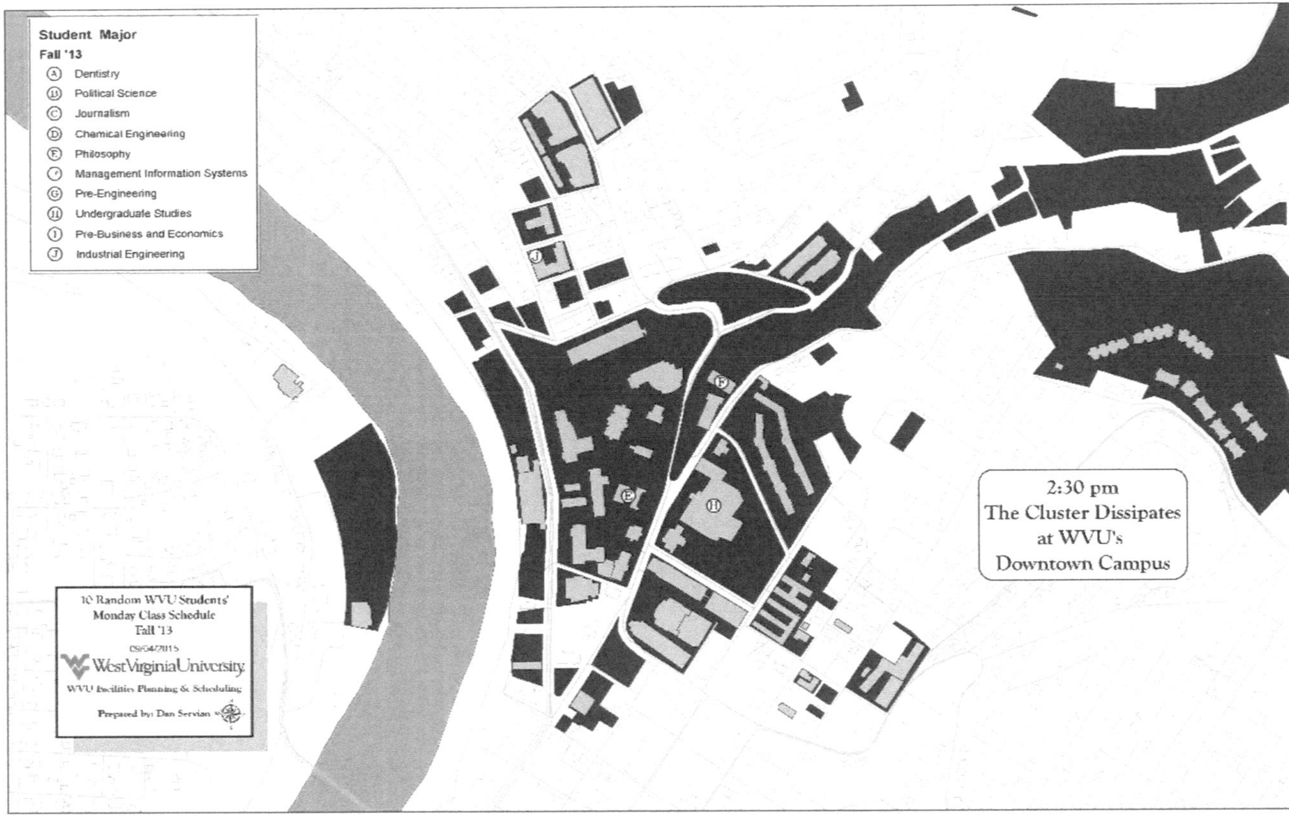


*Figure 9.12* Time lapse for Fall 2013, Monday—2:30 p.m.

## Student Movement Between Regions Methodology

This project builds on the student geocoded data from the proximity methodology. To test our methods, we employed a sample of ten students. To see how class rank and on-campus versus off-campus housing options affected students, the student data was divided into two main groups: students who live on campus and students who live off campus. To accomplish this action, a stratified random sample was utilized. The two groups were then both split into five population segments. The segmentation was accomplished by using the students' class ranking. The five population segments consisted of freshman, sophomore, junior, senior, and graduate. This created ten population segments, five segments from on-campus housing and five from off-campus housing. Once the student populations had been divided into the ten categories, one student was then randomly chosen from each segment. This gave us our sample size of ten shapefiles.

Each student's class schedule was then linked to the shapefile via the unique ID created to protect the student's identity. Every course at West Virginia University has a unique Course ID number. The Course ID number provides an avenue to link into a database containing the course's location via a unique building number, thus providing location.

To observe the movement of each of the ten students, a temporal database was created, divided into 30-minute intervals. Classes at West Virginia University begin at 08:00 a.m. and end at 10:00 p.m. on Monday through Friday, giving us 28 columns dedicated to the student class schedules. To watch the subject's movement to and from their residency, the temporal data table increased by two data columns, which indicated the start and end at residency. Hence, 30 columns were created, with the temporal data beginning at 7:30 a.m. and ending at 10:30 p.m.

Two assumptions had to be made about the movement of students within our study. The first assumption was that if a student's schedule had more than a two-hour break where no classes were scheduled, then it is assumed the student returned to their residence. The second assumption made was that students used West Virginia University's PRT to move between campuses due to the small amount of time between each class as well as limited downtown parking available to students. Each cell within the temporal database was populated with a Course ID number (giving us the building location), or 1 indicating home, or 0 indicating between classes. The data was then viewed via ESRI's Time Slider and observations were made.

## Using GIS for Project Planning and Development

When the West Virginia University–WV Outdoor Education Center was being planned, GIS was used extensively in the planning and development of the site. As can be seen in the Planning Packet, GIS was used for the entire project (Figures 9.13–9.19).

As we can see from the GIS images, GIS was used to overlay and layer everything from satellite imagery to contour elevation maps for construction of the WVU–Adventure WV Outdoor Education Center. Using GIS allows for precise planning to ensure efficiency and effectiveness before construction

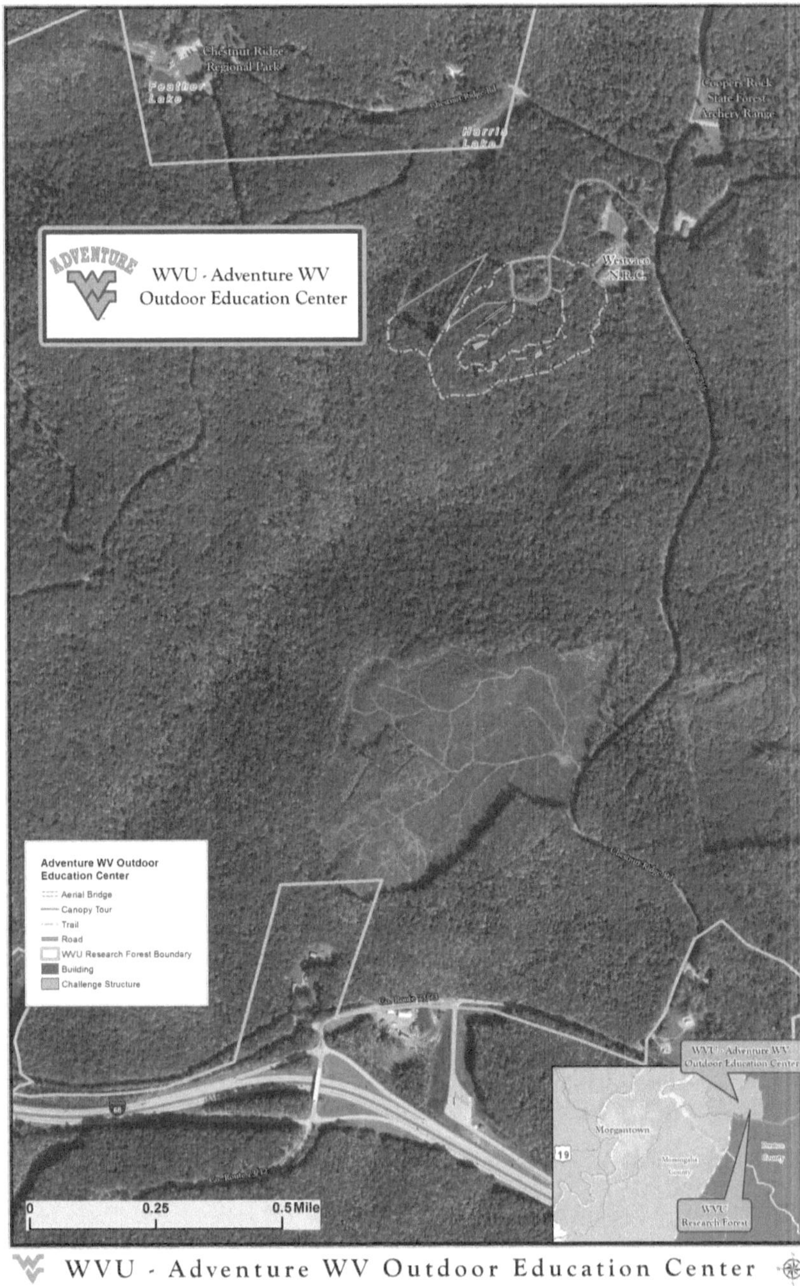


*Figure 9.13* WVU—Adventure WV Outdoor Education Center.

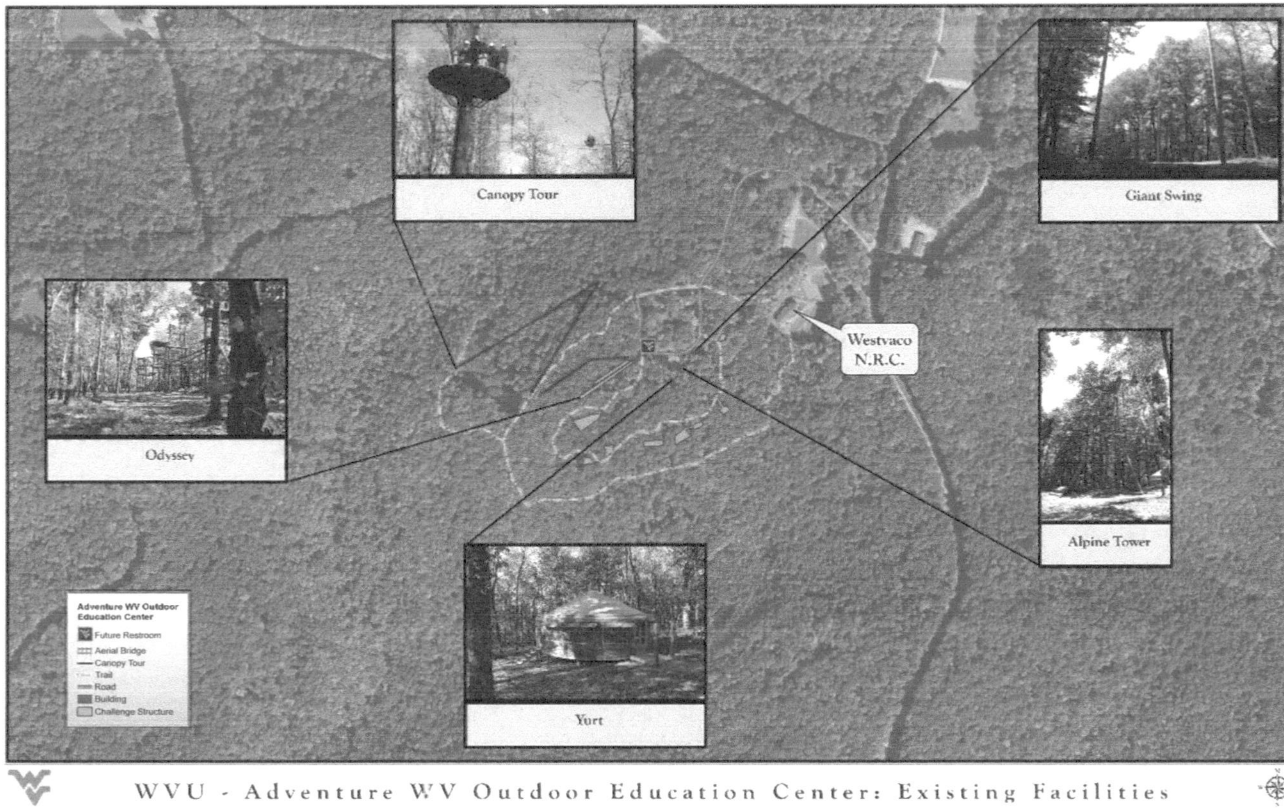


*Figure 9.14* WVU—Adventure WV Outdocr Education Center, existing facilities.

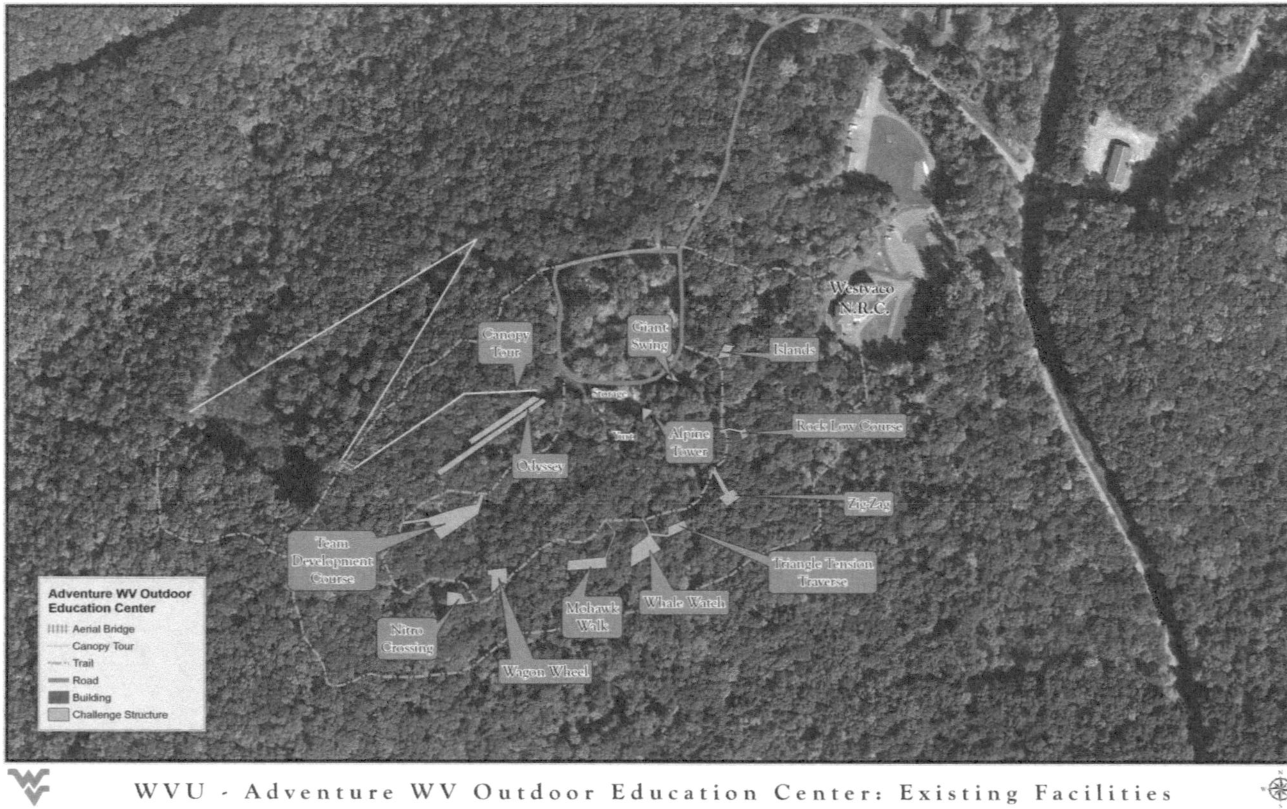


*Figure 9.15* WVU—Adventure WV Outdoor Education Center, existing facilities.

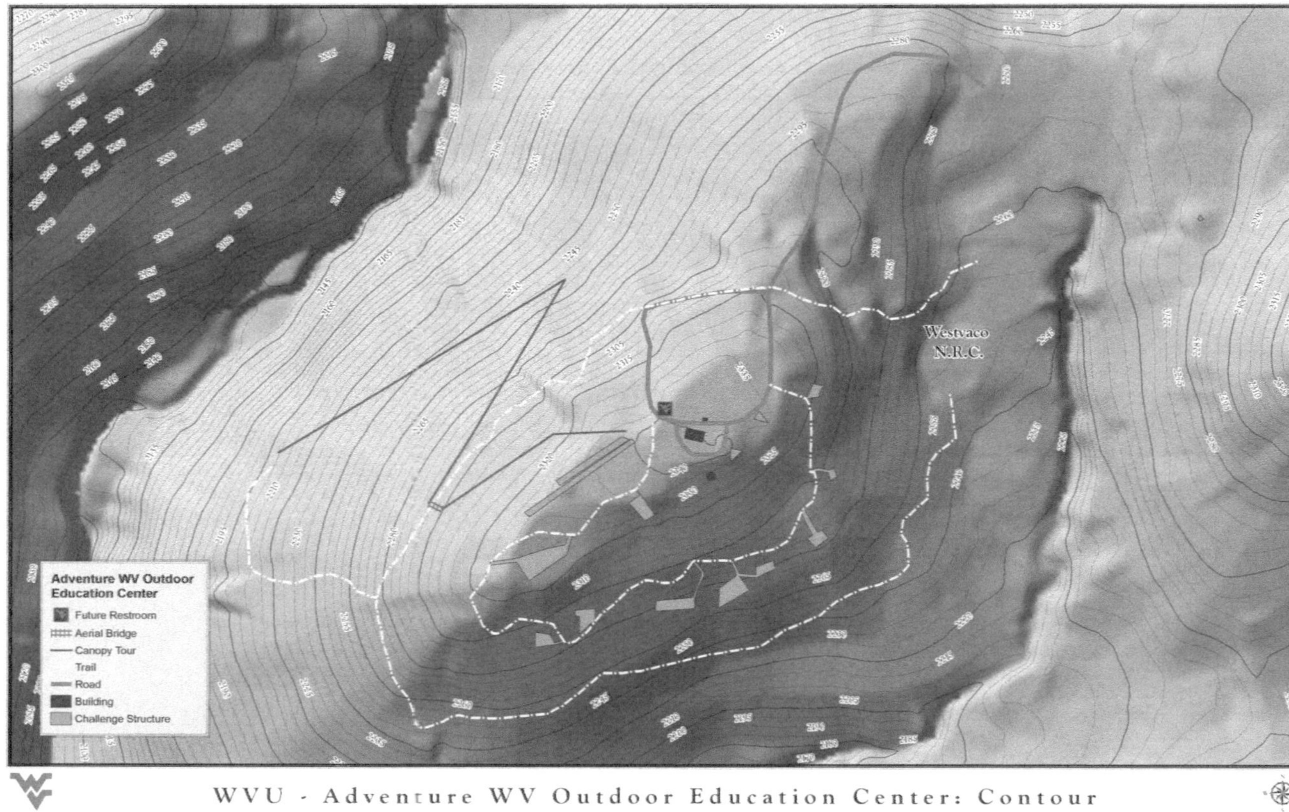


*Figure 9.16* WVU—Adventure WV Outdoor Education Center, contour map.

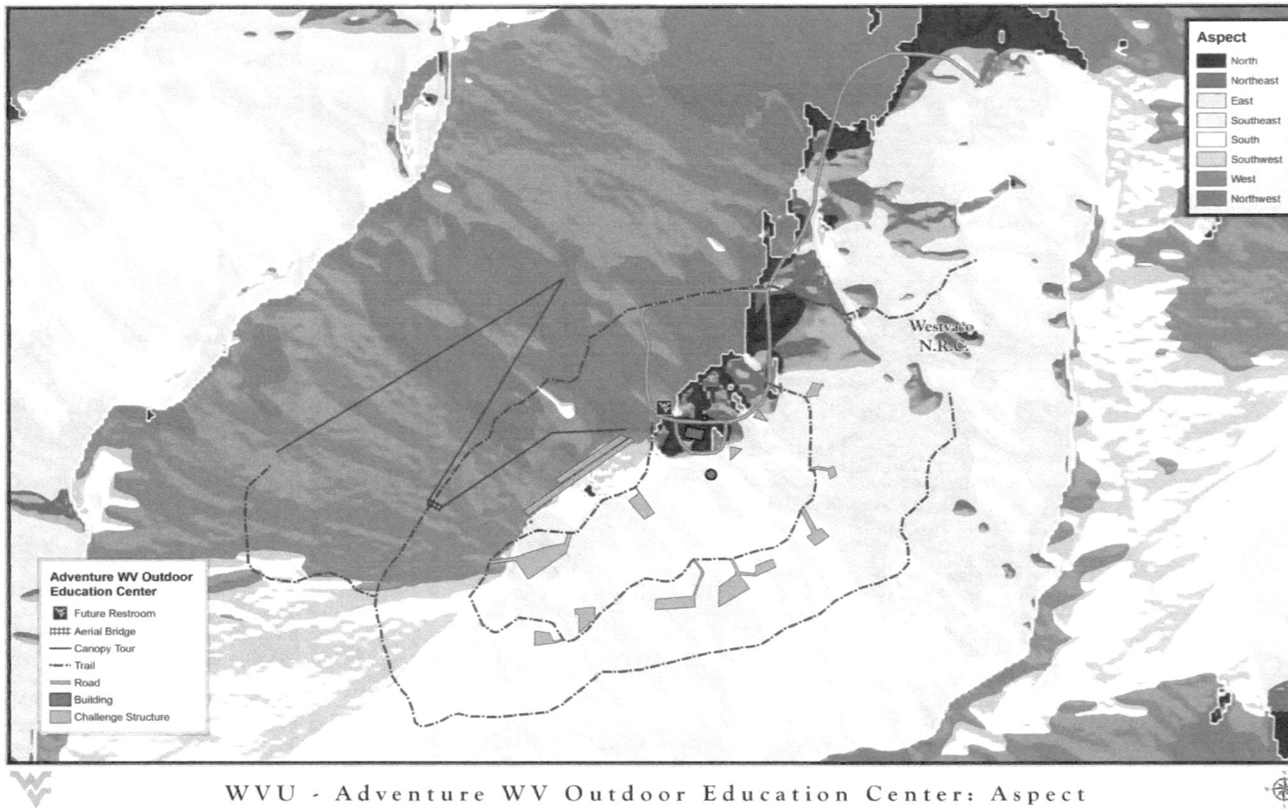


*Figure 9.17* WVU—Adventure WV Outdoor Education Center, aspect.

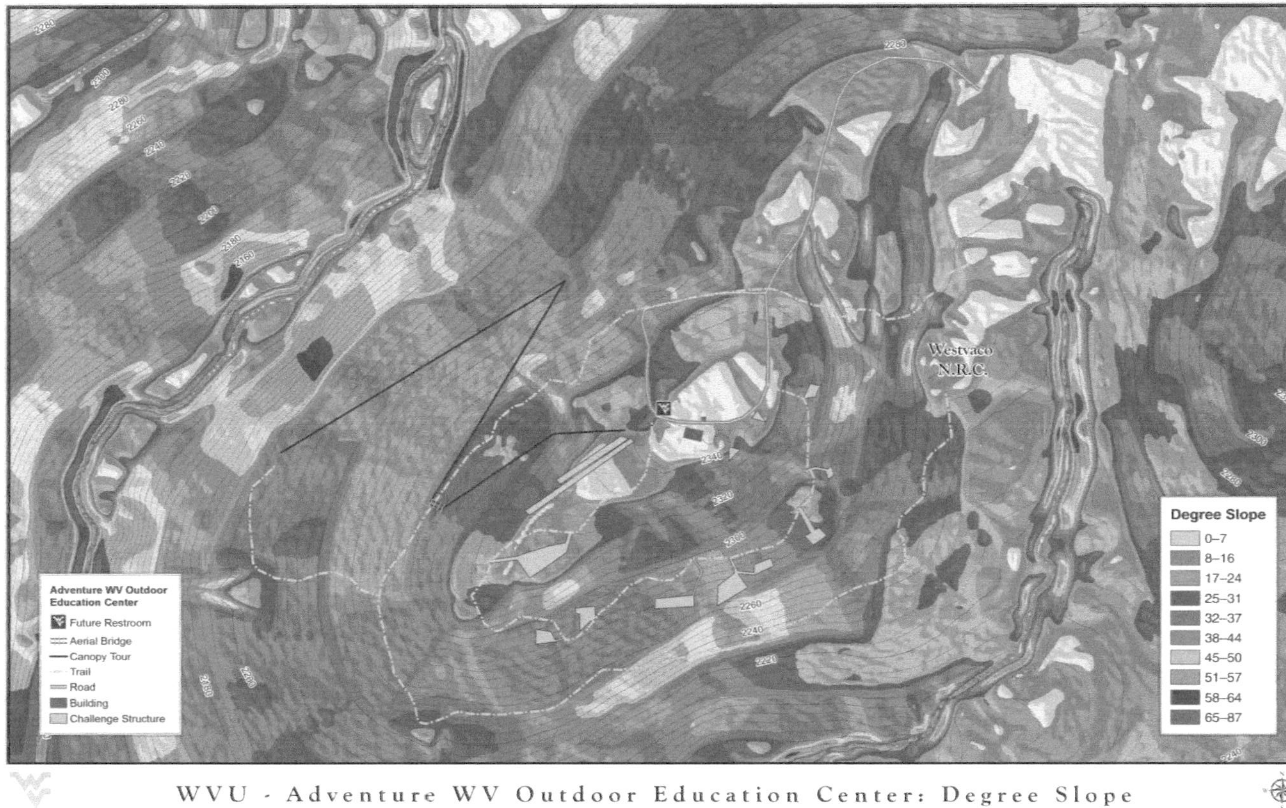


*Figure 9.18* WVU—Adventure WV Outdoor Education Center, degree slope.

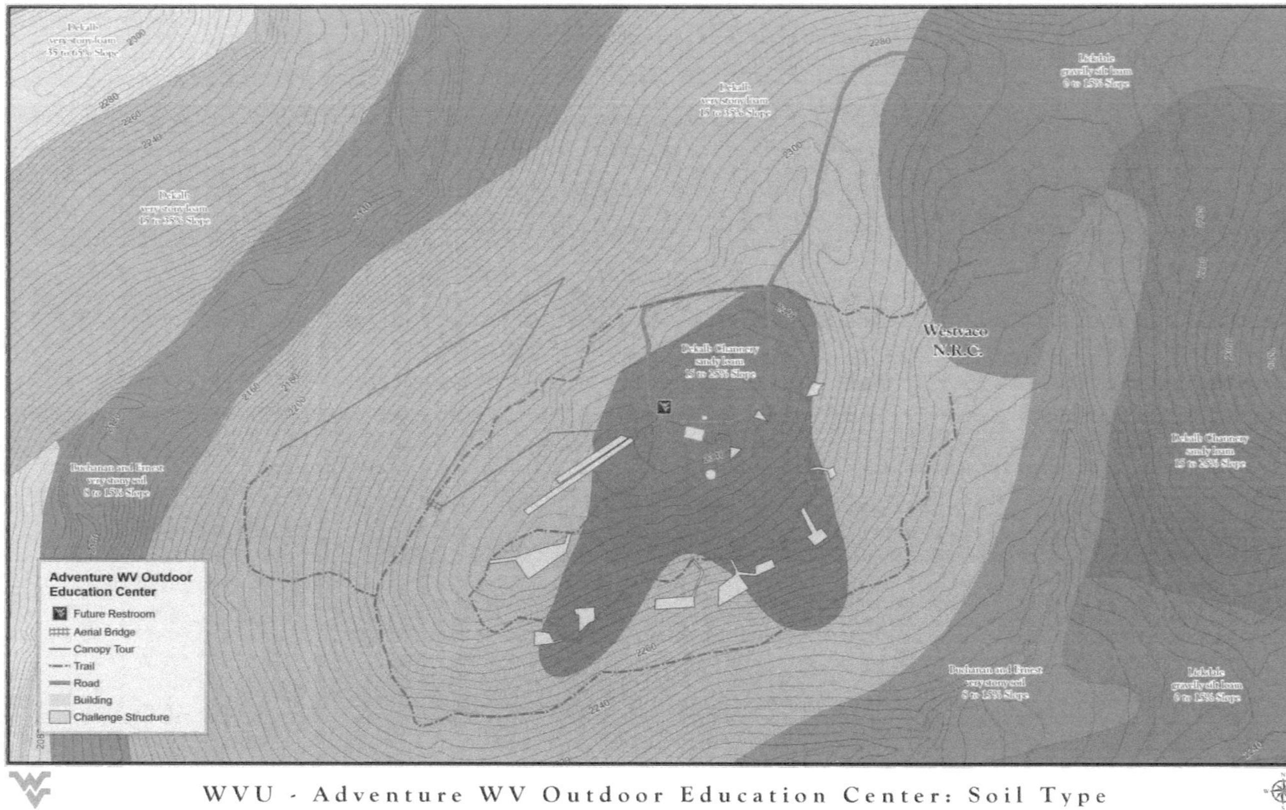


*Figure 9.19* WVU—Adventure WV Outdoor Education Center, soil type.

occurs, which can potentially reduce the man hours spent on the construction of a project as well as materials used for the structures that are to be built.

## GIS Used for Operational Intelligence

Enrollment and retention are two major drivers that determine how many higher education institutions receive their funding through either state appropriations or tuition and fees to support operational costs. For recruiters in enrollment management and academic programs focusing on the success of student retention as well as persistence programs, having operational intelligence on their students is the key to success. GIS adds another dimension of data that can be used to assist staff in the recruitment, retention, and persistence of students by providing a geographic component along with the traditional academic history and demographic makeup of students moving through the institution.

At West Virginia University, enrollment is a major component of how the institution is funded since the state subsidy supporting the institution is only a small percentage of money received into the institution. Therefore, West Virginia University is very dependent upon tuition and fees to operate. In response to bolstering retention and persistence rates, West Virginia University has tried to institute a number of programs to increase retention and graduation rates. One of these programs was the Mountaineer Success Academy (MSA), which proved to be successful when it was evaluated by Institutional Research in 2015. Figures 9.20 and 9.21 show the concentration of students for 2013 and

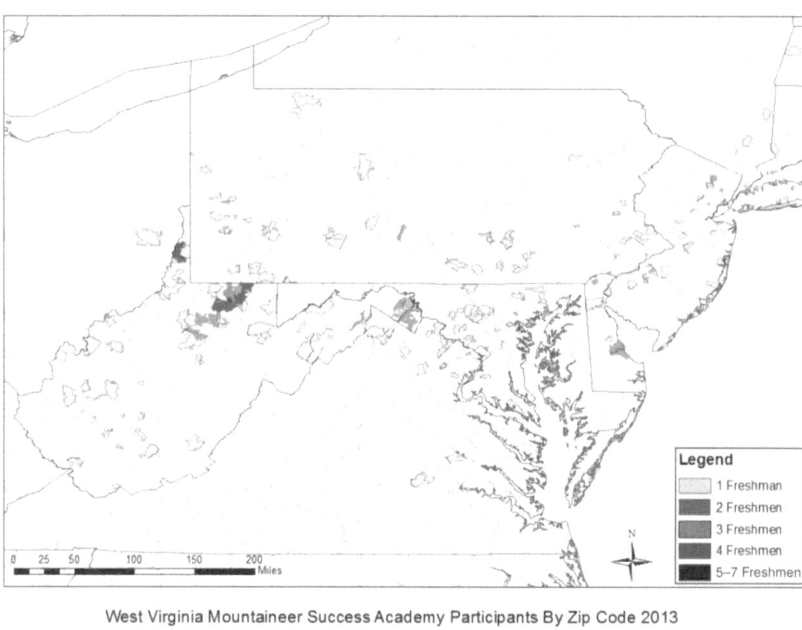


*Figure 9.20* West Virginia Mountaineer Success Academy participants by zip code 2013.

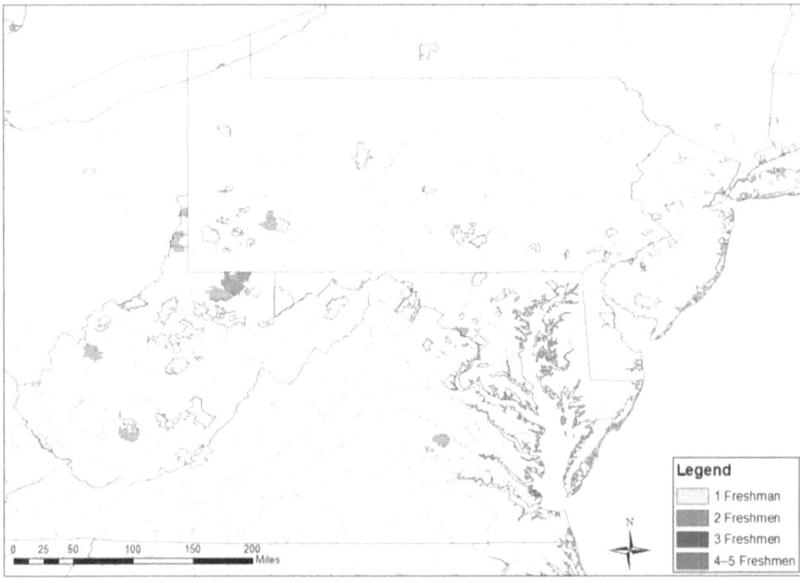


*Figure 9.21* West Virginia Mountaineer Success Academy participants by zip code 2014.

2014, which illuminates where students who enrolled in the MSA program are most likely to come from geographically (Morris-Dueer, Michael, Stoiko, and Jungblut, 2016, Valcik, 2015).

As can be seen between the two figures, the Eastern as well as the Western Panhandles of West Virginia decreased the number of students enrolled in the MSA program, while the southern part of West Virginia began to have more students enroll in the program. In Figure 9.22, another retention and graduation program, Adventure West Virginia for the Explorer Trip, had participants mapped down to their location of origin (Valcik, 2014).

From the GIS map, clusters can be seen in Morgantown, the Eastern Panhandle, and the Pittsburgh area. Since students had to sign up for the Adventure West Virginia program, this provided administrators with a tool to see which students are more likely to sign up for the program by geographic areas.

## Conclusion

This chapter only discusses some of the ways in which GIS can assist university administrators with planning and operational data. Throughout this chapter, a number of different uses for GIS are used in an applied manner for operational purposes. The utilization of GIS is for not only higher education institutions but also public and nonprofit organizations as well as many private

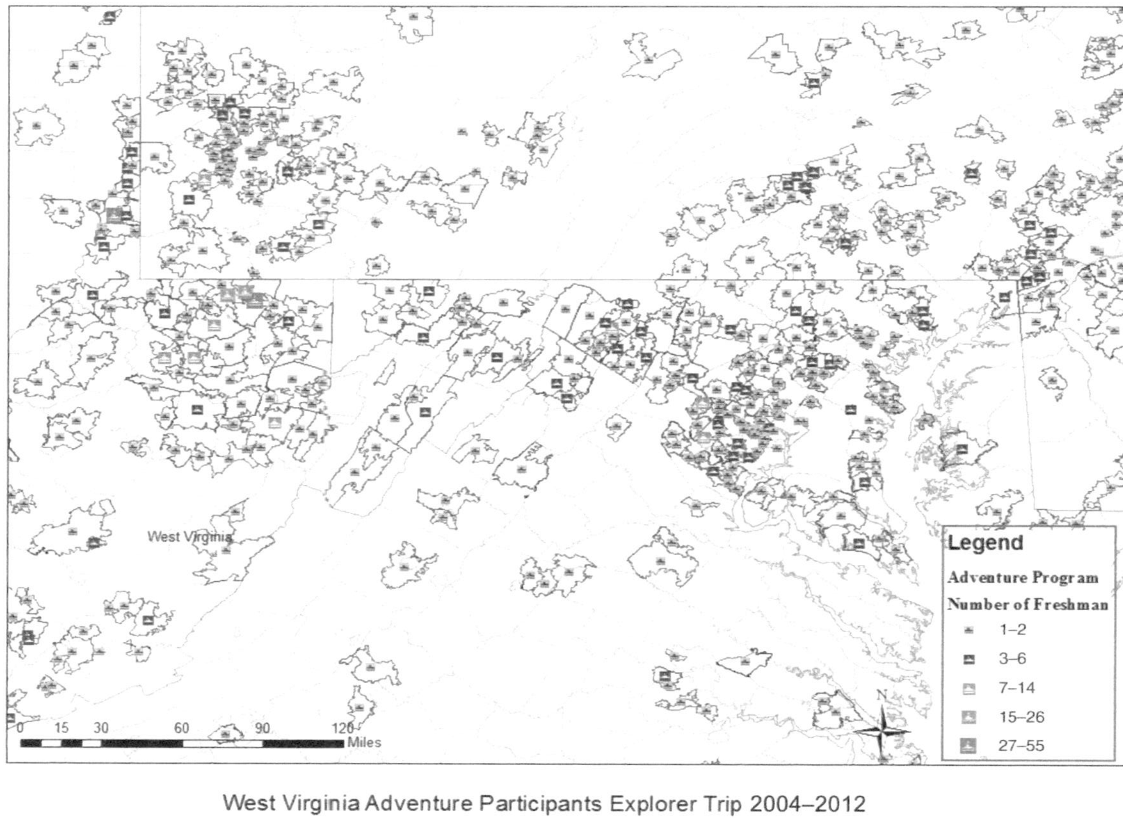


*Figure 9.22* West Virginia Participants Explorer Trip 2004–2012.

industry uses. While data in itself can prove to be useful for planning and operational purposes, without a spatial visualization component, administrators lack a critical reference point that can be used to make informed decisions. Caution must be taken, however, to map the data accurately, since operational decisions will be made from maps produced from the GIS analyst. When better GIS maps are produced, better administrative decisions can potentially be realized by the organization. As the usage of GIS increases, the ability to make decisions based on data will increase accuracy in the decision-making process.

## Acknowledgments


- Facilities Planning and Scheduling, West Virginia University
- Institutional Research, West Virginia University
- Division of Facilities and Services, West Virginia University
- The West Virginia GIS Technical Center
- The Morgantown Monongalia Metropolitan Planning Organization
- Monongalia County Planning Commission
- The University of Texas at Dallas


## References


Blough, David R., 2003. "Integrating GIS into the Survey Research Process", *Using Geographic Information Systems in Institutional Research, New Directions for Institutional Research.* Volume 120, Winter, Jossey-Bass, San Francisco, CA.

Bolstad, Paul, 2016. *GIS Fundamentals: A First Text on Geographic Information Systems, Fifth Edition.* XanEdu Publishing Inc., Ann Arbor, MI.

Burgess and Niple, 2012. "Morgantown Monongalia Metropolitan Planning Organization's 2040 Long Range Transportation Plan", May. Retrieved on November 11, 2015. www.morgantownwv.gov/wp-content/uploads/MCP-Appendix-C4-compressed.pdf

Golledge, Reginald, 2001. "What Is It That Geographers Do?" *Directions Magazine*, July 2. Retrieved on August 18, 2014. www.directionsmag.com/columns/what-is-it-that-geographers-do/129597

Granados, Manuel, 2003. "Mapping Data on Enrolled Students", *Using Geographic Information Systems in Institutional Research, New Directions for Institutional Research.* Volume 120, Winter, Jossey-Bass, San Francisco, CA.

Harvard University, 2015. "Harvard Planning & Project Management". Retrieved on November 11, 2015. http://home.hppm.harvard.edu/pages/property-information

Jardine, Daniel D., 2003. "Using GIS in Alumni Giving and Institutional Advancement", *Using Geographic Information Systems in Institutional Research, New Directions for Institutional Research.* Volume 120, Winter 2003, Jossey-Bass, San Francisco, CA.

Kukaswadia, Atif, 2013. "John Snow—The First Epidemiologist", *Public Health Perspectives.* Retrieved on February 9, 2013. http://blogs.plos.org/publichealth/2013/03/11/john-snow-the-first-epidemiologist/

McCormick, B. Grant, 2003. "Developing Enterprise GIS for University Administration: Organizational and Strategic Considerations", *Using Geographic Information*

*Systems in Institutional Research, New Directions for Institutional Research.* Volume 120, Winter, Jossey-Bass, San Francisco, CA.

Mora, Victor J., 2003. "Applications of GIS in Admissions and Targeting Efforts", *Using Geographic Information Systems in Institutional Research, New Directions for Institutional Research.* Volume 120, Winter, Jossey-Bass, San Francisco, CA.

Morris-Dueer, Vicky, Michael, Jessica M., Stoiko, Rachel R., and Jungblut, Bernadette J., 2016. "West Virginia University Mountaineer Success Academy (MSA) Program Report", March 29, Office of Institutional Research.

Pilesjö, Petter, and Mårtensson, Ulrik, 2009. "Integration of Geomatics in Research and Development", *SAPIENS. Perspectives*, Volume 2, Number 2 Special Issue. Retrieved on August 18, 2014. http://sapiens.revues.org/836

Space Daily, 2012. "$3.7 Billion Reasons Why GIS Technology Is the Future", *Space Daily*, August 29. Retrieved on August 18, 2014. www.spacedaily.com/reports/3_point_7_Billion_Reasons_Why_GIS_Technology_is_The_Future_999.html

Titus, Ree, 2001. "A Career in Geography or the Social Sciences?" *Chronicle Guidance Publications*. CGP Reprint R-200, January. Retrieved on August 18, 2014. http://ejw.i8.com/geog/99/career.htm

Tobler, Waldo R., 1970. "A Computer Movie Simulating Urban Growth in the Detroit Region", *Economic Geography*, Volume 46, Number 2, pp. 234–240. Retrieved on August 12, 2014. www.geog.ucsb.edu/~tobler/publications/pdf_docs/geog_analysis/ComputerMovie.pdf

UCLA, 2014. "Mapping the 1854 Broad Street Pump Outbreak", *UCLA Department of Epidemiology—School of Public Health.* Retrieved on August 18. www.ph.ucla.edu/epi/snow/mapsbroadstreet.html

United States Department of Agriculture Natural Resources Conservation Service, 2006. "Part 641 Drafting and Drawings National Engineering Handbook". Retrieved on August 19, 2014. http://directives.sc.egov.usda.gov/OpenNonWebContent.aspx?content=17761.wba

The University of Texas at Dallas—Office of Strategic Planning and Analysis, 2013.

Valcik, Nicolas A., 2007. "The Logistical Tracking System (LTS) Five Years Later: What Have We Learned?" *Space: The Final Frontier for Institutional Research, New Directions for Institutional Research.* Volume 135, John Wiley and Sons, Inc., Hoboken, NJ.

Valcik, Nicolas A., 2010. "New Hazardous Materials (HAZMAT) Federal Regulations for Higher Education Institutions", *Institutional Research: Homeland Security. New Directions for Institutional Research.* Volume 146, John Wiley and Sons, Inc., Hoboken, NJ.

Valcik, Nicolas A., 2014. "West Virginia Adventure Participants Explorer Trip 2004–2012". West Virginia University, Office of Institutional Research. GIS Map used operationally.

Valcik, Nicolas A., 2015. "West Virginia Mountaineer Success Academy Participants by Zip Code 2013 and 2014". West Virginia University, Office of Institutional Research. GIS Maps used operationally.

West Virginia University—Geography Program, 2014. "Geography", *West Virginia University*. Retrieved on August 12, 2014. http://catalog.wvu.edu/graduate/eberlycollegeofartsandsciences/geologyandgeography/

West Virginia University GIS Technical Center, 2015. "Overview". Retrieved on November 11, 2015. http://wvgis.wvu.edu/about/about.php

West Virginia University—Office of Institutional Research, 2015.

West Virginia University—Personal Rapid Transportation, 2014. "Personal Rapid Transportation", *West Virginia University*. Retrieved on August 18, 2014. http://transportation.wvu.edu/prt

Western Kentucky University, 2014. "PDC GIS/GPS Services", *Western Kentucky University*. Retrieved on August 12, 2014. www.wku.edu/pdc/gis/

# 10 The Logistical Tracking System (LTS) Eighteen Years Later

## What Did We Learn and What Could We Improve?

*Nicolas A. Valcik*

### Introduction

The purpose of this research is to discuss the development of the Logistical Tracking System (LTS©)[1] and evaluate the changes in processes and procedures at UT-Dallas due to implementation of a new type of technology. The chapter will elaborate on the positive and negative aspects of designing and constructing a software application in-house and illustrate the changes in organizational procedures and policies that must occur to implement a new application. In addition, the chapter will discuss how the use of LTS allowed for different calculations for projection of space to occur at the university. The research utilizes qualitative research methods to gather data on the evolution of the facilities information systems at UT-Dallas. The role of the Office of Strategic Planning and Analysis (OSPA) in the construction and implementation of LTS will also be reviewed and evaluated.

### Evolution of the Facilities Information Issue

In 1998, when the researcher was originally introduced to facilities information systems and state reports, he perceived that by automating processes, such as converting floor plans to CAD files, the university could report data to the state more accurately and efficiently. This hypothesis was expanded in 2002 to include technology capable of performing automated tasks and to envision the business processes and practices that would be necessary to successfully (and accurately) capture information on facilities. As the LTS project moved forward, the hypothesis evolved further to include two additional factors: streamlining the application for ease of use and requiring a commitment from all involved parties to ensuring the success of the new system and the new business processes designed to make their operations more efficient and effective.

* Note this article has been updated from the 2008 *New Directions for Institutional Research* volume 135, Space: The Final Frontier for Institutional Research, "The Logistical Tracking System (LTS©) Five Years Later: What Has Been Accomplished?"

Because of its role as the reporting agency for the university, OSPA interfaces with various departments such as Property Administration, Admissions, and the Registrar, among others. Due to the technical skill of the staff, access to all major university databases, and good relations with a variety of departments, OSPA has the capacity to view the work processes of the entire university and provide solutions to help different departments operate more effectively. This unique quality placed OSPA in a position to develop LTS and tailor it to the needs of other departments as well as its own.

Although UT-Dallas employs Computer Aided Design (CAD) operators, no interface owned by the university was capable of supporting an application that could read CAD floor plans. However, the university had several Geographic Information Systems (GIS) resources available, including licensing rights, social science professors who used GIS for research, the Bruton Center,[2] a geoscience department that used GIS in its research, degree programs for GIS, and students that could perform GIS work. Furthermore, the team believed GIS to be more versatile and capable than CAD.

The team decided to use Microsoft SQL Server 2000© (upgraded to Microsoft SQL Server 2005) and Microsoft InterDev 6.0© for the new LTS system. Using SQL Server allowed for a cost-effective and powerful database that could interface with GIS. InterDev, a web-based application, permitted multiple users to access the data at the same time and allowed electronic processes to replace paper processes to make university operations more efficient and effective.

### *Functional Areas of LTS*

The original purpose of LTS was to improve facilities management and permit information in government reports to be utilized by OSPA and the Controller's Office. The development process of the software prompted other departments to view the potential of LTS to enhance effectiveness of certain operations. The application added the following capabilities that had not existed previously:

1. Facilities feed for the AD ASTRA application for the Registrar's scheduling purposes.
2. Tracking chemical, biological, and radioactive materials to location.
3. Allowing integration of security systems (camera output is viewable through LTS).
4. Telecommunication infrastructure tracking.
5. Personnel assignments to facilities.
6. Campus resident assignment to facilities.
7. Room equipment tracking.
8. Safety equipment tracking.
9. Physical plant door key tracking.
10. Calculating utility costs for buildings.

Other areas were added to LTS as required. As always, the addition of capabilities is dependent upon resources available for the task.

## Resource and Technical Issues Developing LTS

The biggest challenge faced with the development of LTS was discovering how to program for the GIS integration and the user interfaces. Finding personnel who could integrate these components successfully led to the second greatest challenge the project faced. No new employees, outside of student workers, were hired to complete LTS. One group member was employed in a different department, University Management Systems (UMS), and was expected to complete his primary job responsibilities before working on a new project with a different department.

A student from the School of Engineering and Computer Science was hired as a research assistant to work on LTS. That student would be the first of ten students from UT-Dallas who would work on LTS from 2001 to 2013. Since the research assistant had never worked on a project such as LTS, the learning curve was extremely steep and the assistant required a great deal of training and supervision, at least initially. However, using students who were studying computer science and management information systems proved beneficial for both parties—work was accomplished on the project and the students gained "real-world" experience that assisted them later in their professional lives. OSPA had two personnel assigned to the LTS project, a database developer (project lead) and a GIS analyst. These employees were required to complete their primary responsibilities to OSPA first and work on LTS as their schedules permitted. At one point in the LTS development, a post-doctoral employee and another student worker were contracted to map down the campus in GIS so all of the floor plans would be available to import information to LTS. As LTS evolved, previous interfaces and reports were updated and their appearance refined so that LTS was easier for non-technical employees to use.

The project needed a server to provide a stable platform for the project. An immediate answer to this challenge was to utilize a surplus personal computer and install Microsoft Server 2000 as its operating system. This machine gave the development team an inexpensive platform to develop LTS to verify that the concept would work. Once the concept had been proven, OSPA purchased a dedicated rack-mounted server to house LTS. One of the bigger technical issues that the development team faced was installing ESRI ArcSDE, which would permit GIS to interface with the Microsoft SQL Server 2000. Not only were the installation instructions inadequate, but the new rack server required a different type of Sentinel Key in place of the SCSI hardware key that had been used previously.

## Process Issues

When the decision was made to develop LTS, OSPA was, at the time, unfamiliar with what the police department, environmental health and safety, telecommunications, student life, or the Controller's Office would require from the system. OSPA interviewed departments that were going to use the new system to understand their operational requirements for mandated state and federal reporting. From these interviews, OSPA gained insight on how to proceed on development for the different sections on LTS.

The existing mainframe systems had no validation techniques that could reject erroneous or illogical data entries. Within character length restrictions, anything could be input into the fields provided. This resulted in the need for constant auditing by programmers and correction by data owners. To minimize data entry errors, LTS was designed with pull-down menus with pre-selected options chosen and updated by the functional areas. Building codes, room numbers, and other infrastructure codes were tied to GIS floor plans to narrow data entry choices to only the most valid ones.

UT-Dallas has relied on mainframe technology for its primary administrative systems, which requires programmers to develop reports, update database elements, and run programs. Departments become dependent upon a centralized entity to produce reports for them. With LTS, the departments can generate their own reports and adjust their own database codes as requirements change.

## Decentralized Data Streams and Empowered Users

Until recently, the administrative systems were kept in "silos", with student data completely separate from human resource data, which is separate from financial data. Programs that were written before 2012 had to be rewritten to connect information among the systems. A major difference between LTS and the previous mainframe systems was that LTS could allow multiple departments to see the same data. LTS could also track changes by user so the person responsible for their area was held accountable for keeping their data maintained. This results in improved communication between departments and ensures updates to the database occur on a regular and timely basis. The reports could be generated from a user-friendly query system and then downloaded to Microsoft Excel without the assistance of a programmer. Processes such as the Facilities Inventory Report, which previously took up to three months to audit and correct, were reduced to a month and a half. Most of the time was due to the necessity of matching data in LTS to the more error-prone data contained in SIS+ (older mainframe system). Even after UT-Dallas converted to PeopleSoft, data still had to be reconciled with LTS to ensure accuracy of facility data in the student information system.

## New Platforms Allowed for Use of New Technology

With new platforms and interfaces, new technology empowered each department with new capabilities. For example, IP addressable cameras enabled first responders to view live camera feeds inside facilities through LTS. LTS allowed users to access the system through a web browser that can be used with a Tablet PC or Pocket PC linked to a wireless network. This allowed users to be mobile (on site) and access large amounts of data quickly. In addition, LTS uses barcodes, digital signatures, and photos to track items, actions, or personnel. These improvements in capability increased safety and made processes more effective than previously. For example, hazardous materials (HAZMAT) were tracked and inventoried in LTS with a barcode. As soon as HAZMAT is delivered to campus, a container ID number is assigned that will keep track of the item as it is transported to the responsible person at its final destination. Prior to the implementation of LTS, HAZMAT was not tracked to location or person and was recorded on index cards for inventory purposes only. LTS permits this information to be quickly and correctly stored in a centralized database that is accessible to auditors and even to first responders during an emergency situation. LTS even has a feature that enables first responders to issue group emails based on HAZMAT location should an emergency arise.

## Improved Processes by Using GIS

GIS eliminated the need for employees to visit each room to measure its dimensions. This alone was a cost savings and increased the accuracy of the measurements for the facilities. When development of LTS began, CAD files for the university were incomplete and had to be converted into GIS. Where CAD files did not exist, blue line drawings were scaled and then input into GIS. OSPA sometimes had to make decisions on how to code areas of blue line or CAD files that were not defined (such as corridor space) without much guidance. This process took six months to complete. However, UT-Dallas's situation was not as bad as that of other universities. One university had framed their blue line drawings on the wall and had no CAD files. Another university was still measuring rooms by hand and completing its facilities inventory reports to the THECB on paper forms as late as 1997. Furthermore, UT-Dallas had a unique resource at its disposal: a geoscience department whose students and faculty had the ability to gather GPS coordinates on the university's facilities and infrastructure. This not only saved the university from having to hire a surveyor, it also enabled its students to apply their skills towards a "real-world" project.

## Advantages to Developing an In-House System

At the time LTS was developed, a commercial software application did not exist for what the university required. To this day, LTS is still considered innovative and was until 2013 continually upgraded and modified to meet new university requirements and needs. The project garnered UT-Dallas a National Safety Council Award of Recognition from CSHEMA for unique or innovative practices.[3] Over the initial three-year development period (FY 2001–FY 2003), the university also recorded a $1,683,205 million in cost savings.[4]

Additionally, LTS was customized to UT-Dallas's operational requirements to provide accurate information on facilities and their contents.

LTS has allowed work processes to be re-engineered through automation. Processes that used to be performed by hand, such as measuring classroom space, were programmed into the system. Paper forms were converted into an electronic format to expedite data entry. Logic checks and data audits were programmed into the system to reduce data entry errors, thereby freeing personnel from devoting wasted time to error detection and correction. By automating such tasks, the university saves time and money in the long term. Additionally, LTS provides capabilities to different departments (such as HAZMAT control) that can potentially save lives or prevent catastrophe from occurring. In short, LTS has added capabilities to the university's data systems that were previously unavailable.

## Training Students to Work With LTS

Between 2001 and 2013, ten students have worked on LTS, each bringing to the project a new vision and set of skills that have enabled LTS to evolve. This project provided the students with a real-world perspective on an application that was used by employees in real situations. The students were informed that the LTS project operated just like a project at a private company. This forced these computer science and management information system students to hone skills often not required in their classes. For example, one student was instructed to improve their verbal communication skills commensurate with what private industry would expect. Another student was asked to produce written memos at the end of each week to succinctly describe what work had been accomplished on the project.

In the business world, there are no grades; the software application either works or it fails, and the result can ultimately affect one's employment. The students were often informed that when developing software, getting a function to work was not enough. One had to be mindful of the type of customer—in this case, university employees—who would be interacting with the software application and to construct it around their needs and skill levels. In addition, students were told to create deadlines for completion of certain tasks and to abide by those estimates. In the classroom, students have some flexibility with how the application they developed works and when the application is completed. There is no such luxury in the business world.

The project proved beneficial for all the students who worked on LTS. All the students who worked on the project were employed in good private industry jobs soon after graduation. One student stated that the work he did on LTS was instrumental in securing a job after graduation. Employing students to work on LTS benefited the students, whose education was supplemented with "real-world" experience, and the university, which received top-notch work on a high priority project with a nominal investment in personnel costs. Students from the computer science department were generally found to have more advanced skill sets to work on LTS than those coming from the management information systems program since those students were (as of 2013) not found to be strong in computer database architecture and network security protocols. After 2011, computer science students were hired to work on LTS instead of management information systems students.

## Intellectual Property Rights

An important advantage that should be considered when building a software application is institutional ownership of intellectual property rights. A software package that can be used by several different organizations can be licensed to an entity, which in turn generates funds for the university. In 2003, the university had LTS licensed by a corporation for the rights to sell the software application to different organizations. Furthermore, developing an application that is not only needed but also innovative resulted in the university winning the National Safety Council/CSHEMA Award of Recognition in 2006. This not only is good for the university in terms of recognition, but also generates potential marketing interest from other organizations. LTS has also enabled the university to apply for two federal research grants. LTS was also licensed to UT-Tyler in 2011, had a provisional software patent in 2009, and had copyrights filed for both the software and training manual in 2011. The intellectual property rights allowed the university to license the software, which can generate revenue.

## Understanding the Data Streams

Another advantage to constructing one's own system is it results in a deeper understanding of how the data flows though the university's system and how it impacts other applications. At UT-Dallas, LTS fed the Astra course scheduling module with building codes and room numbers. If room numbers were incorrect in LTS, inaccuracies would occur in Astra and ultimately in the Student Information System (SIS). With LTS, security has been arranged so only certain employees can input data into certain areas of the system. For instance, only Property Administration can input, modify, or delete information on building or room attributes. Having functional areas tied to areas in the system provides accountability to those specific individuals responsible for inputting data in their areas of control.

## Challenges in Developing an In-House Software System

In order for LTS to become a reality, it first had to gain the confidence and support of many stakeholders before the project could go forward. Winning support from the various departments LTS was designed to assist took longer than the actual development of the system. Department heads had difficulty conceiving of such a system and how it could help to improve their work processes. Several meetings were held to demonstrate the system's capability and how LTS could be expanded to accomplish other tasks to benefit the organization. Many times, OSPA personnel diagrammed proposed developments on white boards. Once development was underway and the system was operational, implementation and training became the next big challenge. Some departments were enthusiastic about the system, while others saw LTS as another "chore" they had to contend with in addition to their regular job duties. In some cases, personnel would leave and their replacements were grateful to be able to use such a user-friendly system that required minimal training. By 2003, LTS was declared operational and was used to report federal, state, and operational data.

## Issues of Resources

As the proportion of the university's budget supported by state funding continues to dwindle, finding financial resources to support non-academic personnel becomes more of a challenge. During the 2002–2003 academic year, the LTS project lost its primary web programmer and a student worker when they found lucrative employment elsewhere. In 2004, the project lost its GIS analyst to a municipal police department, leaving the project without a competent GIS analyst until 2006. During that time, no GIS floor plans were updated. To save money while maintaining quality, OSPA hired student workers to modify LTS for the ongoing requirements of the university. However, constant turnover due to student graduation meant continual training to familiarize new students with the system.

Lack of funding can also lead to responsibilities being assigned to unlikely personnel. In 2005, the Vice President of Business Affairs proposed that OSPA assume responsibility for inputting and maintaining information on facilities. This had been the responsibility of Property Administration, but the increasing burden of tracking controlled items such as computers and science equipment left the small office with no additional time or personnel to measure new and remodeled facilities or complete data entry. Unfortunately, OSPA did not receive additional funding or personnel to manage this work and so was unable to comply. Eventually, the Vice President of Business Affairs assigned this responsibility to an assistant vice president under his auspice.

## Conclusions: What Was Learned?

If the personnel and resources are available, a university should seriously consider building their own customized applications for space inventory as a means to get work done accurately, expediently, and within a modest budget. UT-Dallas invested the time of a small team of people and the modest resources of a few small offices and achieved the creation of a customized facilities inventory system. The estimated cost savings to the university during the first three years of LTS implementation was $1.6 million. The development of LTS enabled business processes to be re-engineered, thus permitting an expansion of the kind of data that could be recorded, and allowed for state-of-the-art technology to be implemented at the university. Resources and personnel who were dedicated to a manual inventory process have been freed to accomplish other tasks. Best of all, the new system enables the university to provide highly accurate data to government agencies quickly and efficiently.

However, one should take heed in gaining stakeholder support before beginning such a project. Developers need to account for a long period of design work on the system and plan to take a great deal of time determining what the application is designed to do and who will ultimately use it. If these questions are not answered, the success of the project will be thrown into doubt. The benefit for UT-Dallas has been an increase in capability and the reduction of labor for certain responsibilities. In addition, the university had a data system, which broke down many of the existing silos of operation. This allowed for additional cooperation between departments that had previously operated in a very fragmented manner. Customized applications developed in-house can be very beneficial, especially if the university is willing to devote the time and energy to make it a reality.

That stated, the loss of personnel in 2013 who could work with LTS and GIS prompted the Executive Director to abandon the system for a data warehouse solution without a GIS component or functional ability beyond basic facility information. Without the GIS component, facilities information will once again need to be input manually, opening up the potential for inaccuracies in the operational data, which in turn could impact state approval for new buildings. The lack of a GIS component means the loss of the analytical work that GIS could perform. The new system does not include a central repository or information system for HAZMAT, homeland security information, indirect cost recovery, facility renovation projects, or infrastructure to any GIS floor plans. The main lesson from this experience is that an institution has to invest in systems to gain and maintain capability. Without that investment, an institution risks the loss of capability and credibility and becomes at risk for liabilities for any gaps that may occur due to inaccurate or missing data. Even the best systems need leaders and stakeholders who understand the importance of accurate data to be successful in a higher education institution, and LTS is no different in that regard.

## Notes

1. LTS was developed by Dr. Nicolas A. Valcik, Danald Lee, Dr. Patricia Huesca Dorantes, and Tarang Sethia. Seven student workers—Dinikeshwari Nagaraj, Rajesh Ahuja, Mohit Nagrath, Shalu Agrawal, Priyankar Datta, Rishi Raj Kapoor, and Ajeet Singh—provided additional programming support for LTS during the 2001–2007 timeframe.
2. Burton Center is a research center located at the University of Texas at Dallas.
3. Esequiel E. Barrera and Dr. Nicolas A. Valcik—*National Safety Council/SCHEMA* Award of Recognition (Unique or Innovative Category), UT-Dallas, 2006.
4. Cost Savings Report FY 2001–2003 reported to State of Texas from UT-Dallas. Sizable cost savings still occurred with the LTS project after FY 2003.

# 11 Trends and Challenges for Geographic Information Systems (GIS) Use by Nonprofits

*Todd A. Jordan*

## Introduction

Like their counterparts in the public and private sectors, nonprofits have increasingly utilized Geographic Information Systems (GIS) to improve the work they do in the community. From needs assessment to fundraising, some nonprofits have been early adopters of GIS to enhance their operations and return value to their stakeholders. Unfortunately, there is not a significant amount of literature on the role of GIS in nonprofits, and while an encompassing review of potential uses is beyond the scope of the present work, this chapter will synthesize some of the existing literature, as well as real-world examples, to provide an overview of the ways nonprofits can utilize GIS. We will begin with a brief overview of the nonprofit sector and GIS before turning to the possible uses of GIS within this sector. With nonprofits encompassing a wide variety of services, this chapter will use the existing literature as a guide that will take us towards social service and community development organizations, with some examples of other types of nonprofit operations. The chapter will then turn towards the potential limitations and risks that utilization of GIS technology can have for a nonprofit. While the technology is powerful in its ability to transform an organization, the barriers to adoption and the dangers to the community must be considered. The chapter will conclude with future directions for both practitioners and scholars. This will include ways that some of the barriers to GIS adoption can be overcome as well as strategies to mitigate the risks. Overall, this chapter will demonstrate that the pervasiveness of GIS in many nonprofits shows the promising potential of the technology and warrants serious exploration by the rest of the sector. While adoption and integration may face challenges, nonprofits should build upon the successes of their colleagues and incorporate GIS technology across their organization.

## The Role of Nonprofits in a Changing World

Nonprofits can engage in a wide variety of work across multiple issues, ranging from service delivery, community planning, advocacy, and business development. Typically, a nonprofit organization in the United States will fall under section 501(c) of the federal tax code. The most common category is 501(c)(3), which includes charitable organizations, churches and religious organizations, political organizations, and private foundations. Some nonprofits may fit into 501(c)(4), which is for social welfare organizations (such as a homeowner associations) and local associations of employees, but these organizations are allowed to participate in political lobbying (unlike 501(c)(3)s) and, in the wake of the 2010 Supreme Court "Citizens United" decision, have drastically increased in numbers (Sullivan 2013). There are also 501(c)(6) organizations, which include business leagues and chambers of commerce.

However, when most people hear the word nonprofit, they tend to think about charitable organizations (such as United Way or Salvation Army), a local institution for the public good (e.g. a museum), or a community development organization. This has also been the trend in the literature around nonprofits technology, and in particular GIS use among nonprofits. Not to discount the other types of nonprofits that operate in the United States, but this chapter will largely focus on the work of social service and community development organizations while touching on the role of GIS in business-oriented nonprofits.

We live in a challenging time for the nonprofit sector. Similar to their public sector colleagues, nonprofit workers are expected to meet the increasing demands of their clients while dealing with static or decreasing resources (money, volunteers, materials). The level of giving in the United States has stayed relatively stable at 2% of GDP for the last 40 years (MacLaughlin 2016), but the nonprofit sector has experienced a significant amount of growth. Based on IRS data, in the US "since 1996, the total number of registered nonprofit organizations has grown from 1,085,296 to 1,517,056 in 2016" (MacLaughlin 2016, pg. 10). When combined with the impact of retrenchment in government services, stronger calls for accountability in the wake of major scandals, and new forms of monitoring available to the general public (such as the website GuideStar), nonprofits are in a complicated place (Hackler and Saxton 2007). Yet, the fundamental purpose of nonprofit organizations remains the same: to improve their communities. Though community may be defined as local, regional, national, or international, nonprofits are driven by unmet need in their communities and can lead action(s) to meet that need.

Technology has the potential to help address many of the challenges that nonprofit organizations face or will face in the coming years. Electronic communication allows nonprofits who effectively employ it to engage their stakeholders and donors in new ways. New software and shared data platforms can allow for better monitoring of program operations and lead to improvements in service delivery or the identification of community needs. However, technology can also open the door to new problems for nonprofits such as risks to client or donor data, additional overhead costs, or conflicts with the staff who struggle to adapt to these changes. While the tools of the trade may be changing, the overall mission of the nonprofit remains the same.

> Although non-profit organizations possess significant latitude in determining their missions and constituencies, ultimately they must rely on interactions with community members to provide direction. To develop

> and pursue their service missions, non-profit leaders must recognize and implement a conception of their community to provide the framework for their mission.
>
> (Brudney, Russell, and Fischer 2016, pg. 2)

Technological innovations, such as Geographic Information Systems (GIS), are one tool that can improve nonprofits' ability to envision and shape their community as well as be a platform for interfacing with members of their community. This will only hold for nonprofits that are able to adopt the technology as part of their practices and are able to guard against the potential pitfalls that come with mapping via GIS. But the strength that GIS platforms can bring to the operations of nonprofits and how they can be utilized for significant improvements in communities all across the world warrant experimentation, if not complete adoption, by those in the nonprofit sector.

## A Brief Overview of GIS

Given the focus of many nonprofits, it is fitting that the history of GIS begins with individuals grappling with public health safety. The first documented application of "GIS" was in France in 1832 by French geographer Charles Picquet, who created a map of cholera epidemiology in Paris using color gradients (an early version of a heat map). In 1854, John Snow (now considered the father of epidemiology) depicted cholera deaths in London, with the key difference being that Snow presented an argument (cholera was spread via the water instead of air) developed from spatial analysis displayed on the map (Dempsey 2012a).

The first use of the phrase Geographic Information System occurs in Roger Tomlinson's 1968 article *A Geographic Information System for Regional Planning*. Tomlinson was an English geographer whose early work with the Canada Land Inventory (1966) and subsequent writing earned him the informal title of the "Father of GIS" (Dempsey 2012b). While there is a significant debate regarding the various definitions and meaning of GIS (Chrisman 1999), as well as key distinctions to be made between Geographic Information Systems and Geographic Information Science (Gold 2006), the present chapter will focus on a more common conception of GIS.

> GIS helps to store, analyze, and present data, and assists in turning complex datasets into relatively easy-to-understand visuals including maps and charts. GIS enables creating powerful visuals that inform programs and planning decisions and advocacy. It enables analyzing data across multiple geographic scales, highlighting spatial distribution and patterns. Geographic units can range from a single address, block, census tract, or zip code to a municipality, county, region, state, or the entire country.
>
> (Al-Kodmany 2012, pg. 292)

While the power of visualizations can be incredibly useful and effective for the operations of nonprofits and their engagement with the community, we sadly have very little research on the subject (Brudney, Russell, and Fischer 2016). While the surge in GIS technology in the 1990s led to some research in the field, there has been a significant gap in the literature since 2005 (Al-Kodmany 2012). This may be the result of GIS only slowly becoming a part of the way that some nonprofits engage their community and evaluate their operations. The hesitancy on the part of nonprofits to adopt GIS software is easy to understand, but that is a pattern that has been changing. While GIS used to require significant organizational capacity, including highly trained experts, we have entered a time when open source software designed to be easy on the user enables access to GIS like never before. The ability of GIS software to help assess community needs, improve operations, engage stakeholders, and further mission of nonprofits has spurred some early adopters. The subsequent sections will lay out multiple examples of ways in which GIS software can be used in nonprofits as well as outline the pitfalls that can occur if GIS is improperly managed by organizations.

## Potential Uses of GIS for Nonprofits

As a flexible and adaptable tool, GIS can provide a lot of value to nonprofit operations if properly adopted and utilized. While there are certainly limitations as well as potential dangers to the use of GIS in nonprofit work, the advantages to adapting and integrating GIS into nonprofit operations warrants consideration by nonprofits of all different types. This section will focus on four primary, and largely overlapping, ways that nonprofits can utilize GIS services to improve the effectiveness and efficiency of their work. The four primary areas for this chapter are: assessment of community need, new or improved service delivery, tool for engagement/advocacy, and fundraising.

### *Assessment of Community Need*

As discussed earlier, the fundamental role of a nonprofit is to fill a void in the community that would better the public good. But this is only possible if the community and the nonprofit are able to establish what the needs of the community are, and that requires a great deal of data on areas of concern. Taking this data and mapping it via GIS can provide powerful visualizations that spur attention to new issues as well as help nonprofit organizations understand where they need to be committing resources in order to improve the community. In a study of Chicago area nonprofits, Kheir Al-Kodmany notes:

> The greatest reward of GIS is its visualization power. "It is often easier to explain data visually as opposed to describing it verbally". Interviewees emphasized that "when GIS maps are presented to the public they become elemental in guiding decisions in virtually every planning project".
>
> (Al-Kodmany 2012, pg. 292)

The power of visual presentation can be incredibly important when highlighting the disparities or showing underserved populations because the visual data makes a powerful case for the inequities of the status quo or the shortages that exist in quality services.

One example of the powers of GIS to map needs in a community in order to spur change comes from the work of United Way of Greater Atlanta (UWGA) and their Child Well-Being Index (Figure 11.1). UWGA commissioned research on the conditions of the Atlanta metropolitan area and found that 500,000 youths were living in neighborhoods with the highest poverty rates and lowest chances for economic mobility in the country. The Child Well-Being Index was created using multiple indicators in three key areas of focus and was tied to data based on zip codes. For the Child measures, there were seven indicators, including high school graduation rate, percent of children without health insurance, and percent of children in poverty. The Family measure had three indicators, such as percent of mothers without a high school diploma. The Community measure had four indicators, including percent of adults without a high school diploma and the unemployment rate. These measures created a composite score for each zip code on a scale of 0 to 100. UWGA undertook this project because "they wanted to create a baseline around which to mobilize the community to set goals to improve" (Staples 2017). The index also includes three pillars that are strategies for changing the communities that are struggling and include a focus on strong foundations, opportunities for success, and nurturing communities. Utilizing a GIS platform, UWGA was able to map the data and display it on their website so that community members, nonprofits, and government officials could look at zip code scores, compare them to the region, and track progress. The goal of releasing all this data was to "raise a flag on the issues our children face and issue a call to action to address the needs because all of us will benefit or pay a penalty for failing to improve their circumstances" (Staples 2017).

GIS can play other roles for nonprofit organizations, aside from showing inequities in community needs. Museums and chambers of commerce can map their attendees or members to see where they are drawing business from as well as where they should increase their outreach efforts. Community development corporations or branches of the national body of the Local Initiative Support Corporation (LISC) can perform market studies and gap analysis to attract new businesses or investment to certain areas. Grassroots transportation organizations can use maps to show the current status of biking and walking trails as well as sidewalks in order to show the need for expansion as well as the public health benefits of those projects. The list of uses for assessment of community need is as expansive as the different types of nonprofits, but the important theme is that GIS has a very practical and powerful role to play in visualizing the mission and purpose of nonprofit organizations.

### *New or Improved Service Delivery*

Building off the previous section, the assessment of community needs often generates ways of designing new programs or enhancing existing service

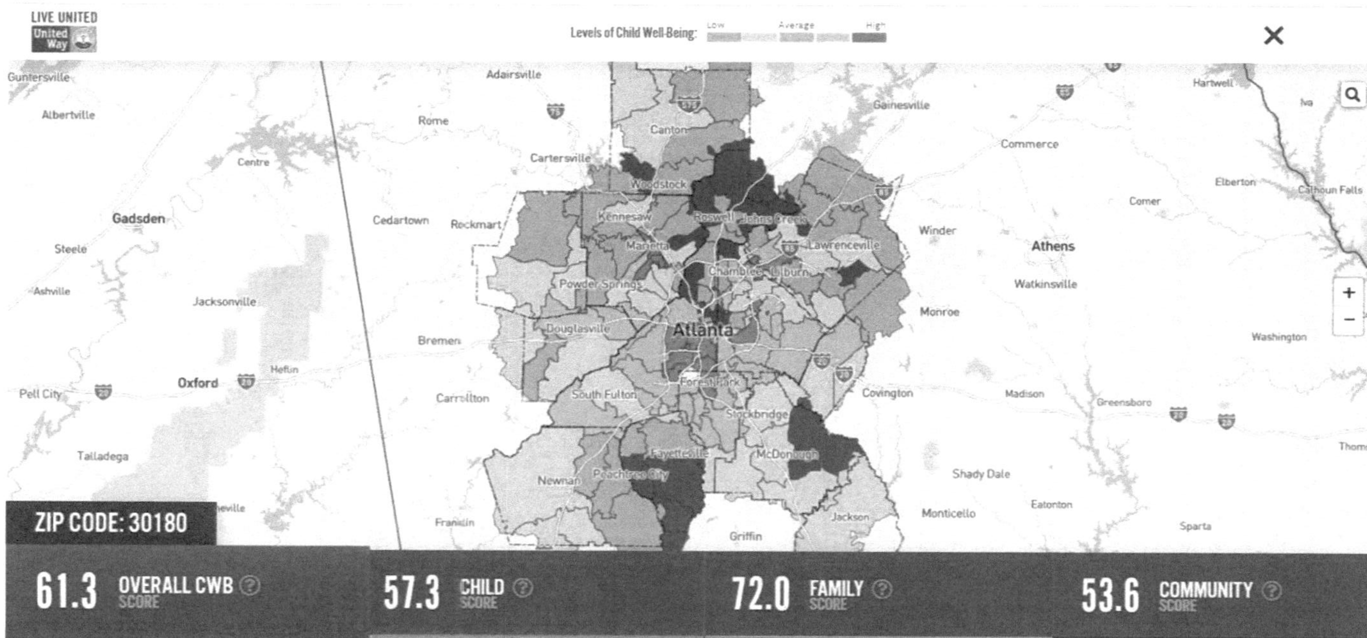


*Figure 11.1* Child Well-Being Index for Greater Atlanta.

Source: United Way of Greater Atlanta Child Well-Being Index, www.unitedwayatlanta.org/child-well-being-map/ (accessed 6/15/2018)

delivery in order to fill gaps or increase effectiveness. Through story-telling, Al-Kodmany (2012) details several different Chicago nonprofits that focus on urban planning. One example comes from the Woodstock Institute (a nonprofit focused on community developed in marginalized neighborhoods), which utilized GIS to map bank branching in Chicago and show disparities in where bank branches were prevalent. By showing where banks were creating new branches (and more importantly, where they were not), the Woodstock Institute raised the profile of the issue, giving local governments the data they required to emphasize policies or programs needed to attract bank branches to underserved communities.

In a similar manner, Vaz and Khaper (2016) show the potential open source GIS can have on food deserts and healthy eating by mapping the Toronto food system.

> With the knowledge of open-source GIS software non-profit organizations and local food retailers can research or coordinate where to locate and expand organizations, or urban agriculture to a neighbourhood. The execution of strategically placing healthy and affordable food retailers not only involves a municipal or environmental planner, but impacts realtors and other businesses in the surrounding area by means of avoiding food deserts, which comprise a serious burden to the health sector.
>
> (Vaz and Khaper 2016, pg. 306)

Similar to the assessment of community need, the scope and potential of how GIS mapping can lead to better service delivery will be as varied as there are types of nonprofits. For example, the North American Grid is the network that generates and distributes electricity throughout the United States, as well as parts of Canada and Mexico. The grid is managed by the North America Electric Reliability Corporation, a nonprofit, and is responsible for the reliability of the bulk of North America's power. Monitoring and maintaining such a massive grid that millions of people depend upon necessitates a significant amount of coordination. "This requires taking real-time measurements of electricity output and usage and making split-second decisions using this big data—which is why one reliability coordinator, Peak Reliability, is beginning to depend heavily on the ArcGIS platform" (ESRI 2018, pg. 1). While not every usage of GIS may be as complicated as ensuring the lights stay on in North America, the potential complexity of major social problems can be addressed through nonprofits utilizing GIS.

For example, high-quality child care is critical to getting children ready to learn as they enter school, can reduce barriers that parents or caregivers may face in maintaining employment, and is especially difficult to obtain for low and moderate income families, who may be in most need of it. The Philadelphia-based Reinvestment Fund, a Community Development Financial Institution (CDFI), tasked their Policy Solutions team with developing an analytical approach to identifying gaps in quality childcare for several major cities, including Philadelphia. Using the Policy Maps GIS platform, they created a map of the city to guide investment, business planning supports, and facilities-related projects for childcare. The result was a platform that allowed providers to determine where they should locate their facilities; it allowed investors and policymakers to target resources to increase access to high-quality childcare, and the platform gave parents a tool to find quality childcare centers near where they live or work (see Figure 11.2). As a result, the City of Philadelphia launched a $7 million Fund for Quality (FFQ) to invest in

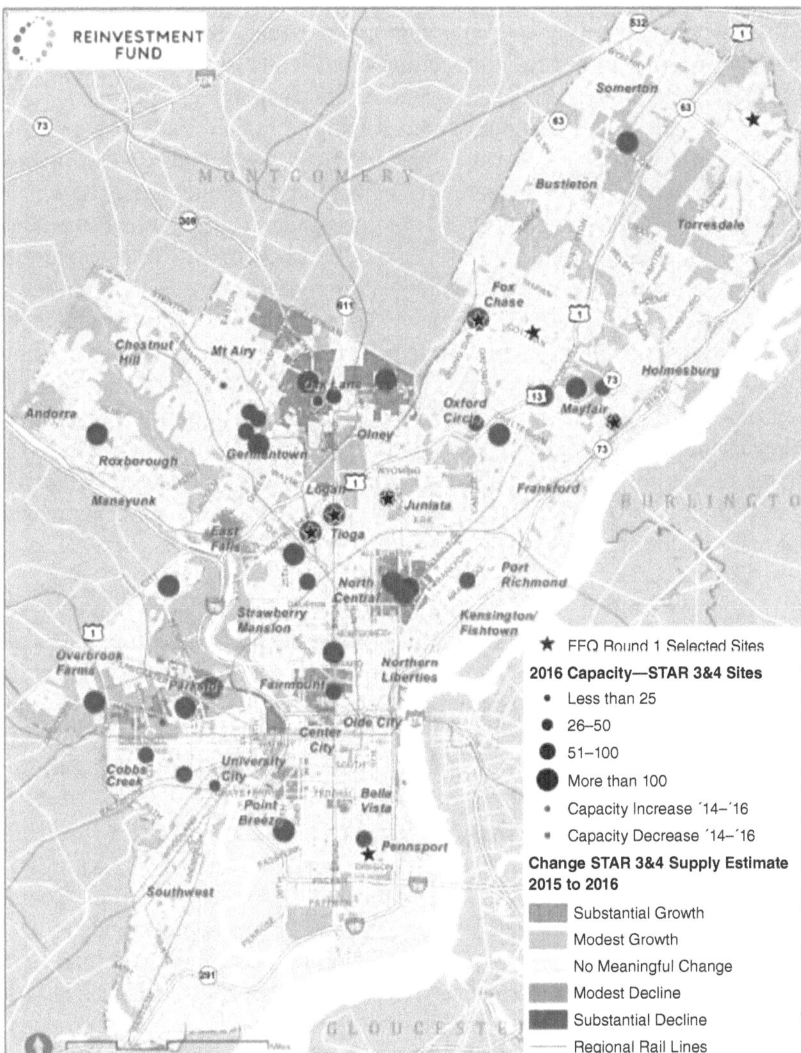


*Figure 11.2* Childcare supply and capacity for STAR 3&4 facilities in Philadelphia, PA.
Source: Reinvestment fund 2016.

high-gap areas (especially those that serve lower income neighborhoods and children of color). In the first two years, the city added 630 high quality spots with 90% being occupied by children from low-income families.

As the examples above demonstrate, the use of GIS can be a powerful mechanism for assessing needs and then developing new or improving existing programs and transforming the communities in which they are employed.

### *Engagement/Advocacy*

On a similar path as the previous sections, GIS can also be a powerful tool to spur advocacy and policy change within communities. Translating an understanding of community needs into action often requires some type of policy change at one or more levels of government. GIS can play a critical role in both engaging people in the community and helping to organize advocacy efforts for change (Brudney, Russell, and Fischer 2016). One framework for this to occur is through Public Participation Geographic Information Systems, which "pertains to the use of geographic information systems (GIS) to broaden public involvement in policymaking as well as to the value of GIS to promote the goals of nongovernmental organizations, grassroots groups, and community-based organizations" (Sieber 2006, pg. 491). Nonprofits can engage with their community members, through a participatory framework, that allows disenfranchised communities to shape the visual representation of what defines their community and in turn use that visualization to advocate for resources or policy changes (Sieber 2006; Bishop 2010).

This process of mapping can be incredibly effective as a form of engagement with people who are often marginalized, but also for uncovering needs that may not surface through traditional mechanisms.

> Maps are effective organizing and advocacy tools because they engage residents in the process of gathering, analyzing, and presenting information about their neighborhoods. GIS provides a way for stakeholders to specify what exists in a community and what they would like to see, and can provide a vehicle for discussions with broader groups of stakeholders.
> (LISC 2002, pg. 5)

One example of how mapping can have a profound impact that reverberates across the country was the Community Benefits Agreement (CBA), which came out of advocacy efforts in Los Angeles. "The Figueroa Corridor Coalition for Economic Justice needed an effective education and organizing tool to respond to the proposed development of an enormous entertainment, hotel, and retail complex adjacent to the Staples Center in downtown Los Angeles" (LISC 2002, pg. 5). Utilizing poster-sized maps, the group was able to show property ownership, and in particular "hot properties" that were targeted as spatial injustices due to their ownership by slumlords, as well as how the proposed development would significantly impact the lives of already marginalized residents.

Leveraging those maps into political advocacy, the coalition won a CBA that included: a developer-funded assessment of community park/recreation needs and $1 million towards meeting those needs, first source hiring for low-income individuals and those displaced by the project, increased affordable housing requirements, and developed funding for residential parking. "This 2001 CBA addressed the interests of low-income residents and now serves as a model for major CBAs across the country" (Saito 2012).

### *Fundraising*

Fundraising and resource development is one of the most under-researched areas for nonprofit use of GIS. Based on the previous sections, where GIS mapping turned into programs, service delivery, and advocacy, GIS can be instrumental in developing new resources for an organization. Most organizations have addresses or some form of geographic information on their individual and corporate donors. Mapping this data can show the dispersion of donors within a community and can be the groundwork for geographically based outreach or donor-appeal efforts. The power of GIS as a visualization tool can be leveraged to show community need or the impact of programs to help with fundraising campaigns. Whether in printed materials, social media, or one-on-one conversations with donors, GIS-based mapping can add another tool to the development officer's tool box that can improve giving.

This is also true for nonprofits that rely on foundation or government support for their operations. "Nonprofit organizations seeking financial resources have increasingly turned to GIS as a tool to enhance grant applications and other requests for support" (Brudney, Russell, and Fischer 2016, pg. 5). One final way that nonprofits could use GIS is to create maps of their service delivery as well as that of other organizations who provide similar programming. These maps not only show the gaps in need and overlap but can also be the groundwork for organizations to partner, which can provide a different twist on an appeal to donors or funders. There is a wide array of potential for nonprofits to utilize GIS in their fundraising or resource development efforts. However, the lack of research on this subject is troubling. Future work around GIS and nonprofits in fundraising could be incredibly beneficial to practitioners as well as scholars.

## Limitations and Barriers for GIS in Nonprofits

While the previous sections laid out the case for the positive potential and benefits of nonprofits integrating the use of GIS into their work, sadly there remain many limitations as well as barriers to the use of the technology. One of the most significant challenges facing GIS adoption by nonprofits is that GIS relies on data, and that data can be hard to come by. The data necessary to generate the map may not exist, or if it does exist, the nonprofit may not have access to it. The data may exist, but it could be in paper copy stored in file boxes that will require a lengthy amount of time as well as accurate data entry in order for it to be useful. Data may be restricted due to legal and/or privacy concerns, especially in the areas of education or healthcare. Even if an organization has the data, there can be issues with too many staff or community partners working with the dataset, which can lead to inaccuracies or inconsistencies.

Also, the data may be available but not at a level that is necessary or useful to the nonprofit. For example, data at the county level might be useful in some regards, but in terms of mapping needs or assets in a neighborhood, zip code or census tract data may be required. There is also a real concern that "problems associated with data sharing do not always stem from technical but, rather, stem from human issues, thus resulting in data hoarding and resistance" (Bishop 2010, pg. 995). Some organizations may be unwilling to share out of fear of competition, as a result of past grievances, or because the data may cast their organization in a negative light. As a result, all of the aforementioned issues with collecting data and maintaining its integrity pose a serious challenge to any organization wishing to integrate GIS into their operations.

Financial issues can also limit the use of GIS. While there are plenty of free data sources and open source GIS software, to use the major platforms an organization will need to be able to afford the subscription cost. GIS software requires staff with some level of expertise, and so nonprofits need to be able to afford training costs or be able to pay a wage that would attract someone with that skill set. Unfortunately, once a staff member is trained to utilize GIS software, they become more valuable and can be recruited away by other organizations. If an organization is able to afford to have a staff member who is proficient with GIS software, but then encounters financial trouble, that GIS staff member might be the first one cut from the staff because their work is not usually direct service delivery or fundraising. Because data collection, staff, and software are not cheap, it can pose a serious barrier to nonprofits and risks creating a system of haves and have nots due to differences in resources.

On a similar note, GIS can be a source of disempowerment for vulnerable communities. "GIS has the potential to exclude and marginalize individuals and communities because of its high cost, technical skill requirements, and reliance on information that lends itself to cartographic and quantitative analysis" (Elwood 2002, pg. 907). The current use of GIS by nonprofits has the potential negative side effect of building assumptions into thinking that the maps people see are inclusive and accurate representations of the community. If the map was created without, or with a poor, participatory framework, or the vulnerable groups cannot create their own map to tell their side of the story, then GIS becomes a way of penalizing marginalized communities who cannot access GIS as a resource.

> The impacts of this technology are contingent on and shaped by complex social and political relationships that constitute the power of different knowledge systems, decision making processes, actors, and institutions. The question is less whether GIS is empowering or disempowering, but

> in what ways does it foster empowerment and disempowerment, and for whom? What is the basis of this empowerment or disempowerment for different actors and institutions?
>
> (Elwood 2002, pgs. 907–908)

Even if a nonprofit or a researcher working for a nonprofit is sensitive to the needs of marginalized groups, they need to understand that they might hold preconceived notions about how the community operates that do not reflect the realities of the community that they are working with.

> Data collection is often dictated by administrative boundaries such as census tracts, zip codes, or catchment areas, but these may not match the areas that residents see as relevant to them. Instead, evaluators need to calibrate the units of measurement with residents' perceptions to the degree that it is possible.
>
> (Coulton, Chan, and Mikelbank 2011, pg. 25)

In relation to fundraising, GIS can be helpful, but it is not a fundraising or development plan by itself. Without the organization having a well-developed method of cultivating donors or resources, then the introduction of GIS-based maps will provide very limited returns to the organization. While GIS can be useful in shaping grant requests, there are still major barriers from funders that prevent its widespread use. Many requests for proposals are explicit in what they will consider as part of a funding request, and if they do not call for a GIS map, then a nonprofit may be unable to submit one. Even with sections for optional attachments, there is no guarantee the funder will utilize a GIS map as part of their scoring of proposals. As mentioned before, while their elements of GIS that can buttress fundraising efforts, a far more comprehensive set of research needs to be conducted to demonstrate the efficacy of using GIS maps in fundraising or grant proposals.

## Potential of GIS and Future Paths

While the barriers and limitations for GIS are not easily dismissed, the technology has a budding ability to make a significant difference in the work of nonprofit organizations. Since GIS is already a ubiquitous presence in our society, nonprofits have little choice but to engage the technology or else stakeholders and community members may pressure them to adopt it. As with any new technology, it will be a learning process for many organizations that will have setbacks as well as milestones. Through careful engagement with their staff, stakeholders, and community members, nonprofits can leverage GIS to drive improvements in meaningful engagement, increase the effectiveness of service delivery, and transform their communities for the better. If there is progress to be made, it will begin with the data that nonprofits collect or acquire. Without solid data on their community, GIS technology is of little value to a nonprofit.

Aside from what they collect internally, there are plenty of third-party data sources (government, universities, regional planning bodies) that can help nonprofits build profiles on the needs of their communities. Since few locales have only a single nonprofit, and since many nonprofits have some overlap in terms of community needs or programming, leveraging partnerships with other nonprofits can be crucial. In her work on the assessment of GIS adoption and usage among several social service nonprofits in Columbia, Missouri, Sheila Bishop noted that

> the presentation of maps indicating target populations, service boundaries, and client characteristics opened up a discussion about where programs overlap and about how nonprofits could collaborate, and even partner together, to better deliver services. Established relationships among these nonprofits might possibly serve as a foundation for future cooperative networks that, in turn, could support data sharing.
>
> (Bishop 2010, pg. 1008)

While turf battles and competition for resources may be a barrier to cooperation, GIS also holds open a new way of presenting needs and services delivery that can return nonprofits to their community-based orientation and spur them to new efforts at collaboration.

While many nonprofits will continue to face tight budgets and have to make difficult choices regarding how to invest the limited amount of money they have for overhead, integrating GIS technology can positively impact every part of the organization and is worth supporting. Here funders and foundation can take on a unique role where they are able to drive the sort of organizational, if not system-wide, change they often seek to create with an award. While capacity building grants can be hard to come by, the unique impact that GIS technology can make, especially for nonprofits that can tackle the complex problems facing our most marginalized communities, is worth funders and decision-makers investing in (Al-Kodmany 2012).

Once an organization makes a commitment to adopting and integrating GIS technology, then they must work to go beyond creating maps that look good on a website and create buy-in around the technology, as well as the implications from the visualizations that it can create.

> A wide range of stakeholders is required to ensure that the work extends to ongoing engagement to build a coalition of potential partners and users. Only with broader buy in can the full potential of GIS be realized as a core tool in the community building work undertaken by non-profit organizations.
>
> (Brudney, Russell, Fischer 2016, pg. 16)

While GIS introduces a new dynamic into the work of nonprofits, the principles of their community orientation at the heart of their mission remain the same. Engage your community through genuine and participatory processes. Leverage what you learn to create new visualizations around the work your organization does, what has yet to be done, and what can be improved. Use that information to improve your practices, provide value to your partners as well as stakeholders, and push for the change in your community that will create an equitable and thriving place for all. When GIS is supported and used in this kind of work, it can be a transformational tool for the betterment of everyone.

## References and Further Readings

Al-Kodmany, Kheir, 2012. "Utilizing GIS in Nonprofit Organizations for Urban Planning Applications: Experiences from the Field", *Journal of Geographic Information System*. Volume 4, Pages 279–297.

Bishop, Sheila Watson, 2010. "Building Programmatic Capacity at the Grassroots Level: The Reactions of Local Nonprofit Organizations to Public Participation Geographic Information Systems", *Nonprofit and Voluntary Sector Quarterly*. Volume 39, Number 6, Pages 991–1013.

Brudney, Jeffrey L., Allison Russell, and Robert L. Fischer, 2016. "Using Data to Build Community: Exploring One Model of Geographically Specific Data Use in the Non-Profit Sector", *Community Development Journal*. Volume 51, Issue 2, Pages 354–371.

Chrisman, Nicholas R., 1999. "What Does 'GIS' Mean?" *Transactions in GIS*. Volume 3, Number 2, Pages 175–186.

Coulton, Claudia, Tsui Chan, and Kristsen Mikelbank, 2011. "Finding Place in Community Change Initiatives: Using GIS to Uncover Resident Perceptions of Their Neighborhoods", *Journal of Community Practice*. Volume 19, Pages 10–28.

Dempsey, Caitlin, 2012a. "History of GIS", *GIS Lounge*. May 14, 2017. Retrieved June 14, 2018. www.gislounge.com/history-of-gis/

Dempsey, Caitlin, 2012b. "Who Coined the Phrase Geographic Information System?" *GIS Lounge*. December 17. Retrieved June 14, 2018. www.gislounge.com/phrase-geographic-information-systems/

Elwood, Sarah A., 2002. "GIS Use in Community Planning: A Multidimensional Analysis of Empowerment", *Environment and Planning A*. Volume 34, Pages 905–922.

ESRI, 2018. Big Data Keeps the Lights On. *ArcNews*. Volume 40, Number 2, Page 1.

Gold, Christopher M., 2006. "What Is GIS and What Is Not?" *Transactions in GIS*. Volume 10, Number 4, Pages 505–519.

Hackler, Darren, and Gregory D. Saxton, 2007. "The Strategic Use of Information Technology by Nonprofit Organizations: Increasing Capacity and Untapped Potential", *Public Administration Review*. Volume 67, Issue 3, Pages 474–487.

Local Initiative Support Corporation, 2002. "Mapping for Change: Using Geographic Information Systems for Community Development", December. Retrieved June 22, 2018. www.neighborhoodindicators.org/sites/default/files/publications/LISC_mapping_for_community_change.pdf

MacLaughlin, Steve, 2016. *Data Driven Nonprofits*. Saltire Press, Glasgow.

Reinvestment Fund, 2016. "Documenting the Influence of Fund for Quality Investments on the Supply of and Demand for Child Care in Philadelphia", March. Retrieved October 12, 2017. www.reinvestment.com/childcaremap/pdfs/ReinvestmentFund-Documenting%20the%20Influence%20of%20Fund%20for%20.pdf

Saito, Leland T., 2012. "How Low-Income Residents Can Benefit from Urban Development: The LA Live Community Benefits Agreement", *City & Community*. Volume 11, Issue 2, Pages 129–150.

Sieber, Renee, 2006. "Public Participation Geographic Information Systems: A Literature Review and Framework", *Annals of the Association of American Geographers*. Volume 96, Number 3, Pages 491–507.

Staples, Gracie Bonds, 2017. "You Won't Believe How Poorly Metro Atlanta Children Are Doing", *The Atlanta Journal-Constitution*. March 2. Retrieved April 4, 2018. www.myajc.com/lifestyles/you-won-believe-how-poorly-metro-atlanta-children-are-doing/ozsXhl2kJeLIZgSGrYOrWL/

Sullivan, Sean, 2013. "What is a 501(c)(4), Anyway?" *The Washington Post*. May 13, 2013. Retrieved June 10, 2017. www.washingtonpost.com/news/the-fix/wp/2013/05/13/what-is-a-501c4-anyway/?utm_term=.c615f918f966

Tomlinson, Robert F., 1966, "A Geographic Information System for Regional Planning", *Papers of a CSIRO Symposium*. Retrieved June 14, 2018. https://gisandscience.files.wordpress.com/2012/08/1-a-gis-for-regional-planning_ed.pdf

Treuhaft, Sarah, 2009. "Community Mapping for Health Equity Advocacy", *Report for the Opportunity Agenda*. Retrieved April 22, 2018. https://opportunityagenda.org/sites/default/files/inline-files/Community%20Mapping%20for%20Health%20Equity%20-%20Treuhaft.pdf

United Way of Greater Atlanta, 2018. "Child Well Being Map". Retrieved June 15, 2018. www.unitedwayatlanta.org/child-well-being-map/

Vaz, Eric, and Monica Khaper, 2016. "New Resources for Smart Food Retail Mapping: A GIS and the Open Source Perspective", *Journal of Spatial and Organizational Dynamics*. Volume IV, Issue 4, Pages 305–313.

# 12 West Virginia Trail Inventory

*David Donaldson and Kurt Donaldson*

## Overview

Starting in 2010, the West Virginia Trail Inventory project has been funded by the West Virginia Division of Highways to inventory, collect, and integrate all publicly accessible trails in West Virginia. Currently there are over 5,000 miles of inventoried trails in West Virginia. An online trail application (www.mapwv.gov/trails) allows users to view and identify recreational trails inventoried in West Virginia. In addition, the online trail application allows trails stewards to validate their trail geometry, attributes (e.g. trail surface, trail use, organization), and contact information. The online trail application can be accessed by users with multiple devices, including phones, tablets, or computers. In addition, the freely available GIS trails inventory can be accessed by the public to make customized print or online trail maps, generate trail statistics, and plan future trails, as well as be used for other purposes. In 2018, the West Virginia Division of Highways provided additional funding to finalize the inventory of all trails in West Virginia and to create smartphone applications for recreational trail users.

## Trail Inventory Phases

The West Virginia Trail Inventory project began in 2010, when the first phase funded the West Virginia GIS Technical Center to develop a State Trail Data Model. The next two phases, during the period 2010–2014, in partnership with the Rahall Transportation Institute, encompassed trail data collection efforts for 41 counties, which inventoried 75% of the trails in West Virginia. During this period, the West Virginia GIS Technical Center developed the desktop version of the West Virginia Trail Inventory (www.mapwv.gov/trails). In 2014, a fourth phase funded the mobile Internet version of the trail application (www.mapwv.gov/mtrails). In 2018, a fifth phase was approved for the West Virginia GIS Technical Center to complete the statewide trail inventory of trails, enhance tool functions of existing applications, and develop standalone mobile trail applications for the Android and Apple smartphones.

## Trail Inventory Process

The trail inventory process involves collecting publicly accessible recreational trails in the field using GPS handheld units, processing the trail data into a standardized trail geodatabase with GIS software, and then validating and publishing the trail information (Figure 12.1).

All the trail information resides in the public domain, accessible by either the State Data Clearinghouse (www.wvgis.wvu.edu) or the interactive West Virginia Trail Inventory application (www.mapWV.gov/trails). The trail information adheres to a standardized trail database schema for the trail *lines, point* features of interest, and contacts *table*. It is important that the trail geometries (points and line features), trail attributes (trail owner, trail surface, trail length, trail use, etc.), and trail contact information are collected and stored in a consistent manner. A critical element of the trail inventory process involves contacting the local trail stewards to validate that their trail geometries, trail attributes, and contact information are correct. Likewise, trail stewards can use the Trail Inventory web application to verify their trail geometries and attributes (Figure 12.2 and Figure 12.3).

In addition to collecting missing trails, often the *existing* trails must be updated to reflect trail re-locations, trail closings, modified trail uses, etc. Consequently, it is important to maintain a current *trail contacts* database of all the state and local trail stewards so trail information can be routinely verified.

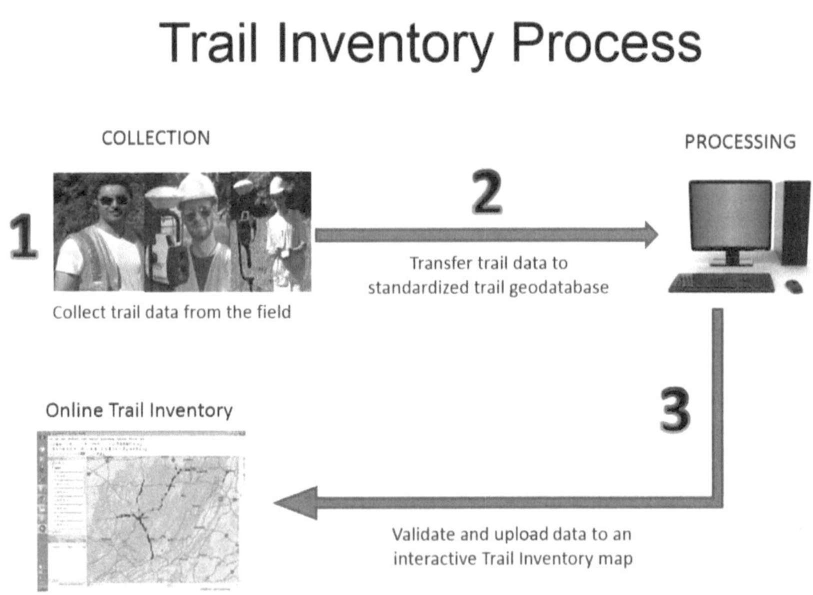


*Figure 12.1* Trail inventory process.

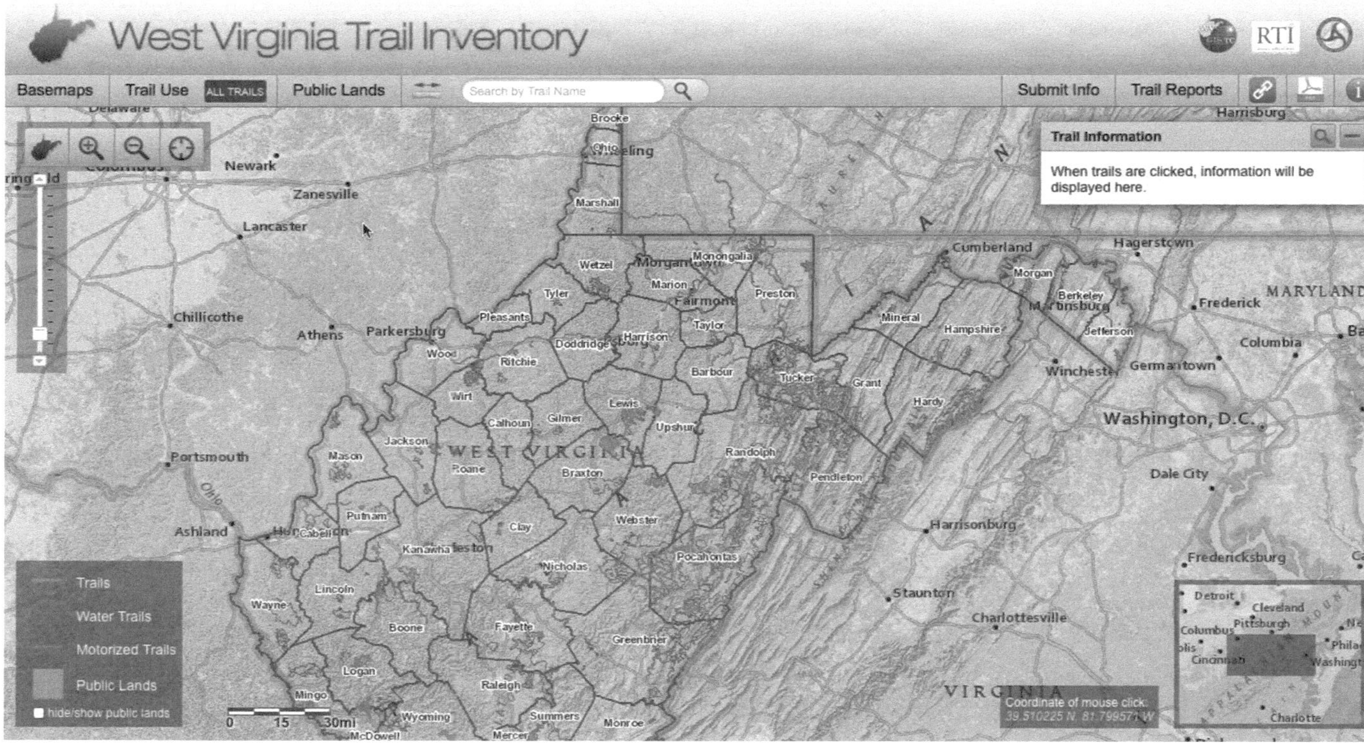


*Figure 12.2* Online trail inventory desktop.

Source: www.mapWV.gov

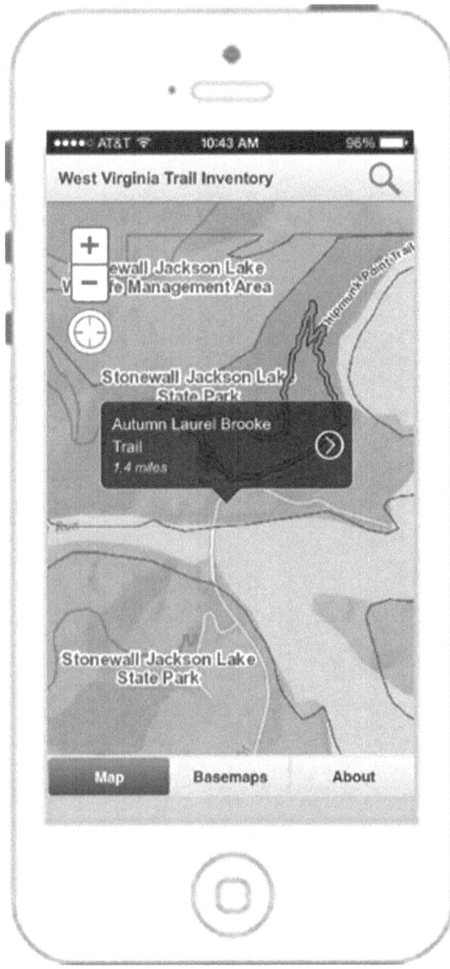


*Figure 12.3* Mobile applications.

Source: www.mapwv.gov/mtrails

## Trail Collection Priorities

High priority trail collection efforts focus on trails located on state and county public lands, nature conservancy lands, designated "blue-water" trails, and motorized trail systems. Lower trail priorities are the National Forests and Parks, which have their own trail inventory programs and are the authoritative sources for national trail inventories. Trails in Wildlife Management Areas (WMA) are maintained by the WV Division of Natural Resources and are primarily designated for hunting and fishing access. WMA trails typically are neither named nor permanent. See Figure 12.4, which depicts state and national data flows for exchanging trail information.

***High Priority***

- State Forests and Parks
- County Parks and City Parks
- Motorized Trail Systems
- Water Trails (blue water or calm water)
- Wildlife and Nature Preserves

***Low Priority***

- National Forests and Parks
- Wildlife Management Areas
- Whitewater Trails
- Adventure Parks (if trails publicly accessible)

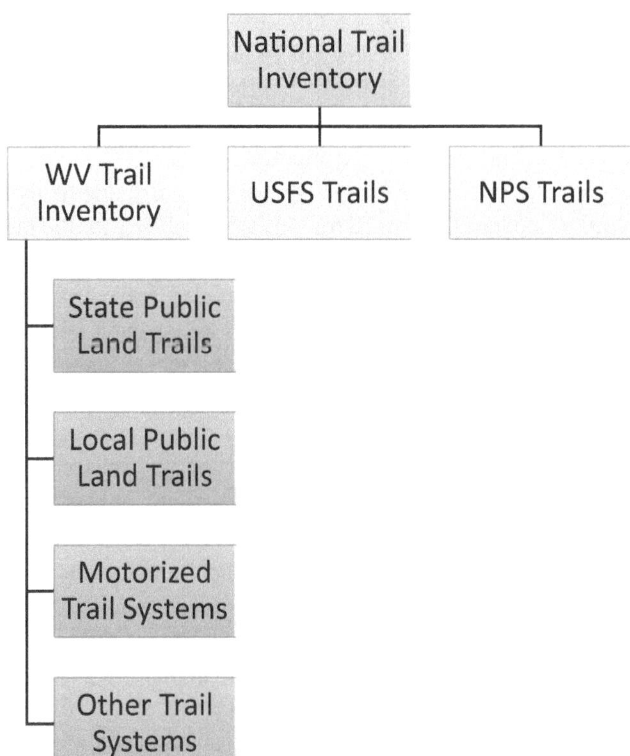


*Figure 12.4* State and national data flows for exchanging trail information.

In 2016, the US Geological Survey consumed the West Virginia Trail Inventory for The National Map. After USGS performed trail analytics, the federal agency commented that the data quality of the West Virginia trails was among the best when compared to other states.

## Trail Inventory Features and Benefits

The trail inventory sponsored by the West Virginia Division of Highways provides many benefits, including the establishment of a comprehensive trail database, trail statistics and reports, static or interactive trail maps, and valuable information for future trail planning. The trail inventory, sponsored and built by public organizations, provides personal and communal benefits to its citizens. It serves the public good by improving our community livability along with providing economic development, recreational, and healthy living benefits.

Features of the Trail Inventory application include a search by trail name and a filter by trail use. Trails can be filtered by non-motorized and motorized trail use. Non-motorized trails filters include hiking, backpacking, horseback riding, fitness, interpretive, cross-country skiing, water, and rail trails. When a trail is selected, a trial information window opens that lists the trail name, trail length, managing organization, management area, trail use, contact information, external trail website link, elevation profile, and downloadable options in GPX or KML formats. A "Submit Trail information" function and share links allows users to exchange vital trail information.

Technologies like GIS allow for the spatial inventory and analysis of the trail inventory. A modern GIS-based trail inventory allows for the public with varying interests and devices to access trail information that was not possible before the digital age. GIS allows virtually limitless trail information to be integrated with map layers. Information such as trail reports, pictures, tables, elevation profiles, and other multi-media can be presented to the trail users.

One of the principal advantages of employing online GIS-based maps is the increased usability and accessibility. A web map can provide information to a wider audience and offers viewers the opportunity to download and customize the data to fit their needs. The trail data can be referenced and overlaid directly with other map applications and web map services. Internet applications also allow for the consumption of valuable map services hosted from different locations and by different publishers, but all seamless to users via a single web map interface.

In the context of trail mapping, these online web services improve data sharing and collaboration among researchers, trail managers, and outdoor enthusiasts who are striving to enhance trail visualization, day-to-day operations management, trail marketing strategies, and the understanding of the impacts trails have on people and their communities. Effectively, many of the shortcomings presented with static trail maps are addressed with the cutting-edge capabilities provided by interactive GIS mapping.

*Table 12.1* Statewide map applications supported by the Center

| *Application* | *Purpose* | *URL* | *State Sponsor* |
|---|---|---|---|
| WV Trail Inventory | Trails | www.mapwv.gov/trails | Division of Highways |
| WV Flood Tool | Flood Hazard Zones | www.mapwv.gov/flood | State Emergency Management Office |
| SHPO Map Viewer | Cultural Resources | www.mapwv.gov/SHPO | State Historic Preservation Office |
| Statewide Addressing & Mapping System | E911 Addresses | www.mapwv.gov/address | State Emergency Management Office |
| Hunting and Fishing | Hunting and Fishing | www.mapwv.gov/huntfish | Division of Natural Resources |
| Highway Plans Locator | Highway Plans | www.mapwv.gov/dotplans | Division of Highways |
| WV Property Viewer | Real Estate Property | www.mapwv.gov/property | Property Tax Division |

## Public Sector Applications

The West Virginia Trail Inventory is part of the mapwv.gov suite of successful web map applications developed and hosted by the West Virginia GIS Technical Center to service the public. Other public-sector applications support hunting and fishing, cultural resources, flood hazards, real estate assessments, and E911 addresses (Table 12.1).

For many of these applications, the Technical Center assists with the state-level integration of important reference data layers like parcels, site addresses, and leaf-off imagery. In 2018, the Technical Center received a Special Achievement in GIS (SAG) Award by ESRI for its important contributions to GIS.

# 13 One Government

## The Enterprise Approach in a Silo Environment

*Cy Smith*

The use of GIS can be very successful in single organizations and for individual projects. However, many important processes, from social service provision to public safety to natural resource management, require multiple organizations across jurisdictions and levels of government, and often including non-governmental organizations, to work closely together. It is often more difficult to implement GIS successfully in that kind of environment. Collaboration is usually required at both operational and policymaking levels. As with an orchestra (Figure 13.1), it is not enough for everyone to have, and to be highly skilled at playing, an instrument.

In addition to a conductor, there must be a piece of music to be played and an agreed-upon process to follow. Every musician must understand the objective of the entire orchestra and their role in achieving that objective for each piece of music. To implement GIS successfully across an enterprise of multiple organizations, it is essential to have a collaborative governance structure, an organizational structure in which collaboration can take place.

Collaborative governance has been studied academically for some time now, but formal studies have increased dramatically in the last decade or so. A recent publication by Emerson and Nabatchi contains a very good history of the academic study of collaborative governance, which also integrates the different pieces of collaborative governance into a dynamic system (*Collaborative Governance Regimes*, Emerson & Nabatchi, 2015). Such systems are very important to the success of GIS in government, and to government in general, but the full importance of collaborative governance is not widely recognized. Simply put, collaborative governance is an organizational structure within which partners can make decisions together.

Collaboration is necessary when the partners have no authority over one another and do not fall under the purview of the same governing body. In other words, no single entity is in charge of their activities, and yet they need to work together to solve a problem or improve a process because it is in their shared interest to do so. There are many examples of collaborative governance processes related to GIS in government, as well as in other organizations. Many state governments have GIS councils that provide a collaborative governance structure for decision-making by a group of state agencies, local governments, universities, tribes, private sector organizations, etc.

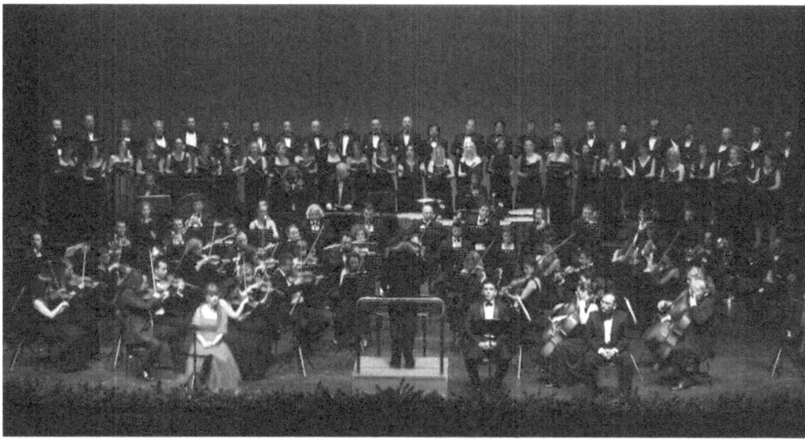

*Figure 13.1* Orchestral collaboration.

The Coalition of Geospatial Organizations is an example of a collaborative governance structure at the national level related to GIS. This coalition is a group of 12 geospatial professional associations that collectively represent over 170,000 GIS practitioners (Coalition of Geospatial Organizations, 2015). The coalition includes such organizations as the American Association of Geographers, the International Association of Assessing Officers, the National Society of Professional Surveyors, and the American Society of Civil Engineers. They have many shared interests and need to develop agreement on a wide range of policy issues in order to enact change and improve the use and potential of GIS nationwide. One of the key contributions made by the coalition is the Report Card on the status of the US National Spatial Data Infrastructure (NSDI), published every three years (Coalition of Geospatial Organizations, 2015).

All 12 coalition member organizations have to agree on every aspect of this extensive report card. The Report Card plays an important role in driving improvements in the NSDI at the national, state, and local levels. Collaboration is necessary for this coalition, and a collaborative governance structure and processes are essential to achieve agreement. There are many processes where organizations from multiple levels of government, and sometimes nongovernmental organizations, are already working separately on public policy issues like childhood trauma, workforce development, emergency response, public health, stream restoration, and much more. But significant progress on those issues is often difficult and sometimes fails because there is no collaborative governance structure that enables the organizations to form effective partnerships to make decisions together on an authoritative, consistent basis. The lack of a formally recognized method for making collaborative decisions results in inefficiency, inconsistency, and waste.

When organizations cannot work together on a consistent, reliable basis, each organization operates on its own to achieve its mission, and duplication of effort is nearly always the result. Multiple organizations develop and maintain road centerline data, or address data, or any number of other necessary datasets. And multiple organizations create applications and web-based tools to use that data. The development and maintenance of the data and tools could be shared if a collaborative governance structure was in place. Additionally, the kind of processes involving cross-organizational effort are almost always comprised of tasks that simply cannot be performed by or within a single organization. Without collaborative effort and decision-making, those processes fail.

There are problems across the United States with drug abuse of one kind or another. Those problems often adversely affect children of drug abusers and have significant societal impact (Figure 13.2).

Methamphetamine abuse has been a serious problem for the children of abusers and suppliers. The Sheriff of Umatilla County in rural northeast Oregon, John Trumbo, said:

> Rarely have I served a search warrant on a meth house where there were not children present. Many times there are babies in diapers crawling through trash on dirty floors, inhaling the toxic fumes from in-house production of methamphetamine by their parents. The future will bring on another epidemic of medical issues for those children related to second-hand exposure to meth chemicals.
>
> (Sheriff Trumbo, 2004)

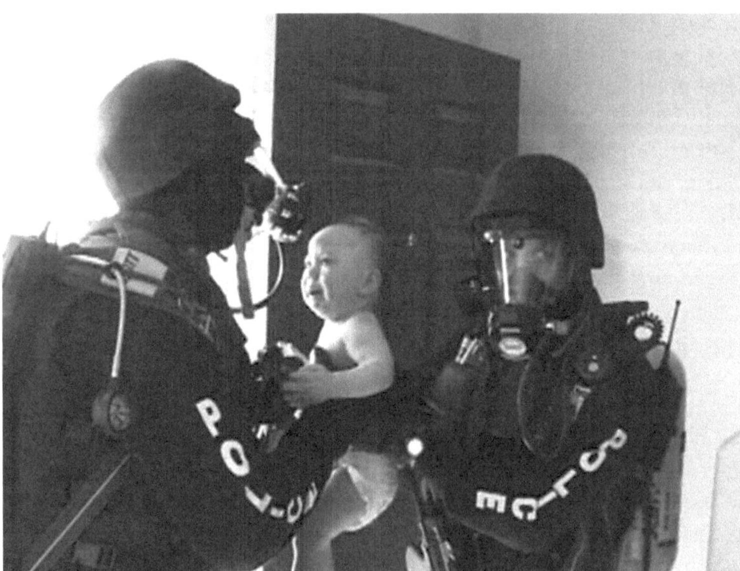

*Figure 13.2* Adverse effects of drug abuse.

Children from homes torn apart by drug abuse often enter the foster care system at a very young age. In 2012, nearly half the children entering the foster care system in Oregon came from homes where the parents were arrested for meth abuse, and a large number of those were under age 4 (OHSU Center for Evidence-Based Policy, 2012). Entry in the system before the age of 4 has a much greater negative, long term impact on a child, resulting in health problems, poor performance later in school, and a much higher rate of incarceration than the societal norm.

Map 13.1 shows the hot spots in Oregon in darker shades where more children entered the foster care system under age 4 (OHSU Center for Evidence-Based Policy, 2012).

Childhood trauma from this and other causes is very expensive in the long term. Investment in children and their families to avoid childhood trauma is worthwhile. There are literally thousands of government and non-government organizations working in this space in Oregon. There are 10,429 nonprofits working in the early childhood space in Oregon, a state with only 1.3% of the US population (John Kitzhaber, 2017). Of course, there are also hundreds of government organizations in the state in this same space. There is very little collaboration or information sharing between these organizations, resulting in duplication and wasted effort. A collaborative governance structure would enable them to work together on solutions to avoid childhood trauma, which would likely save the state and taxpayers a significant amount of money.

A governance structure is a formal recognition of decision rights—who makes which decisions, how those decisions are made, what triggers the necessity for a decision, who sits at the table, who has a say, etc. Governments at all levels are traditionally set up in silos, with funds pushed down those silos by a governing body, like a legislature, commission, or council, to perform discrete functions. But they almost always have to work with other, autonomous organizations in other silos to effectively complete their tasks. The mechanism that can make collaborative work possible, consistently as part of the genetic code of government, is a collaborative governance structure. Collaborative governance is useful between any silos, but when the silos are controlled by separate governing bodies with their own elected or appointed officials, collaborative governance is essential.

GIS is a transformational technology that enables visualization of information, evidence-based decision-making, and more effective performance management. Government often struggles to use information to make decisions because there is no comprehensive governance structure across all levels of government that enables collective decisions and follow through. GIS has been used across a large swath of the western United States in the last few years related to natural resource conservation and mitigating the economic impact of such conservation. This activity involved collaborative governance among a large range of government and non-governmental organizations that do not answer to the same authority but are nevertheless important stakeholders in the decision-making process.

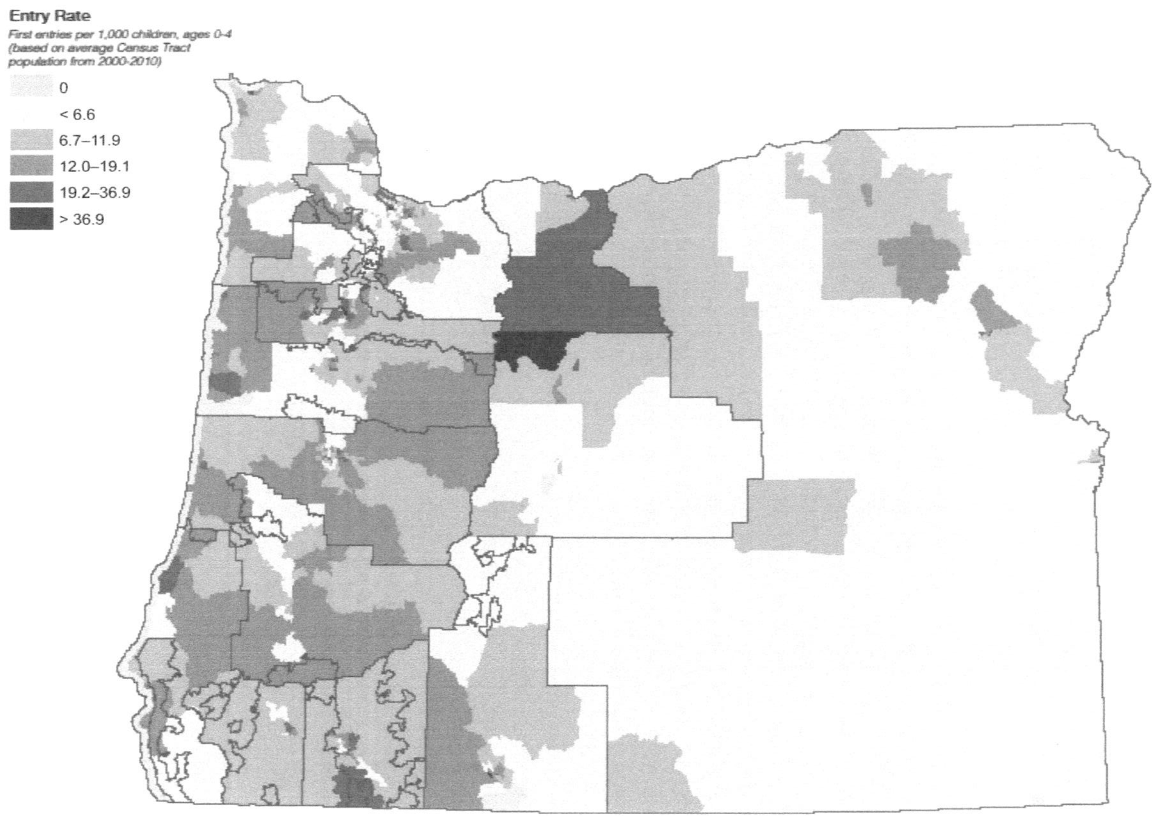


*Map 13.1* Children in Foster Care.

Infrastructure development and renewal normally must go through a permit review and approval process. That process is often time-consuming, difficult to navigate, and expensive, increasing the cost of infrastructure development significantly, if not stymieing it entirely. Finding ways to streamline the permitting process can make a big difference. Geospatial technology and data are important parts of that effort.

Sage grouse habitat stretches across the Pacific Northwest and Northern Rockies, in Oregon, Idaho, Montana, Nevada, and Wyoming, and to a lesser extent Washington, Utah, and northern California. Sage grouse conservation is shorthand for a host of complex issues related to public lands, roles of various levels of government, rural community sustainability, energy and economic development, wildfire, outdoor recreation, and vast ecosystems supporting unique and important wildlife. Sage grouse habitat covers some 175 million acres in that part of the country (Map 13.2) (U.S. Fish and Wildlife Service, 2014).

Habitat protection measures have been developed collaboratively across the region, focusing on core areas that are the highest priorities for the majority of the bird's population. Strengthening land use rules has limited and controlled development in those core areas and requires compensation for impacts on sage grouse habitat through conservation investments. Such investments are designed to provide a net conservation benefit for sage grouse. The stronger land use rules combine habitat protection with greater flexibility to accommodate needed development. The rules also address the potential for a small set of

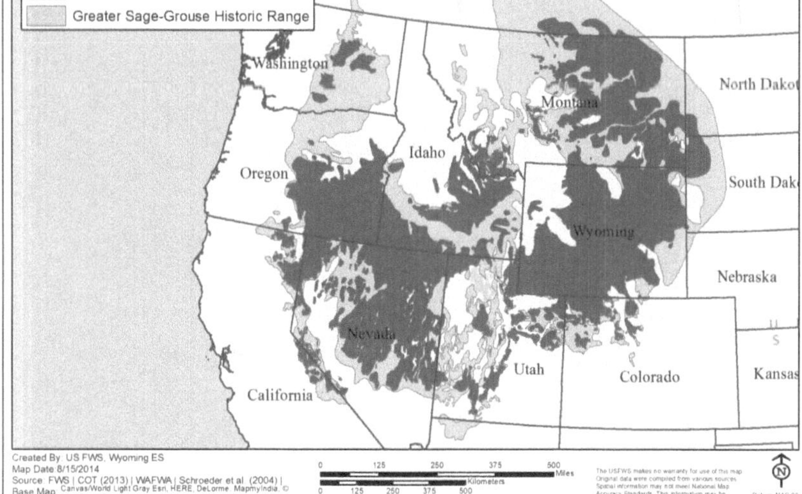


*Map 13.2* Greater Sage Grouse Range.

large-scale development activity that could occur in sage grouse habitat. Local governments retain responsibility for permit evaluation and approval, following standards set at the state level.

Energy development (Figure 13.3), including oil/gas and mining operations, major electrical transmission lines, and renewable energy projects, as well as new or upgraded roads associated with such development, are examples of infrastructure projects that must be evaluated for permits.

A group of ranchers, farmers, developers, utilities, environmental groups, and government agencies used a collaborative governance process to find methods for permitting development in such ecologically sensitive areas. Their work has streamlined the process, significantly shortened the time required for permit approval, and halted the potential listing of sage grouse as a threatened and endangered species, which would have further complicated the permitting process.

Maps and geospatial data provide a tool for planning and identifying appropriate mitigation in the event of human development in sage grouse habitat. Large-scale infrastructure development and renewal is potentially some of the most disruptive for sage grouse habitat. The collection, modeling, and mapping of biological data using geospatial technology allows government agencies to determine species densities and calculate age ratios, sex ratios, peak hatch dates, and proportion of successful hens. Blood samples from harvested birds has enabled tracking and research on West Nile virus.

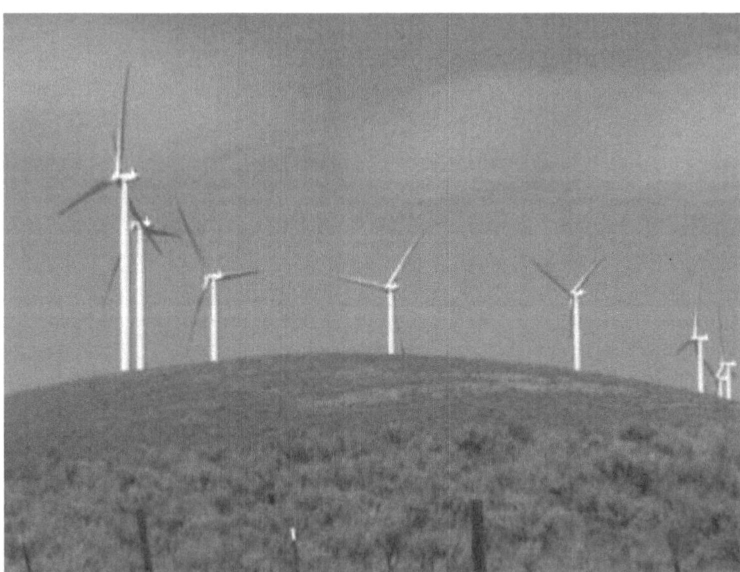

Elkhorn Wind Farm (Baker County)

*Figure 13.3* Infrastructure in ecologically sensitive area.

Breeding density data combined with legal and administrative boundary lines and overlaid on National Agricultural Imagery Program (NAIP) aerial imagery enabled the collaborative stakeholders to evaluate habitat and topography in establishing the initial core areas for protection. A series of other maps and geospatial analyses of the core areas, including oil/gas development sites, mining permit boundaries, permitted wind development, sage grouse breeding areas, and base data (roads, surface water, etc.), provided the necessary understanding to hone the core area boundaries and establish the initial land use rules to guide the permitting process.

The land use rules and associated permitting processes were further refined and streamlined with the use of sagebrush habitat maps, sage grouse observation data, human footprint data, updated sage grouse breeding density data, and many other supplemental geospatial datasets and geospatial analyses. In addition to the creation and refinement of the core areas, geospatial technology and data were also used to identify "connectivity" habitat corridors to support sage grouse movement and genetic connectivity between populations in the various states.

The hurdles to permit streamlining are not primarily related to geospatial technology and data. The collaboration necessary to achieve such streamlining is exceedingly difficult and requires far-sighted leadership at all levels and among all stakeholder communities. There are more than just environmental issues at play in the permit process, of course, and each issue presents its own set of challenges that takes significant leadership and collaboration to overcome.

The challenges that are related to geospatial technology and data are funding and collection or acquisition/sharing of appropriate data. Technology and data require significant short-term funding for development at the required levels and long-term funding to continue to support the permitting process. Even with sufficient funding, challenges related to collecting or acquiring data, and with sharing data between jurisdictions, can be significant problems that have to be carefully managed over time. Collaboration is difficult, even under the best circumstances, and requires the development of an appropriate collaborative governance structure, great leadership, and continuous effort and investment.

Work was done in Oregon by the state government a few years ago to design a collaborative governance structure to enable evidence-based policymaking, as visualized in Figure 13.4.

It was based on the collaborative governance structure for GIS that has been used in Oregon for over three decades to make decisions among federal, state, local, tribal, and regional government organizations. The governor's desired outcomes related to health, safety, the environment, the economy, etc., underpinned the approach. Key organizations that represent 96% of the state budget were identified as stakeholders in each of the governor's policy areas (Oregon Chief Financial Services Office, 2014). Those stakeholder groups identify or articulate activities and programs that collectively achieve desired outcomes. The Enterprise Leadership Team develops definitions of desired

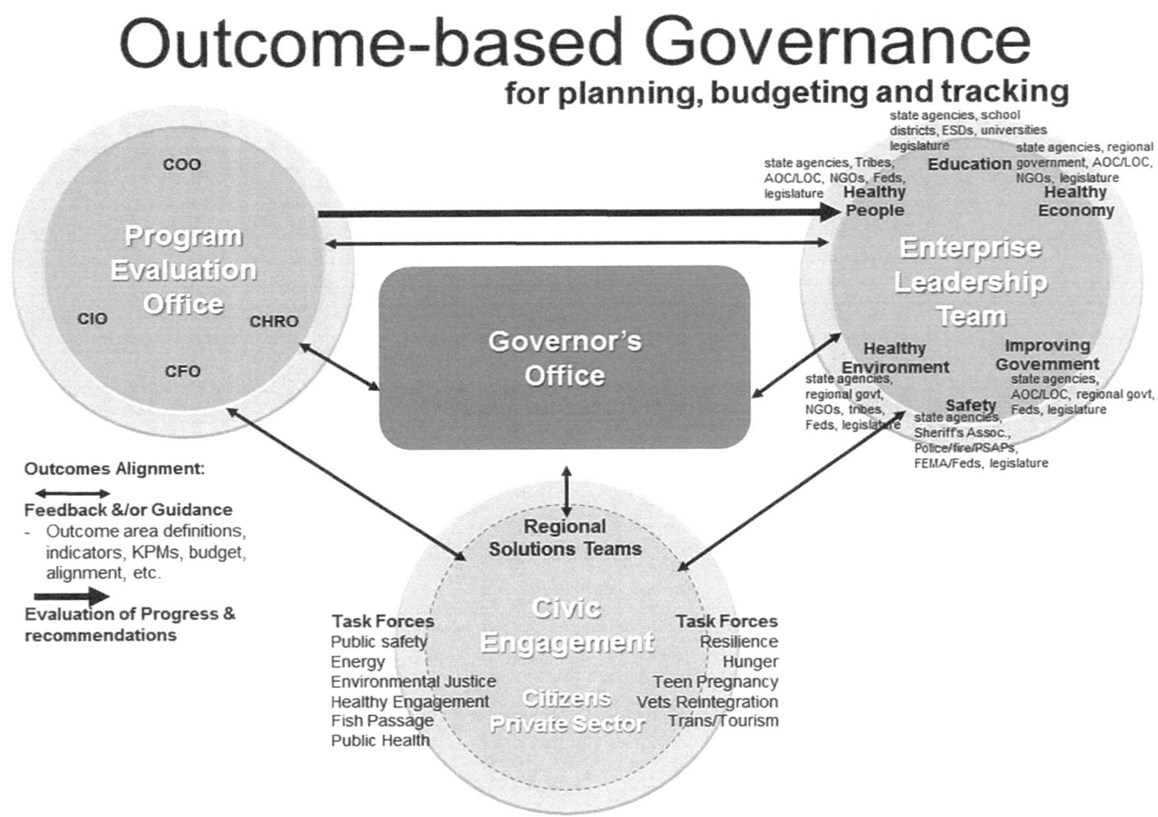


*Figure 13.4* Outcome-based governance.

outcomes, including indicators that are outcome-based and measurable, and works with the stakeholder groups to refine those outcomes and measures.

The Program Evaluation Office, comprised of staff from the offices of the State's Chief Operating Officer (COO), Chief Financial Officer (CFO), Chief Information Officer (CIO), and Chief Human Resources Officer (CHRO), provides guidance and feedback to the stakeholders and Enterprise Leadership Team on outcomes. The public is involved in the collaborative governance process through the Civic Engagement task forces, most of which existed prior to the development of the proposed governance structure. The proposed model is not intended as a replacement for the existing silo structure of government. It is a formal collaborative model designed to connect the silos in a persistent manner, to enable government business processes to be conducted and prevent those collaborative processes from breaking down when people move around within and between silos. When operating at full maturity, it would engage all the government and non-governmental organizations in decision-making related to collaborative processes, and envisions civic engagement in a constructive way through focused task forces.

In part, the work put into this aspirational model prompted a fresh look at ways to overcome barriers to geospatial data sharing among and between all public bodies operating throughout Oregon. Despite significant progress over the 35 years since the Oregon Geographic Information Council was established by Governor's Executive Order, struggles have continued with a problem common to government organizations worldwide: inability or unwillingness to share data with partners. Instead of sharing data, government organizations often duplicate data development, update, use, and storage at great cost.

The Oregon Geographic Information Council (OGIC) commissioned a study ten years ago and found that Oregon state and local government spent $5 billion annually on geospatial data development, management, and use, and that they collectively wasted $200 million annually on those activities. Approximately 80% of the expense and waste was related to personnel costs for duplicated data development and update (PlanGraphics, Inc., 2007).

To combat these seemingly intractable data sharing issues, OGIC decided to seek statutory authorization for the collaborative governance structure of the Council and its mission, and a mandate for public bodies to share at least the base, or reference geospatial data, called Framework data. Prior to this effort, the Governor's Executive Order that formed OGIC's authorization was only able to provide authority over executive branch state agencies. In the 2017 Oregon legislative session, the Council's effort was successful. The new legislation establishes OGIC as a collaborative governance body representing all public bodies in Oregon: state, county, city, special district, and regional government (State of Oregon, 2017).

The effort to enact the Oregon collaborative governance statute is instructive. At the direction of the Legislature, OGIC established a 24-member, multi-jurisdictional stakeholder group to draft the legislation. This stakeholder group worked for nine months to craft an agreed-upon statute prior to legislative introduction of the agreed-upon bill (HB 2906). The new law mandates that all public bodies in Oregon share geospatial Framework data with each other free of charge. The regional, tribal, and local government stakeholders demanded, in exchange for their support, that the legislation include the necessity to share the Framework data securely, meaning that the data is not all simply placed in the public domain.

That provision sets the stage for the State CIO's Geospatial Enterprise Office to set up a secure data hub from which all public bodies will share Framework data with each other. This approach has created a new partnership between all public bodies and a collaborative governance structure to make decisions about how that partnership will be managed. The new OGIC collaboration gives all public bodies an equitable seat at the table and should result in significant savings and/or cost avoidance over time. It will also lead to more consistent, effective, and efficient government services across the state, as most government services rely on geospatial data.

The public utilities, public universities, federal agencies, nonprofit organizations, and citizens are also represented on the new governance structure. The Council is tasked with making a recommendation to the legislature to establish a sustainable funding mechanism to help local governments and other public bodies pay for development and maintenance of standardized Framework data statewide. The collaborative governance approach has already generated a renewed discussion with the public utilities about sharing geospatial data with public bodies in Oregon.

The reluctance of utilities, like electric, gas, and telecommunications, to share geospatial data with public bodies has had serious consequences (Figure 13.5).

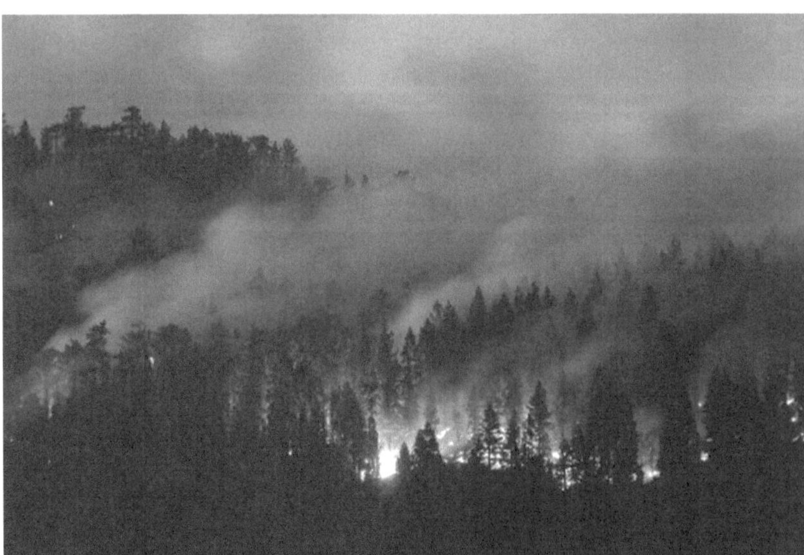

*Figure 13.5* Wildfire in Oregon.

One of the most serious in Oregon occurred in 2004 during a heavy wildfire season. To fight wildfires, emergency responders from many different jurisdictions must come together in areas with which they may be unfamiliar. They often use helicopters to search for nearby ponds and lakes from which to gather water to fight the wildfire. They send planes back to scoop the water from bodies large enough and open enough to accommodate such activity. The planes then drop the water on the fire to extinguish it and return for more water.

But the helicopter pilot looking for water sources to fight a wildfire near The Dalles in north central Oregon in 2004 (Figure 13.6) did not have data about the location of electric lines.

The helicopter pilot clipped a line and crashed, killing himself and a state forester riding with him. This situation still exists today, but discussions are finally underway to solve the problem based on the establishment of the improved collaborative governance structure for GIS. This is not simply a data sharing issue. It is, more importantly, a collaboration issue. If the public utilities have a seat at the table and are able to participate in how, when, and for what purpose their data will be shared, the problem can be solved in a way that persists beyond an agreement reached between a few people or organizations.

To effectively address wildfire risks, or childhood trauma, or development in sensitive environmental areas, or any of the myriad other problems in which GIS can play an important and enabling role, we must have consistent, trustworthy data when and where it is needed. In order to make that happen, we also must have more effective methods for collaborating on these and all our other shared problems. We must have collaboration across the silos of government,

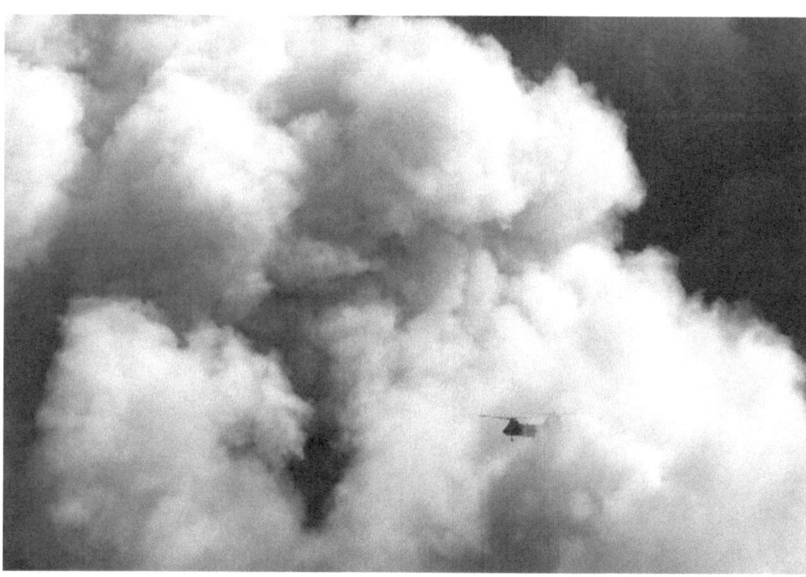

*Figure 13.6* Seeking water for a wildfire.

collaborative governance structures that persist in the same way the silos persist, regardless whether specific people come or go.

## References

Emerson & Nabatchi, 2015. *Collaborative Governance Regimes*. Washington, DC, Georgetown University Press.

Coalition of Geospatial Organizations, 2015. *National Spatial Data Infrastructure (NSDI) Report Card*, February 6, 2015. Retrieved on June 5, 2018. http://cogo.pro/uploads/COGO-Report_Card_on_NSDI.pdf

Kitzhaber, John, 2017. Governor of Oregon John Kitzhaber, 2017 presentation at Oregon GIS in Action conference.

OHSU Center for Evidence-Based Policy, 2012. *Foster Care Impacts in Oregon*, Portland, OR.

Oregon Chief Financial Services Office, 2014. *State Budget Summary*, Salem, OR.

PlanGraphics, Inc., 2007. Business Case for the Development of a Statewide GIS Utility, Salem, OR.

State of Oregon, 2017. Oregon Revised Statutes 276A. 500–515.

Trumbo, John, 2004. Sheriff of Umatilla County.

U.S. Fish and Wildlife Service, 2014. U.S. Fish and Wildlife Services, Wyoming Ecological Services, 2014.

# 14 GIS Practices for Best-Run County Governments

*Greg Babinski*

## Introduction

A Geographic Information System should be designed, managed, and operated to support the business case of the entity that it serves. There is extensive literature on generic GIS program management (Tomlinson 2013; Croswell 2009). The URISA GIS Management Institute was established to help develop best practices related to GIS operation and management (Babinski 2018).

This chapter will focus on key challenges, opportunities, and *good practices* related to managing and operating a Geographic Information System (GIS) for a county government. Good practices for county GIS management and operations can be classified conceptually in three categories: first, GIS for local government functions that are usually performed only by county governments; second, GIS for local government responsibilities that are shared between county and municipal governments; and third, GIS functions that could be shared by both county and municipal governments.

This chapter will also outline how the URISA GIS Capability Maturity Model can help GIS managers and stakeholders systematically evaluate the management of their GIS and incrementally improve their operational practices.

### *Business Case of Counties*

Counties are a form of municipal government, but with aspects of their business case that differentiate them from city, state, and provincial government entities. The business case for any governmental jurisdiction can be thought of as a moral imperative to maximize the potential benefits from its assets to the benefit of the jurisdiction's stakeholders. In many cases, the stakeholders and key assets are one and the same. Key assets that also represent stakeholders include the citizens and residents of the jurisdiction. Businesses and educational and cultural institutions also can be both assets and stakeholders. The natural resources within a jurisdiction represent assets. However, while we would not think of natural resources as stakeholders, they should be considered as held in trust to optimize their sustainable usefulness. Likewise, the future generations that will populate the jurisdiction, either as descendants or as immigrants, are not usually thought of as stakeholders. Nevertheless, all the assets of the jurisdiction should be considered to be held in trust for these future generations. Another asset is the jurisdiction's brand, or reputation—is it a good place to live, work, study, raise a family, start a business, or retire? One last asset is the jurisdiction's geography. The site and situation of a location describe the geographic factors within the jurisdiction's boundaries (site), and the jurisdiction's locational geography (situation) relative to the broader region, state, province, nation, or global environment (Abler et al. 1971). Best-run county governments leverage GIS to maximize the current and future potential of the jurisdiction's assets.

### *The Unique Nature of Counties*

Counties in the United States, Canada, and many other countries are a form of intermediate municipal government. For this chapter, counties are defined as a first-tier subdivision of a state or provincial government. Counties also usually include other government subdivisions within their boundaries. For example, in the United States, counties (or parishes in Louisiana and boroughs in Alaska) are typically chartered by the state. Within US counties are usually found second-tier subdivisions, including cities, towns, villages, townships, boroughs, etc. Most provinces in Canada also have counties or regional districts as first-tier jurisdictional subdivisions, with second-tier municipalities contained within counties.

There are some exceptions to the normal intermediate nature of county governments. Two states (Rhode Island and Connecticut) have abolished counties as functional entities. Within some states and provinces, city and county governments have merged (the City and County of San Francisco, for example). In Virginia, where counties do exist, all cities are independent of their county, reporting directly to the Commonwealth government. Nevertheless, for most of the 3,142 counties in the United States and for most of the counties and municipal districts in Canada, the intermediate nature of their governmental responsibilities impacts the nature of their Geographic Information System.

For this chapter, I will use the term *county* to refer to counties, boroughs, parishes, and municipal districts in the United States and Canada that serve as first-tier subdivisions of their state or province. I will use the term *municipality* to refer to second-tier municipal subdivisions (cities, towns, villages, townships, etc.).

### *Basic Principles and Finites of Nature*

In addition to the preliminary discussion about the nature of counties and municipalities, above, there are a few basic natural law-related principles that validate the need for GIS and create an imperative for its use by any governmental jurisdiction. These principles are related to a small number of *finites* that impact every life.

First, while the universe is infinite, the space that we humans share on this Earth is finite. And when we focus on our local county or municipality, space in the form of real estate is truly limited and its value is derived from a variety of locational factors. Related to the concept of finite space is location within space. Second, within the shared space on Earth, non-renewable natural resources are finite. Also, non-human communities compete for a share of the global ecosystem. Third, while from a universal perspective we assume that time is infinite, from our human perspective, it is finite. The finite nature of time at the human scale is limited by the span of a life, by an age of life, by budget years, project schedules, loan terms, monthly reports, weekly meetings, daily to-do lists, commutes, alarm clocks, and ever-present deadlines. Lastly, money is finite. Availability of money determines many of the mundane personal decisions of life. Money drives business decisions. Human demand for a share of finite space, for preferred location within space, for natural resources, and for time are all expressed in monetary value. For counties and municipalities, budgets determine social priorities for the limited financial resources that taxes and other funding sources provide.

Why do these *finites* matter? Counties and municipalities work because they concentrate people, resources, ideas, industries, and markets. Places where people come together are the centers of innovation. With exceptions, cities generally are the place where individuals come together to build better lives for themselves and their descendants. Cities work by enabling the easy circulation of people, services, ideas, and innovations. Within this exciting environment of municipalities, counties play a key role in partnership with the cities.

However, concentration with municipalities puts a premium on the best locations. Suburbs form to move some of the housing, business, and schools to lower-cost real estate. Also, concentration and increased circulation invariably result in friction within the transportation infrastructure in the form of traffic congestion, crowding, strained utility networks, and increased cost and lost opportunity. Circulation of people, products, and services across space takes time, and time is money. Finite space, resources, time, and money are inter-related. And GIS is a proven tool to understand the inter-connection of these factors and to enable optimal urban and regional development, planning, and management.

The author has proposed a moral imperative for the GIS profession related to these finites (Babinski 2012):

> The GIS profession uses geographic theory, spatial analysis, and geospatial technology to help society manage the Earth's finite space, with its natural resources and communities, on a just and sustainable basis for the benefit of humanity.

## Thinking About GIS for Counties

GIS managers, operators, and stakeholders need a framework to analyze the business needs of county GIS and the suitability of the Geographic Information System resources available to meet those business needs.

A sustainable GIS requires that management and stakeholders periodically assess key risk factors. GIS factors include lack of adequate resources, lack of staff redundancy/capacity, deferred maintenance, and ad-hoc or, at best, repeatable but non-documented processes.

The GIS Capability Maturity Model provides a framework to assess the key components of any Geographic Information System. It can be used to analyze GIS for local government functions. The GISCMM can also help us think about GIS functions that could be shared by both county and municipal governments in a GIS-utility environment.

### *The GIS Capability Maturity Model*

The URISA GIS Capability Maturity Model (URISA 2013) allows GIS stakeholders to examine and assess an individual Geographic Information System in sufficient detail to draw conclusions about its developmental status, suitability to support business needs, and operations, maintenance, and management practices. This model examines both the capability of a GIS (hardware, software, data, staff resources) and its process maturity (operations, maintenance, usage, and management).

The GIS Capability Maturity Model (GISCMM) identifies 23 enabling capability components of a Geographic Information System. Enabling capability is described as "the technology, data, resources, and related infrastructure that can be bought, developed, or otherwise acquired to support typical enterprise GIS operations. Enabling capability includes GIS management and professional staff" (GIS Management Institute 2013). The GISCMM rates each component against a developmental scale progressing to full development sufficient to meet the business needs of the entity that the GIS supports.

The GIS Capability Maturity Model also identifies 22 execution ability components of a GIS. Execution ability is described as "the ability of the [GIS] staff to maximize the use of the available capability, relative to a normative ideal". The "normative ideal" assumed by the GISCMM is that the operation, maintenance, and management of a GIS is most effective when based on defined and document procedures, supported by performance metrics, and periodically reassessed to apply improved processes and practices (GIS Management Institute 2013).

One note about the term *best practice* as related to GIS. Ask a group of GIS managers if they use *best practices* to operate their GIS, and invariably hands will raise. However, without a means to validate that a GIS management practice warrants the superlative *best*, what most are really using are *good* GIS management practices. The URISA GIS Management Institute has proposed a process to develop a body of thoroughly researched, vetted, and peer-reviewed GIS best practices that would correspond to the components of the GIS Capability Maturity Model. Nevertheless, best-run county governments should continually strive to improve their operational practices.

### *Generic and Shared Responsibilities of County Governments*

While there are many variations across specific states and provinces, there are several key governmental responsibilities that are usually delegated to counties. These often include responsibilities for regional policing and jails, E911, superior courts, elections, public defense, property assessment, tax collection, regional highways, regional transit, regional parks and trails, regional planning and zoning, regional emergency management coordination, and so on.

Other responsibilities may be shared with or exclusively the purview of municipalities. While there are many exceptions, these can include municipal utilities, municipal policing, fire protection, and emergency medical. Other governmental functions that are more municipal-focused include but are not limited to urban planning, city streets and street addressing, permitting, schools, and local parks.

### *GIS ROI and GIS Effectiveness*

A number of basic principles support good county GIS management practices. Society expects good value from the portion of its financial resources that it provides for GIS. While the ROI from county GIS has been proven (Zerbe et al. 2016), GIS managers should understand and be prepared to communicate the basis for good return on investment. Local agency elected officials and administration leadership will consider ROI for any new capital project investment or program funded from ongoing operational sources. GIS competes for funds with every agency program. The mere fact that a GIS program or a major enhancement to the GIS provides a return on investment may not guarantee the needed funding. Other major investments, new programs, or expanded services within an agency will be developing its own ROI forecast. A new GIS imagery acquisition project may compete for funds with a public works proposal for a new utility excavation machine, a new public safety forensic system, a proposed traffic decongestion project, or an expanded environmental health service. A GIS manager must understand how to determine GIS program ROI and communicate its value within this environment of competing needs for funding.

In its simplest terms, GIS ROI is derived by minimizing costs and maximizing financial benefits (see Figure 14.1). Minimizing GIS development, implementation, operation, and maintenance costs is difficult. But it is these costs that represent hard dollars in county budgets. GIS managers should be rigorous in looking for opportunities to minimize or even reduce costs. The first-tier subdivision nature of counties can provide opportunities to reduce agency costs by sharing or collaborating the components of the GIS.

GIS ROI is also derived by maximizing benefits. Fortunately, most of the GIS operations, maintenance, and management costs are fixed in nature. GIS benefits from the fact that most of the expensive components of GIS can be used by an almost unlimited number of users with little incremental cost.

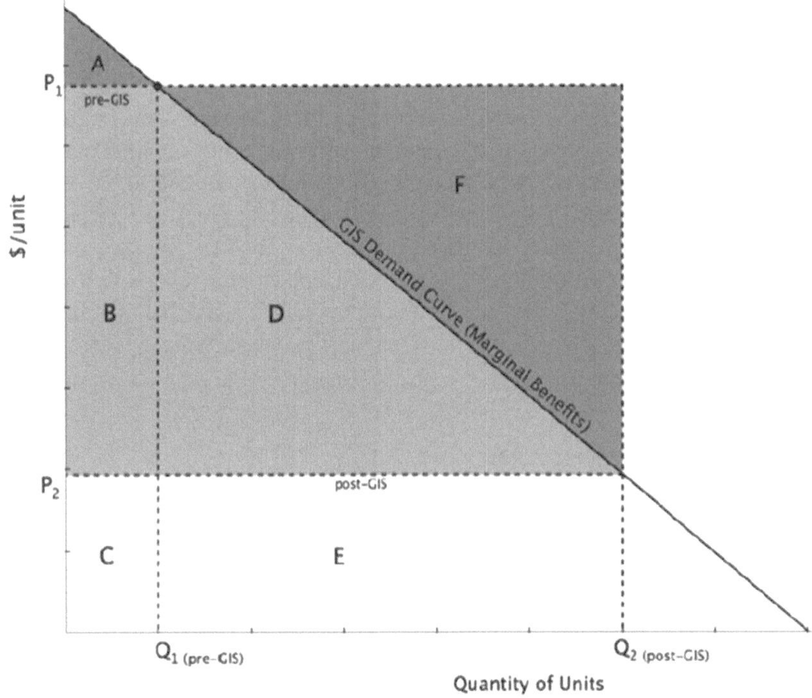


*Figure 14.1* GIS ROI is derived both by reducing operational costs ($P_1$ to $P_2$) or by increasing quantifiable benefits ($Q_1$ to $Q_2$).

Source: Zerbe et al. (2016)

A regional water utility might justify development of its GIS with as few as 5% of its staff being GIS users. But the same utility could easily put GIS tools into the hands of 25% or more of its staff for a minimal increase in costs. GIS is a "build it once and use it many times" system.

In addition to ROI, GIS provides many other benefits. GIS can enable more effective government services and better decision-making. GIS can also help agencies respond efficiently to unfunded mandates from the national and state/provincial government levels. GIS can help agencies implement policy priorities from their elected leadership. County GIS data and resources, when open for use by citizens, researchers, students, nonprofits, and businesses, can provide regional economic benefits and more informed participation in democratic processes.

There are some basic principles that apply to both municipal and county governments and their GIS operations. First, citizens expect their levels of government to cooperate and coordinate their activities. While most citizens do not think about how GIS is organized and operated, an appropriate question for GIS managers to ask is, "how would citizens and journalists judge our use of financial resources for GIS in the context of potential cross-jurisdiction cooperation and cost savings?" When the author worked as GIS Mapping Supervisor for East Bay Municipal Utility District in Oakland, California, this was a question that served as a filter for conceiving, designing, developing, and implementing new projects or services.

Second, citizens expect their government agencies to focus on value-added functions and services. While a well-designed and adequately resourced GIS is critical, GIS managers should focus on the value that GIS provides for their agency and the citizens and other customers that it services. Back-office GIS functions are a critical foundation, but they do not add value. GIS managers should understand and minimize costs while maintaining capability and ensuring sustainability of their GIS. GIS managers should maximize utilization by promoting low-cost access to GIS tools and data by as many staff as possible. And GIS managers should put GIS tools and data into the hands of citizens, businesses, and other government agencies.

### *County–City GIS Coordination*

There are many common areas where counties and municipalities cooperate. A good practice for a county GIS manager is to establish a strong relationship with the GIS leadership in all the jurisdictions within the county boundaries and with nearby jurisdictions. Shared geography, citizens, businesses, and taxpayers between the county and the cities, tribes, special districts, and state and federal agencies provide special opportunities to seek out and implement GIS-related resource and services sharing. This can both reduce costs for participating agencies and enable enhanced and more sustainable GIS services. King County, the thirteenth most populous county in the US, includes 39 cities, two tribes, a regional planning agency, a regional transit agency, an E911 agency, and a port within its boundaries. Twenty-two of the 39 cities operate GIS (see Figure 14.2).

What competencies should the county GIS manager develop to be effective at regional GIS coordination? The URISA Geospatial Management Competency Model (GIS Management Institute 2012) was adopted by USDOLETA as tier 9 of the Geospatial Technology Competency Model in 2012. The GMCM identifies a number of key GIS-related management competencies that are relevant for the regional GIS coordination function of a county GIS Manger. These include:

1. Foster and environment conducive to teamwork.
2. Develop and maintain relationships with other organizations to promote mutually advantageous partnerships and best practices.
3. Develop and maintain strategic partnerships.
4. Build consensus.
5. Identify collaborative opportunities to achieve project goals.

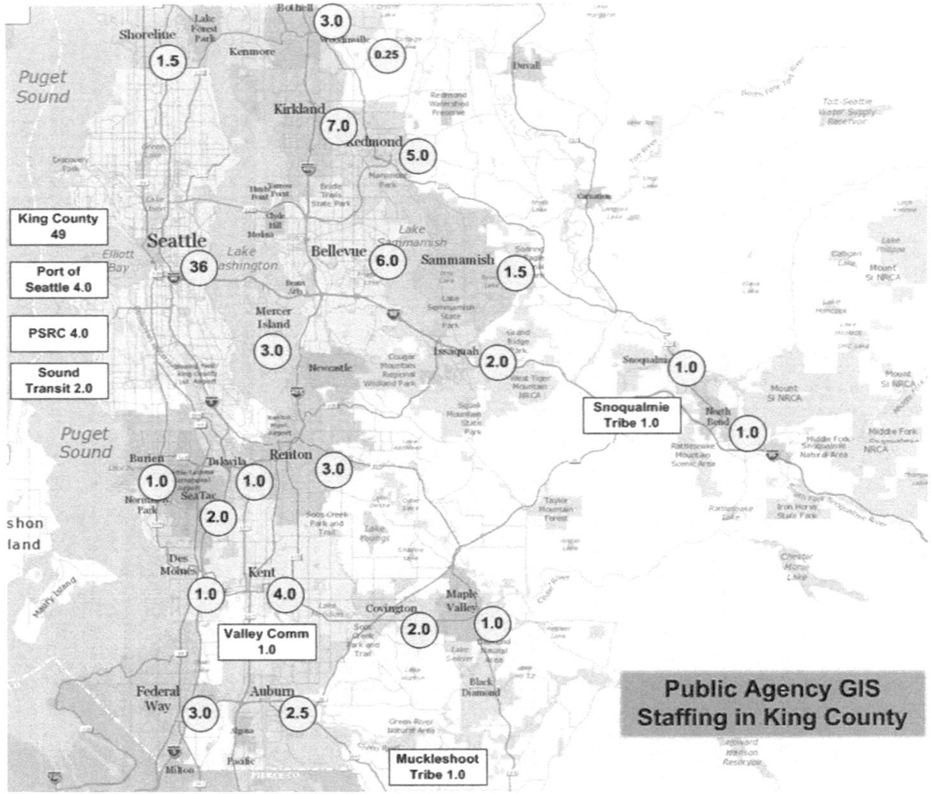


*Figure 14.2* 2016 Public agency GIS staff within King County (does not include public utility and special districts).

Source: Babinski (2016a)

6. Cooperate within political and professional organizations.
7. Pursue goals tactfully in context of particular organizational cultures and governance structures.
8. Respect jurisdictional responsibilities.
9. Develop service level agreements.
10. Identify funding sources and obtain funding, including collaborative opportunities.

## The GISCMM and Good County GIS Practices

A key concept for good GIS operations is that counties, because of the intermediate nature of their governmental responsibilities, are typically in an excellent position to *acquire* key components of their GIS from outside sources. Acquired resources usually save considerable cost. Counties are also well positioned to share their GIS components, both up to the state/provincial level and down to the municipal level of government.

Within the GISCMM, Enabling Capability GIS data is covered by four specific components: framework GIS data, framework GIS data maintenance, business GIS data, and business GIS data maintenance. The assumption is that each key data component includes both an acquisition/development stage and an ongoing maintenance stage. Framework data corresponds to the seven FGDC-defined NSDI framework data types. Business GIS data is defined by the county or other agency itself. This agency-defined key business data should support the priority business functions of the jurisdiction. In 2016, King County GIS completed a GIS self-assessment report against the GISCMM (see Figure 14.3).

### *Geodetic Control Data (EC1a)*[1]

Geodetic control is included as an NSDI framework dataset because good, accurate survey control is the bedrock foundation for all other GIS data layers. Good county GIS management practice is to work with the county surveyor to compile and make available all regional recorded monumentation. A good example is DuPage County, IL GIS. County GIS should also coordinate with other survey groups that do work within their jurisdiction. These could include city engineers and surveyors, the state, provincial, or national highway department, or private survey firms that record their survey work. A countywide geodetic control database can both benefit from this regional coordination and provide a valuable regional resource that provides ROI for other government agencies, business, and citizens.

### *Cadastral Data (EC1b)*

In the United States, most states delegate private property assessment and property-based taxation to counties. The system of property parcel mapping

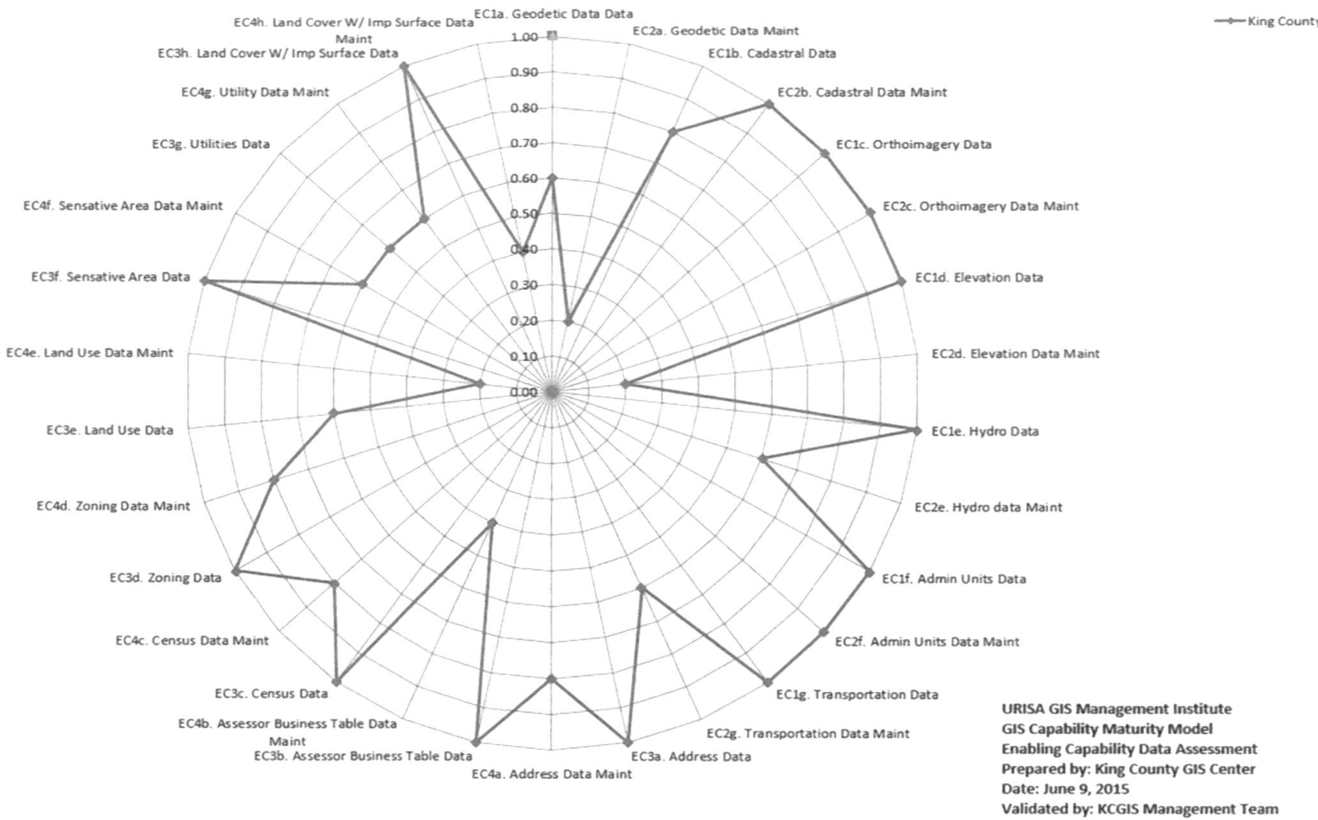


*Figure 14.3* King County GIS data assessed against a portion of the GIS Capability Maturity Model.

Source: Babinski (2016b)

and information is referred to as a cadaster. As early as 1980, the key role of a digital multi-purpose cadaster was recognized as a key requirement for an effective local government agency GIS (Somers and Eichelberger, 1987). In Canada and in some US states (Oregon), cadastral property parcel data can be provided by the province or state to counties and other subordinate jurisdictions. In most US counties, however, cadastral data development and maintenance is a key data responsibility.

A good practice for county GIS operations is to make highly accurate and up-to-date cadastral data available for use by the municipalities within its boundaries. A good relationship with cities is important because property splits and subdivisions usually originate in municipalities. For example, the South Central Regional Council of Governments both consumes GIS-based cadastral data and makes it publicly available via an online portal. King County GIS property parcel data is viewable on two versions of a public-facing web application. More than half the 39 municipalities within King County include links on their web sites to these King County GIS parcel data viewers. These two King County applications are used more than three million times annually by outside agencies, businesses, researchers, and citizens.

### *Orthoimagery Data (EC1c)*

Orthoimagery (and other remotely sensed data like LiDAR) is an expensive component of a GIS. And because the data becomes out of date as soon as the sensor platform lands, it must be updated periodically for maximum utility and relevance.

A key responsibility of a county GIS manager is to determine and document the business requirements for imagery data within the jurisdiction. This requires an understanding of the variations in remotely sensed data types, and of the possible variations in data quality. Variations in business requirements for remotely sensed data type and quality within a county can vary considerably. For example, within dense urban areas with extensive public and private built infrastructure, higher resolution natural color imagery is needed more than in rural agricultural districts. Agricultural areas within a county may need infrared data but with much lower resolution requirements.

Good county GIS practice is to assume a leadership position in the multi-agency acquisition and maintenance of orthoimagery. Often, medium-resolution data can be acquired at the state or provincial level from the transportation department or agriculture department. A GIS manager should have a good working relationship with the GIS leads for these state departments related to their imagery acquisition projects. In addition to acquiring this data at reduced costs, the county GIS manager can eliminate the considerable effort and expense for project management of an imagery acquisition project. Other key contacts for keeping informed about acquiring data in the US include the regional USGS National Map Liaison and the USDA National Agricultural Imagery Program.

However, for the higher resolution imagery required for many county and municipal GIS applications, a local imagery acquisition program may be warranted. King County GIS (WA) was able to partner with 53 agencies for its 2012 imagery acquisition program, and with 88 agencies for its 2015 imagery acquisition. These partnerships spanned parts of multiple counties and resulted in significant cost savings for all participating agencies. The Los Angeles Regional Imagery Acquisition Consortium (LAR-IAC) includes the county as well as municipalities and local educational institutions to pool funding to acquire geospatial imagery for the region.

### *Elevation Data (EC1d) and Hydrography (EC1e)*

Elevation data and hydrographic data are inter-related in that high-accuracy hydrography utilizes elevation data to validate possible changes to the stream network. The primary source for modern, highly accurate, and up-to-date elevation data is LiDAR. Changes to the hydrography of a county can be either man-made, through development, faming, and forestry activities, or a result of flooding, landslides, or seismic activity. With climate change, flooding in many areas is more frequent and intense, which can change stream networks.

Elevation and hydrographic data are also critical for flood plain mapping. Accurate and up-to-date flood plain maps can result in lower flood insurance rates for many property owners by lowering risk for insurance carriers. They can also inform property owners of these same risks so that they can make better-informed decisions about development of their property. There are many instances in the professional literature and popular media of city and county councils acknowledging the value of the investment in GIS-based flood insurance mapping. For example, the group Taxpayers for Common Sense reported on the benefits of a flood plain mapping program in North Carolina. Calgary, Canada publicizes its flood mapping program, which is used both for zoning regulations and to provide flood risk information to both insurers and property owners.

What is the county GIS role in elevation and hydrographic data acquisition and maintenance? Topography and watercourses cross jurisdiction boundaries. Just as states and provinces take the lead in acquisition of this type of data at a scale and level of accuracy appropriate for their purposes, counties have an important role at the local level. One exemplary program is the Puget Sound LiDAR Consortium. This is a group of counties, regional agencies, and utilities in the Central Puget Sound area in Washington State. Kitsap County, Washington was the original lead agency and still serves as the jurisdiction that procures, contracts, and pays for LiDAR projects. The Consortium is an informal contacting and cost-sharing consortium. It has no formal structure but has operated since 1999. Other uses of LiDAR data include landslide risk analysis, earthquake fault research, archeology, and change detection.

### *Administrative Boundaries (EC1f)*

As the primary subdivision of states and provinces, counties have a critical responsibility for delineating boundaries of administrative units. And because of their responsibility for administering elections, counties have an interest in the boundaries of all the jurisdictions and legal districts within their boundaries. In many cases, counties are also responsible for approving new legal administrative boundaries through a boundary review board or similar entity.

County GIS operations should establish close working relationships with their boundary board, as well as with the cities, school districts, utility districts, other special districts, tribes, ports, and state and federal agencies that have a presence within the county. Even within these separate and overlapping jurisdictions, boundary mapping is required for taxation areas, census tract boundaries, and election precinct boundaries.

The term administrative boundaries has additional meaning for county GIS operations. GIS is often called upon to help delineate purely internal administrative boundaries to help counties manage their work. For example, the public works department of a large county might have multiple maintenance yards where equipment and material are stored, maintenance work is conducted, and crews are dispatched. Typically, each will have an area of responsibility. Periodically, changes in workload related to variable maintenance workload or changes to resources will require GIS to help adjust these service area boundaries.

There may also be boundaries that are created by county code that must be delineated as conditions change. For example, states often have ordinances that restrict how close to a school or park a liquor store or retail marijuana outlet can be located. GIS will often be called up to assist with delineating this type of administrative boundary. For example, King County Washington has a no-shooting ordinance that uses GIS to interpret locations within and outside this boundary.

### *Transportation Network (EC1g) and EC3 Business Data—Street Addresses*

The last NSDI framework category is transportation network data. In addition, a key business data for most counties and cities is street address data. Counties usually share responsibility for the street network with state or provincial government and with the cities within their boundaries.

Because road networks are all interconnected, counties have an interest in the transportation data of both neighboring jurisdictions and of all of the cities and other jurisdictions within their boundaries. Transportation network users are interested in commute times, road use restrictions, planned and unplanned road closures, and capital project planning. The county GIS shop can coordinate acquisition of data from all regional jurisdictions to create a regional spatial data warehouse that supports regional transportation reporting and business needs and public applications. There are many third-party applications that assist commuters and transportation companies with real-time road traffic conditions, which can relieve counties of the need to develop and maintain traffic condition applications.

However, a good practice for counties is to coordinate both transportation network and street address data with the cities and other responsible jurisdictions within its boundaries. Types of non-real-time traffic data that can be coordinated include planned road closures, planned utility work, unplanned road closures, special event-related road changes, and traffic camera feeds. Planned closures can also include priority snow removal routes across jurisdiction boundaries.

Unplanned road closures can include emergency utility work, public-safety actions, and flooding, snow, ice, seismic, and wind-related events. Citizens and businesses will expect this regional approach. And, of course, counties will have an interest in transportation network conditions in neighboring counties as well.

While street address data is not an NSDI framework data layer, URISA has proposed to FGDC that it be included in the future. URISA, along with NSGIC and NGAC, has also proposed the development of a national address database (NAD) that would be a single authoritative and open source for address data across the United States (URISA 2016). Within the GISCMM, street address data would be considered a business data. Another good practice for counties related to address data is to align their standards with the URISA Street Address standard that was adopted by FGDC (URISA 2011).

The GISCMM assumes that "individual GIS operations have access to adequate business data (non-framework GIS data) to meet its business needs. [The] need for [business] data is based on agency business needs, therefore this data will vary from agency to agency" (GIS Management Institute 2013). The author has never encountered a county GIS operation that does not consider street address data as a key, mission-critical GIS dataset. Because many county business functions fall within cities, tribes, and other jurisdictions within its boundaries, a comprehensive address database is critical. Types of address-critical functions include property assessment and taxation, elections, transit services, regional emergency management, and county sheriff police functions.

The coordination of street address data is closely related to transportation network data. Good practice for a county GIS operation is to establish a staff responsibility to establish and maintain coordination with city and tribal public works, planning, and permitting departments to ensure that proposed, new, and revised transportation and street address data is communicated and incorporated into the GIS on a timely basis.

A more ambitious approach to regional spatial data management is an integrated multi-agency database approach. The King County Department of Transportation developed TNET—a county–city consortium for collaborative editing and maintenance of a countywide GIS-based transportation network. TNET was designed to be

> a consortium of regional cities, county agencies as well as public/private partnerships participating in maintaining a seamless database of transportation related spatial and attribute datasets. These datasets are housed centrally and maintained by transportation planners, city and county engineers, Emergency Response personnel and GIS analysts. This cooperative arrangement permits the availability of a high-accuracy, up-to-date transportation network suitable for a variety of transportation planning, operations, and related business functions throughout the region.
>
> (TNET Consortium 2010)

While TNET never became fully functional on a regional basis, the TNET concept is being revisited as part of a current regional GIS study being conducted by King County, Seattle, and several other medium and small cities and tribes in the region.

The Federal Highway Administration GIS in Transportation Program provides a clearinghouse for good practices, policies, and procedures related to GIS for transportation data. One useful example is a report titled *Development of a Regional Public Transportation GIS Architecture and Data Model*. This report details a regional transportation GIS data infrastructure developed for the Florida Department of Transportation Region 7. It provides specifics of a regional GIS transportation data approach that could be replicated by counties and other regional agencies.

A good example of regional GIS address data maintenance and dissemination is the San Diego Geographic Information Source. SanGIS is a formal joint powers authority that allows the City of San Diego and San Diego County to collaborate on the development of a common GIS data source. SanGIS manages and maintains a situs address GIS database linked to APNs (Assessor Parcel Numbers). Source data is provided by the addressing authority in each of 18 cities within the county, as well as by San Diego County itself. The advantage is a more accurate GIS address database that is of use throughout the region.

### *GIS Data Coordination (EC5), Metadata (EC6), Spatial Data Warehouse (EC7), and Data Backup and Security (EC12)*

Data is one of the key foundations for an effective GIS. The first four GISCMM capability areas focus on foundational spatial data. Without it, there are no maps, no analysis, no end-user applications, and no GIS ROI. But with few exceptions, GIS data does not directly provide a financial benefit or enhance end-user effectiveness. Indeed, data should be thought of as the primary capital asset of the GIS. Some public agencies include GIS data in their financial asset inventory. Even a small city or county GIS can easily have an investment of more than a million dollars in its GIS data.

And yet data acquisition, development, and ongoing maintenance is one of the highest cost labor items for GIS. The GISCMM also identifies a variety of high-level data management functions. These include data coordination (EC5), metadata development and management (EC6), operating a spatial data warehouse (EC7), and critical data backup and security (EC12).

Data coordination (EC5) includes both internal and external functions. A well-run GIS will rely on data maintained by subject matter expert data stewards. These might be in the county assessor's office for property parcel data, in the roads or transit department for street centerline and pavement data, the survey office for geodetic control data, etc. The key function for an enterprise GIS is to manage data from many different sources and to compile it into a centralized spatial data warehouse. A single authoritative data warehouse is more efficient and effective than relying on multiple datasets in end-user departments. Data coordination also should include ensuring that enterprise metadata standards (EC6) are established and followed, so that end users and application developers know the appropriate use and limitations of the data they encounter.

Data coordination activity for a county is not only an internal function. It should also include the development of comprehensive data sharing agreements and practices with all the regional spatial data sources. A county is the ideal location for this coordination and for a spatial data hub infrastructure. The county data hub should be the location where each agency uploads a copy of the datasets for which it is the designated data maintenance steward. The county data hub should also be the location where each agency can access data provided within the data hub collaborative structure.

Management of a spatial data warehouse (EC7) should be the responsibility of database administrators and system administrators who are knowledgeable about geospatial data. They should work closely with the GIS data coordinator to ensure timely updates to mission-critical framework and business GIS data. A common question is whether a GIS DBA should be assigned to GIS or within IT. The key factor is ensuring that the DBA and system administrator have good working knowledge of GIS data and of the types of analysis and end-user applications that the data is intended to support. URISA publishes Model GIS Job Descriptions (Butler 2013), which should be the minimal basis for defining the competencies of DBAs and system administrators responsible for GIS infrastructure.

Data security (EC12) is another key factor for well-run GIS operations. In addition to appropriate login credentials to access, read, and/or edit GIS data, security procedures should be in place to protect the integrity of the GIS database. Many agencies consider GIS data to be mission critical.

Spatial data security should consider risk factors. The primary data risk mitigation practice is to have a data backup plan. The primary data risk is failure, damage, or destruction of the data servers. Redundant datasets should be backed up and stored in a remote location to allow data restoration within minimal data loss. GIS operations in buildings located in certain risk areas require special consideration. If the GIS operation is in a flood hazard area, a seismic risk area, a wind-storm risk area, a landslide area, etc., the backup location should be outside the same risk area.

A GIS data backup and restore exercise should be performed periodically, with a goal of a quick restoration process in the case of a catastrophic data failure. A complete data restore process for a GIS with terabytes of data can take as long as a week. This is unacceptable for a mission-critical system. The end users can suffer critical impact on their business functions from a lengthy restore process. This impacts ROI and critical public safety services. An emerging threat is a crypto-virus attack. The GIS data coordinator and spatial data warehouse team should have a plan in place for shutting down its GIS in case of a crypto-virus attack, physically isolating servers and computers, and restoring GIS services from unaffected data and software.

## County GIS Coordination Opportunities

The GIS for cities, special districts, and tribes within a county's boundaries also have a need for these same data-related GIS functions described above. While GIS data can be easily copied and shared at little cost, the real opportunity is to share the spatial database and related coordination and support functions. With simple GIS data sharing, there remains a cost for each agency to store, maintain, and administer the duplicate data.

A county GIS is a logical location to provide regional GIS data sharing coordination and infrastructure for the jurisdictions within the county's boundaries. Cloud computing creates emerging opportunities for sharing of many back-office GIS functions. Agencies that share geography should also look for opportunities to share non-value-added GIS functions. Within a county's boundaries, local agencies also have an interest in GIS data from neighboring jurisdictions. Each city is impacted by its neighbors' development and demographics, traffic and crime, natural resources, policies, and planning. Sharing data between neighboring agencies should proceed with a view towards development of a single authoritative spatial database. Development of such a collaborative, centralized authoritative database should be a key strategic goal of every GIS.

### *GIS Software Maintenance (EC11)*

Similar to data, GIS software should be selected, maintained, supported, and coordinated to support the defined end-user business needs of the agency. GIS-CMM EC11 supposes that the GIS will ensure that adequate GIS software is available for the needs of the agency that it supports. But how do end users know the appropriate GIS software to meet their business needs? This informing of end users is a key role for the GIS operation management. Counties and other agencies that utilize the most common types of commercial GIS software typically have a variety of capabilities to choose from for their software portfolio. For example, only a small cadre of GIS professionals and super users will require the most powerful GIS software. High-production data stewards will require powerful editing software. A sizable middle tier of power users should be able to meet their needs with standard GIS software. The largest group of typical county end users will meet their needs with web-based mapping applications or simple data visualization software. King County GIS serves 14,000 employees with about 30 professional GIS staff. About ten of the GIS professional staff use the most powerfully GIS software functionality. About ten use powerful data editing licenses. About 650 county staff use standard desktop GIS software. At least 6,000 county staff use web-based GIS mapping capability on an annual basis (see Figure 14.4).

A good practice for managing GIS software within any medium to large county is to pool all GIS software licenses. King County GIS can serve all its power and desktop GIS users with a portfolio of licenses that is a fraction of the total number of users. The key factors for efficient software license management is to understand hourly, daily, weekly, and seasonal patterns of use. King County GIS uses a license management system that monitors normal daily demand. Even with spare licenses under maintenance for very high peak demand periods, the total licensing is a fraction of the total 650 users. This provides a significant cost saving to the county.

Centralized software management also ensures that all GIS software is under appropriate license to minimize agency liability and risk. Centralized management also supports cost-effective contract administration, version control and upgrade planning, and helpdesk support. Centralized software GIS management by a county also has potential for a regional GIS service by providing spatial software access to cities, utilities, and other regional agencies.

An emerging issue for GIS operations within both cities and many other types of agencies is the emergence of SAAS-based special data visualization services. What is the role of open source GIS software, Google Maps, Tableau, and other non-traditional spatial data visualization systems? GIS managers need to understand these tools and educate end users of their benefits and limitations, which are many. A key factor is to ensure that well-vetted data and GIS software are used for critical public agency analysis and decision-making.

### *GIS Application Portfolio (EC13), GIS Application Portfolio Management (EC14), and GIS Application Portfolio O&M (EC15)*

These components of the GISCMM focus on targeting the highest value GIS applications. These deliver the highest ROI. They are typically designed for unique mission-critical agency functions. They address three inter-related aspects of GIS ROI. First, does the agency even have a portfolio of GIS applications (EC13)? Second, is the portfolio managed (EC14), meaning is there a common architecture with common standards? Is the portfolio managed so that code is developed to common standards that support interoperability and reuse? Do the resources (staff and time) exist to operate and maintain the application portfolio (EC15) to meet the defined end-user business needs?

The county GIS operation should also look for opportunities to develop or acquire and maintain applications that can be shared across the region. This

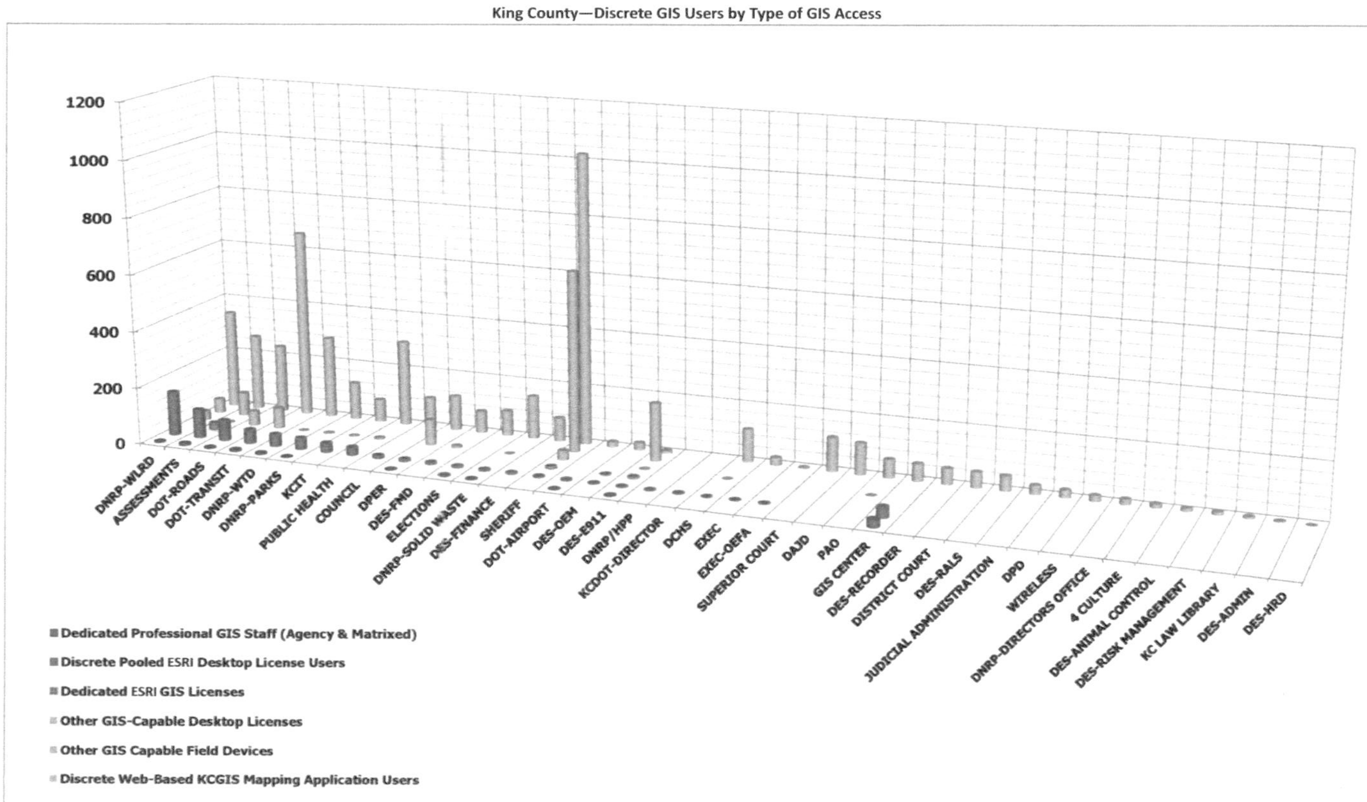


*Figure 14.4* 6,000 GIS users in King County by county agency and type of GIS user.

happens by default within many counties, when their parcel data web mapping application is used by cities and utilities within its boundaries. But this also provides an opportunity to use this web mapping framework and the management and O&M functions to develop and maintain additional web mapping functionality to meet city, utility, or special district needs. This sharing of resources puts tools in the hands of end users in many subordinate agencies that might otherwise be beyond their capability. It also helps to create a more cost-effective and sustainable environment for long-term O&M.

### *Training and Professional Staff Development (EC18)*

Another good practice for counties is to take the lead in regional training and professional staff development. For 20 years, King County GIS has run a GIS training program that has helped GIS end users improve their skills and abilities and also helped deliver enhanced ROI for the departments that use GIS. Not many counties will be able to manage their own GIS training program, but even medium-sized counties can play a key GIS professional development role.

Types of activities might include hosting monthly user group meeting open to all regional agency staff. As GIS use matures and the sophistication of GIS professionals and users becomes more specialized, specialized user group meetings can be scheduled. Types of specialized meetings could include those targeted for GIS developers, GIS data stewards, GIS analysts, etc. User group meetings are a low-cost way to discuss problems, share lessons learned, and coordinate activity within the countywide region.

The county GIS can also coordinate access to more formal GIS-related classroom training. For example, the foundation of the King County GIS training program is a variety of free one-hour hands-on classes. A one-hour introduction to GIS workshop is targeted at those with no familiarity with GIS or GIS concepts. This workshop has been attended by many new employees, mid-level and senior managers, and even elected officials, as well as citizens and people from schools, businesses, and other jurisdictions. Other free one-hour workshops focus on doing property research with publicly available GIS tools, introduction to understanding GIS metadata, using ESRI's ArcGIS Online, using Pictometry data, etc.

The cost of attending face-to-face, hands-on GIS training is prohibitively expensive for students who must travel to a remote training center. But if the county GIS can coordinate providing basic desktop GIS training in its own facility or a local computer training lab, and then making the training available to interested students from other regional jurisdictions, the per-student cost can be a fraction of the alternative. Qualified instructors might come from within the county GIS itself, or from the academic community, or commercial GIS training services providers.

A GIS training and professional development program provides dual benefits. It leads to enhanced ROI for the agencies deploying GIS. It also provides the continuing education that professionals working in a knowledge industry like GIS need for long and successful careers.

## Regional GIS and Good Practices for County GIS: GIS as a Utility

Near the end of the nineteenth century, thousands of counties, cities, universities, and businesses scrambled to implement a new technology that was delivering tremendous ROI and enhanced effectiveness. This new technology was distributed electrical energy. Many entities believed that the way to harness this technology was to design, build, and operate their own electrical power generating stations and distribution networks. History proved this approach to be unsustainable. Small redundant electrical power plants suffered from lack of scale, high cost to operate, poor technology choices, and rapid obsolescence. What electrical power users wanted, and still want, is to flip the switch and have the lights come on, heat or cool their environment, cook their food, and make the wheels turn. A variety of public and private utilities proved better positioned to provide the benefits of electrical power to all comers.

What do GIS end users want? It is to activate their GIS tools, to access GIS data, and then to display, analyze, manipulate, model, and map the data. For 50 years, most GIS operations have evolved like the late nineteenth-century electrical power model—everything GIS-related self-contained to the greatest extent possible. But 50 years of GIS history have demonstrated that small and even some medium-sized GIS are at significant risk for long-term viability.

A clear understanding of the key role of local government agency GIS and of what delivers ROI and enhanced public services should help GIS managers and the agencies that employ GIS make good decisions about how their GIS is organized and resourced. GIS-enabled applications in the hands of end users provide the benefit to society that justifies the investment in GIS and its continued operation. Non-value-added core functions are candidates for centralized operation and maintenance. These types of functions have been described throughout this chapter.

Core GIS-related functions should be thought of as utility functions. Indeed, regions like counties should work towards development of core GIS utility infrastructure. Where should the GIS utility function reside? There are many candidates. In addition to counties, the core GIS utility infrastructure could be operated by a large regional city, a regional planning agency, a local university, or a standalone special purpose semi-public agency. Other possible models could include the state or provincial government or a special purpose private entity. But counties will always have a key role in initiating, participating, and managing a regional approach to GIS.

County GIS has the potential to lead the development of regional GIS infrastructure that starts approaching the utility model. This chapter makes the case that county GIS operations are well positioned to collaborate with other regional agencies to develop, operate, and maintain sustainable GIS for all comers. Should GIS infrastructure evolve into a utility-like regional service? What is the role of county GIS operations in such an evolution?

A recent survey (Croswell 2015) of multi-organizational GIS programs found that of 38 programs studied, for 65% of the programs a county was a lead agency. A handful of regional GIS entities originated at a time when GIS was a new technology and it seemed logical for a county with nearby cities, utilities, and other agencies to band together for coordinated and collaborative GIS development, operation, and maintenance. But in environments where counties and cities launched their own GIS programs in parallel, there are few instances where all the benefits of regional collaborative GIS have been achieved. Recently there have been a few efforts to bring well-established GIS operations together to create new county/city/utility collaborative GIS entities.

County GIS operations and those who manage them should be attuned to pursuing the regional collaboration opportunities outlined in this chapter. And all local GIS operations should periodically consider establishing a regional collaborative GIS infrastructure to reduce risks and help create a more sustainable and cost-effective regional Geographic Information System.

## Note

1. The alpha-numeric designation within parentheses refers to a specific component of the GIS Capability Maturity Model.

## References

Abler, R., Adams, J.S., and Gould, P. *Spatial Organization: The Geographer's View of the World*. Englewood Cliffs, NJ: Prentice-Hall, 1971.

Babinski, Greg. *Is There a Moral Imperative for GIS*. The Summit, Summer 2012, p. 21: https://waurisa.wildapricot.org/resources/Documents/TheSummit/TheSummit_Issue28_2012_Summer.pdf

Babinski, Greg. *Proposal for an Integrated Regional, Collaborative, and Sustainable GIS*. Seattle: King County GIS Center, 2016a.

Babinski, Greg. King County GIS Center 2015 GIS Assessment Report. *URISA Journal*, Vol. 27, No. 2, 2016b, pp. 21–36.

Babinski, Greg. *Supporting Professional GIS Management: A Vision for the GIS Management Institute*. Edmonds: Orzel Books, 2018.

Butler, J. Allison. *Model GIS Job Descriptions*. Des Plaines: URISA, 2013.

Croswell, Pete. *The GIS Management Handbook*. Frankfort: Kessey Dewitt Publications, 2009.

Croswell, Pete. *Report on National Survey of Multi-Organizational GIS Programs*. GIS Management Institute, 2015.

DuPage County, IL, Geographic Information System. Geodetic Control Overview: www.dupageco.org/GIS/GPS/

GIS Management Institute. *Geospatial Management Competency Model*. URISA. 2012: www.urisa.org/clientuploads/directory/GMI/Advocacy/GMCM%20final.pdf

GIS Management Institute. *GIS Capability Maturity Model*. URISA. September 2013: www.urisa.org/clientuploads/directory/GMI/GISCMM-Final201309(Endorsed%20for%20Publication).pdf

Los Angeles County GIS Imagery Consortium: https://egis3.lacounty.gov/dataportal/lariac/

Somers, R., and Eichelberger, P. The Development of an Integrated Cadastral Database, Papers from the 1987 Annual Conference of the Urban and Regional Information Systems Association. URISA, 1987.

South Central Regional Council of Governments: http://scrcog.org/regional-planning/gis/parcel-data-summary/

Taxpayers for Common Sense (North Carolina): www.taxpayer.net/infrastructure/case-study-north-carolina-floodplain-mapping/

Tomlinson, Roger. *Thinking About GIS*. Redlands: ESRI Press, 2013.

URISA Policy Paper. Support and Recommendations for the Proposed National Address Database (NAD), 2016. www.urisa.org/clientuploads/directory/Documents/Advocacy/FINAL_URISA_NationalAddressDatabase06062016.pdf

USDA National Agricultural Imagery Program: www.fsa.usda.gov/programs-and-services/aerial-photography/imagery-programs/naip-imagery/

USGS National Map Liaison: http://nationalmap.gov/

Zerbe, R., Fumia, D., Reynolds, T., Singh, P., Scott, T., and Babinski, G. An Analysis of Benefits from Use of Geographic Information Systems by King County, Washington. *URISA Journal*, Vol. 27, No. 1, 2016, pp. 13–28.

# 15 Using GIS for Enrollment Management and Campus Management at a Public University

*Rebecca Rose and Jonathon D. Henderson*

## Mapping Student Data

### *Introduction*

There is an increased push to recruit and retain more students using limited resources while competing with other universities facing the same challenges. One way to combat this challenge is the application of enrollment management. When applied successfully, enrollment management can help bring a university's goals and mission to reality through careful planning and implementation (AACRAO, 2004). One of the key components of the successful execution of enrollment management is the effective use of data.

Data can help leaders make informative decisions and create realistic goals that will help avoid pitfalls. As you would expect when there is no use of data, enrollment management is no longer strategic (as it is intended), but rather tactical (AACRAO, 2004). How do Geographic Information Systems (GIS) contribute to enrollment management? GIS is a powerful tool that provides another way to communicate data that may get lost in tables and graphs. By showing a visual of a university's strengths and weaknesses, it can help the enrollment management team (which often includes admission and recruitment officials) make impactful decisions.

### *Data*

It is important to consider what information is going to be gathered and how it affects students' privacy rights. It is also important to ensure that any information used does not violate the Family Education Rights and Privacy Act (FERPA). Students who indicate that they do not wish to have their information used are "flagged". This means students are removed from reports where they could be identified or contacted.

Most maps provide aggregated results when the total number of students is large; however, when the total number is smaller, personal identifiable information can be unintentionally revealed. The more information that is included in the map, the more identifiable a student can become when the total number is smaller, as can happen in rural communities, for example.

### *Internal Data Sources*

At Central Washington University (CWU), the Department of Institutional Effectiveness and Information Services maintains a data warehouse that contains all student records and information. Students' physical home address, city, zip code, county, state, gender, race/ethnicity, and admit type can be used for mapping purposes. If the admissions and enrollment department were interested in where first-time, full-time freshman (FTFTF) were coming from, then physical home address would be used.

### *External Data Sources*

The Washington Geospatial Open Data Portal was selected as the external data source to accurately map student information. This portal provided the bulk of the information needed to map major highways and interstates, cities and city boundaries, zip code boundaries, census block data, population density, and K–12 school districts. Addresses were geocoded with ArcGIS after student data had been collected. This allowed for accurate geographical coordinates of physical addresses on GIS maps.

## ***Mapping***

There are many approaches to mapping information; however, for the purposes of mapping student data, proximity and choropleth maps were used.

### *Proximity Maps*

Proximity maps are useful to understand where students live in relation to campus. It is a great visual aid that helps administrators see where their student population is coming from. When proximity maps are used broadly, as shown in Figure 15.1, identifying students is difficult. However, when counties and regions are examined individually, students' physical locations can become more identifiable, especially in rural areas with limited road access. In these instances, it is important that there is careful consideration of who the maps are for and the total number of students in each county and/or region.

Proximity maps are also useful when determining how far students are traveling to a university center or main campus. CWU has a main campus, six university centers, and two instructional sites in Washington. By mapping student data and then filtering further based on campus type, this creates a clear visual of how far students are traveling in relation to main campus or centers they are attending. To get a better idea of student points of origin, 5-, 10-, and 15-mile buffer rings were included around CWU campus and centers in Figure 15.2. This is especially helpful if there are a number of students that travel from one area with a center to a different area with another center. This provides clues to officials for evaluating the courses being offered at either center and making appropriate changes based on need.

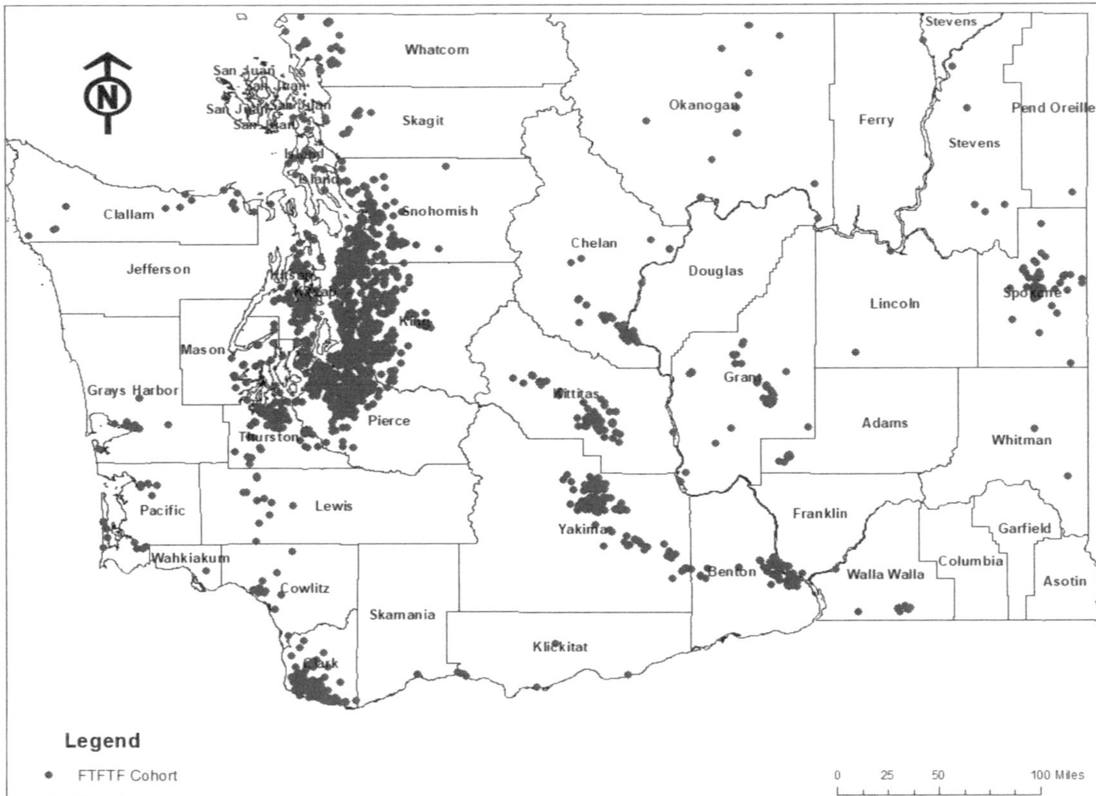


*Figure 15.1* Each point represents one FTFTF who was a Washington resident in fall 2017.

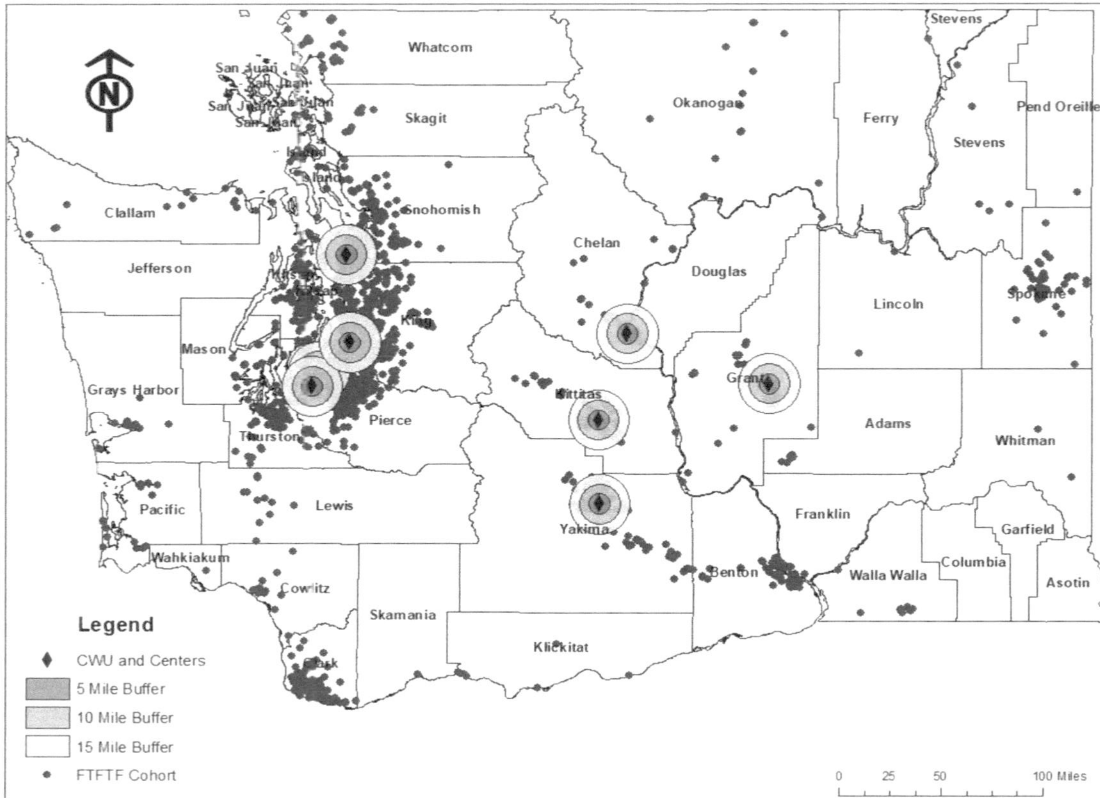


*Figure 15.2* Buffer rings were included to show how far students live in relation to main campus and centers.

*Choropleth Maps*

Choropleth maps provide a colored representation of a particular set of variables of interest in a shape (i.e. polygon) such as a county, census block, zip code, or districts. These maps are most commonly used to communicate data visually such as population density in a particular area (Figure 15.3). Using choropleth maps addresses the concerns that proximity maps fail to address by presenting student data in aggregated form. Student data must be joined to an established choropleth map in order to create student choropleth maps, and this can be done by utilizing ArcGIS tools. This chapter only shows the final output in the following section and does not review joins in ArcGIS.

## *Exploring the Tools*

ArcGIS provides a plethora of data tools. By combining the Washington Geospatial Open Data Portal, it is possible to create specific maps tailored to an audience's needs. In this case, the audience is the Admissions and Enrollment Department. What are they interested in and how does it help them with decision-making? The goal is to show where first-time, full-time freshmen (FTFTF) are from in Washington State. There are several ways to answer this question and all of them are right; it just depends on what they need. Using county boundaries to show where FTFTF are from provides a broad view of which counties have the most students (Figure 15.4). However, areas with a small number of FTFTF could be attributed for a number of reasons not shown unless a geographical base map is included (Figure 15.5). Counties with lower numbers can be attributed to rural areas and mountain ranges that consume a large portion of the county.

Census blocks is another tool that can be used to create choropleth maps. Census blocks are created by man-made features such as roads and railways, by topographic features such as rivers and mountain ranges, or by "invisible" features such as townships, city limits, county limits, and poverty lines. When comparing a rural area to an urban area, census blocks can differ greatly in size and does not account for population size (Figure 15.6). Additionally, census blocks can change year to year depending on available features. Census blocks can help narrow the scope; however, it is best applied in smaller urban areas as compared to rural areas, as shown in Figure 15.6. Understanding where FTFTF are coming from can be evaluated more narrowly with the use of zip codes and K–12 school districts.

City limits allow administrators to see where students are coming from in metro and urban areas; however, this application does not capture students who live outside of city limits. A way around this limitation is by using zip codes because it captures the entire area of interest without losing any information (Figure 15.7). Although this information is beneficial to administrators, it still does not answer the question of where FTFTF are coming from and how it benefits admissions and recruiters. One way to capture this is by mapping where

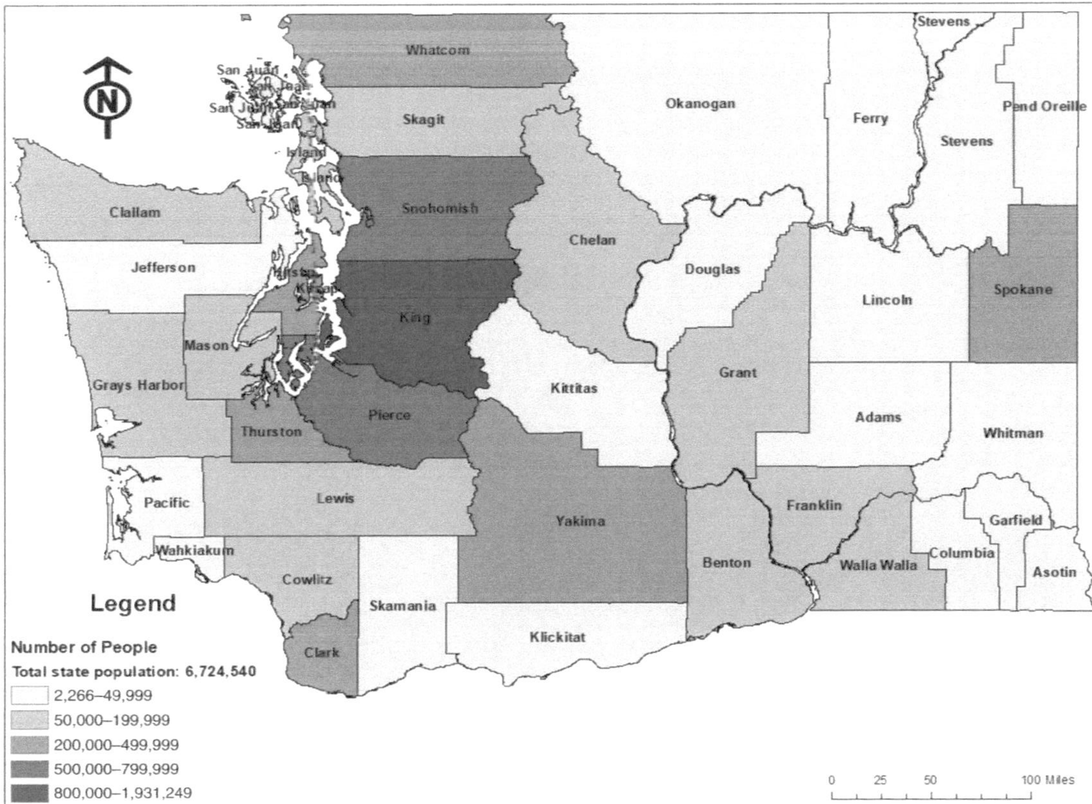


*Figure 15.3* Washington 2010 census report. Choropleth map to show population density by county.

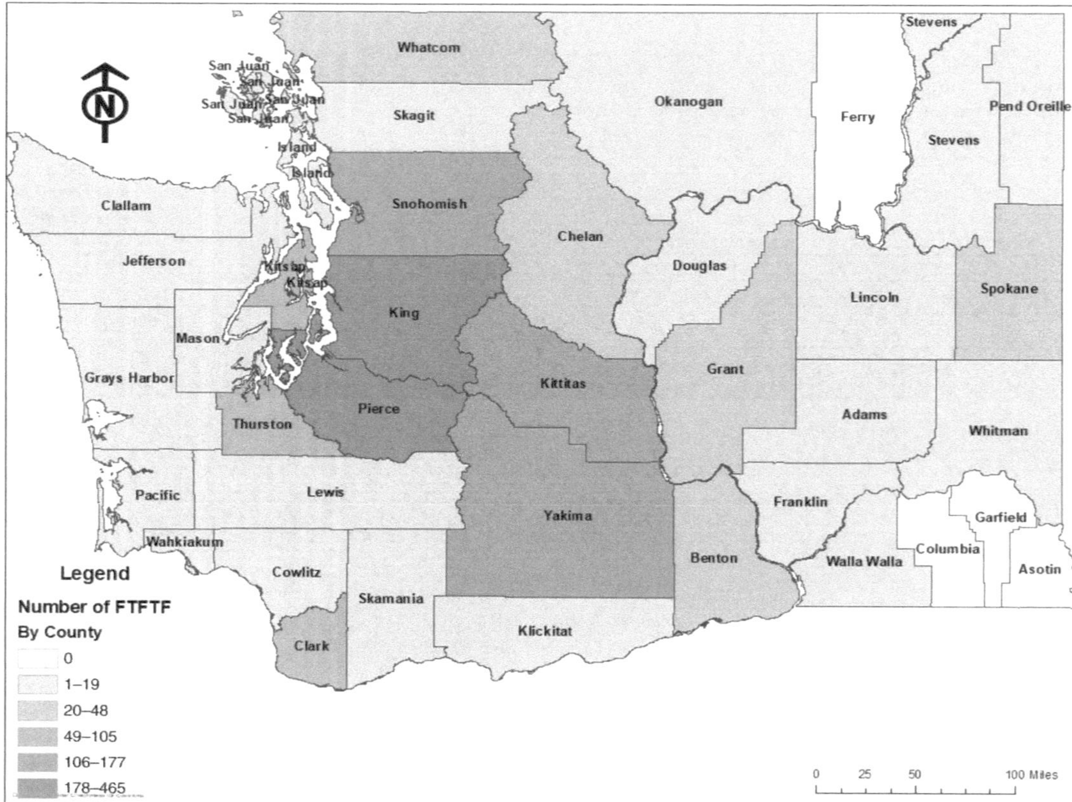


*Figure 15.4* Student geocoded address file joined to county shapefile to produce a choropleth map.

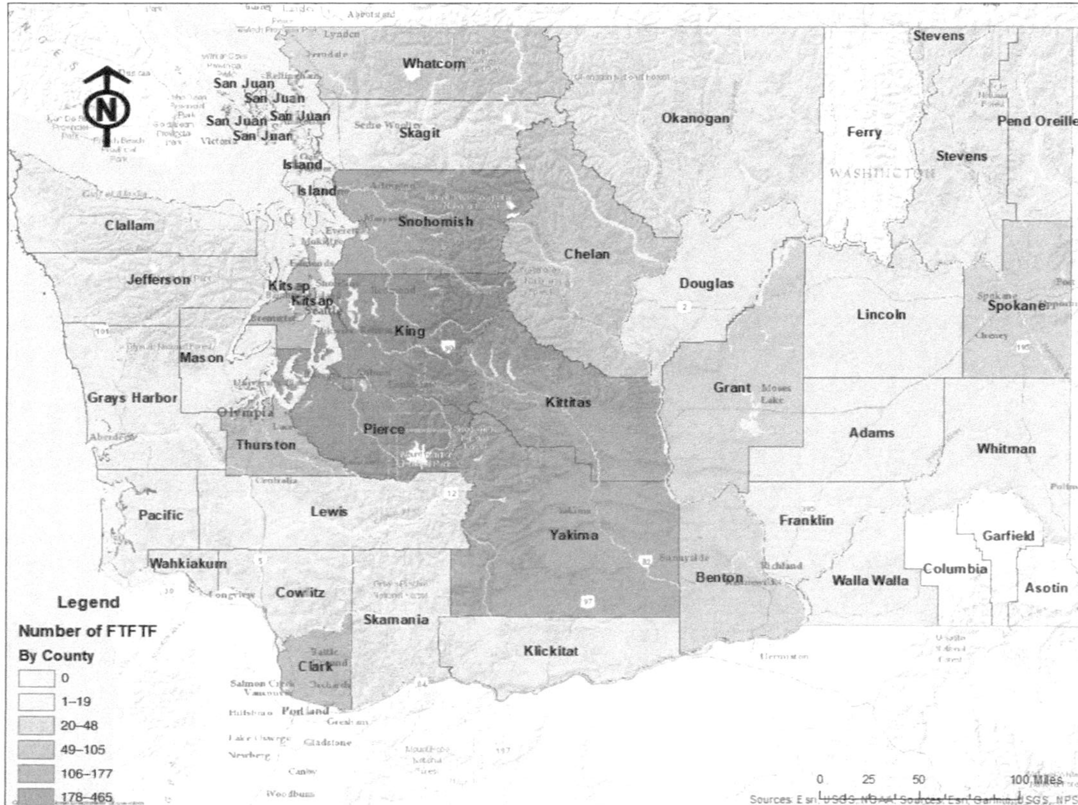


*Figure 15.5* Student geocoded address file joined to county shapefile to produce a choropleth map with a geographical base map. This helps explain low numbers in some counties like Ferry, Columbia, Garfield, etc.

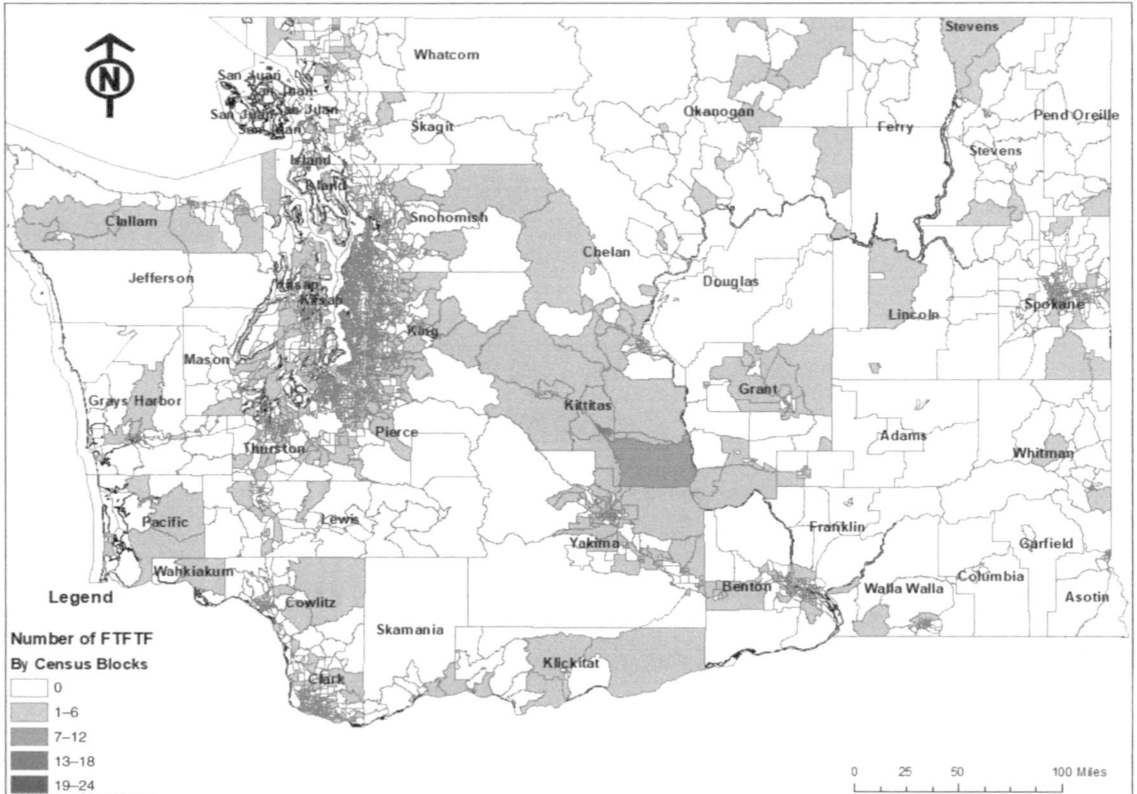


*Figure 15.6* Census blocks used to explain where students reside. They vary in size for a multitude of reasons and can change yearly.

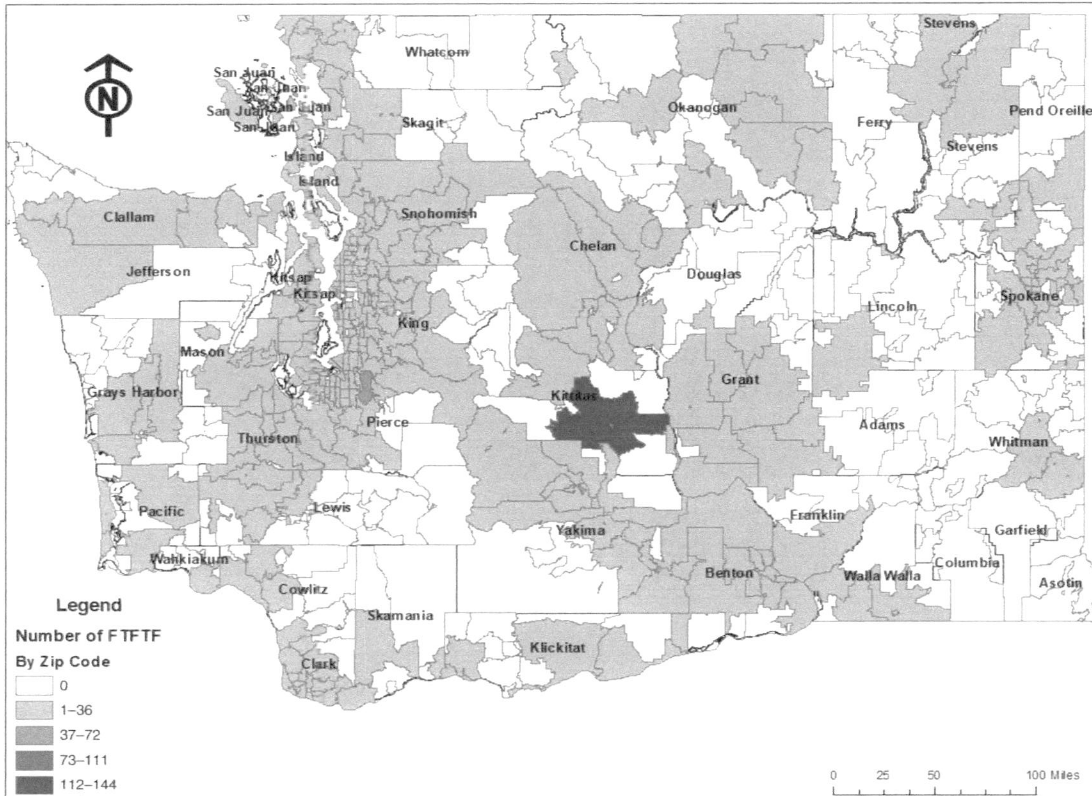


*Figure 15.7* Zip codes capture students who live outside of city limits, providing more information than using city limits and census blocks.

students have attended high school. By using open source K–12 shapefiles provided from the Washington Geospatial Open Data Portal and internal sources, CWU mapped which high schools FTFTF attended (Figure 15.8). This type of map is especially helpful for recruiters targeting schools for future recruitment; unfortunately, this map is only applicable to first-time freshman.

Mapping student data is an excellent way to understand where students are coming from by examining distance to main campus (or centers) based on their physical location. It can also help with recruiting efforts by showing which school districts are producing the most yield. Lastly, it can show university officials what the student profile is like and the geographical challenges that students face.

### *Limitations*

As many academic professionals know, student data can be difficult to organize. At CWU, student data is collected through PeopleSoft and then transferred and stored in a data warehouse. Any time a student updates their address, phone number, etc., the change is recorded in the warehouse. The trouble begins when a student updates their information to reflect that they are living near the main university or center where they are attending classes. Unfortunately, this overinflates the number of students who are "from" Ellensburg, Washington, for example. Additionally, post office boxes do not provide a clear and accurate indication of where the students are traveling from. As a result, those students were removed and the total number of students is reduced.

## Classroom Utilization

Mapping can be a powerful tool to ensure that campus resources, such as classrooms, labs, and office space, are being used effectively. Ensuring effective use of space is an important part of resource cultivation. As a public university, Central Washington University works to achieve continual improvement through the increasingly effective use of resources. Visualizing space utilization through mapping allows university leadership to quickly assess the status of resources, which is important when a university's needs are constantly changing based on enrollment and retention. Central Washington University uses several different mapping methods to assess office, classroom, and office space utilization.

### *Campus Choropleth*

One method of mapping utilization is the campus choropleth. In the campus choropleth, CWU took the different buildings around campus and changed the visuals denoting them based on the following criteria: Students in Class, Classes in Session, and Efficiency of Space Usage (Figure 15.9). This type of object manipulation is called a spatial join. Spatial joins can be used for any feature on a map to combine multiple data points into one. Spatial joins can

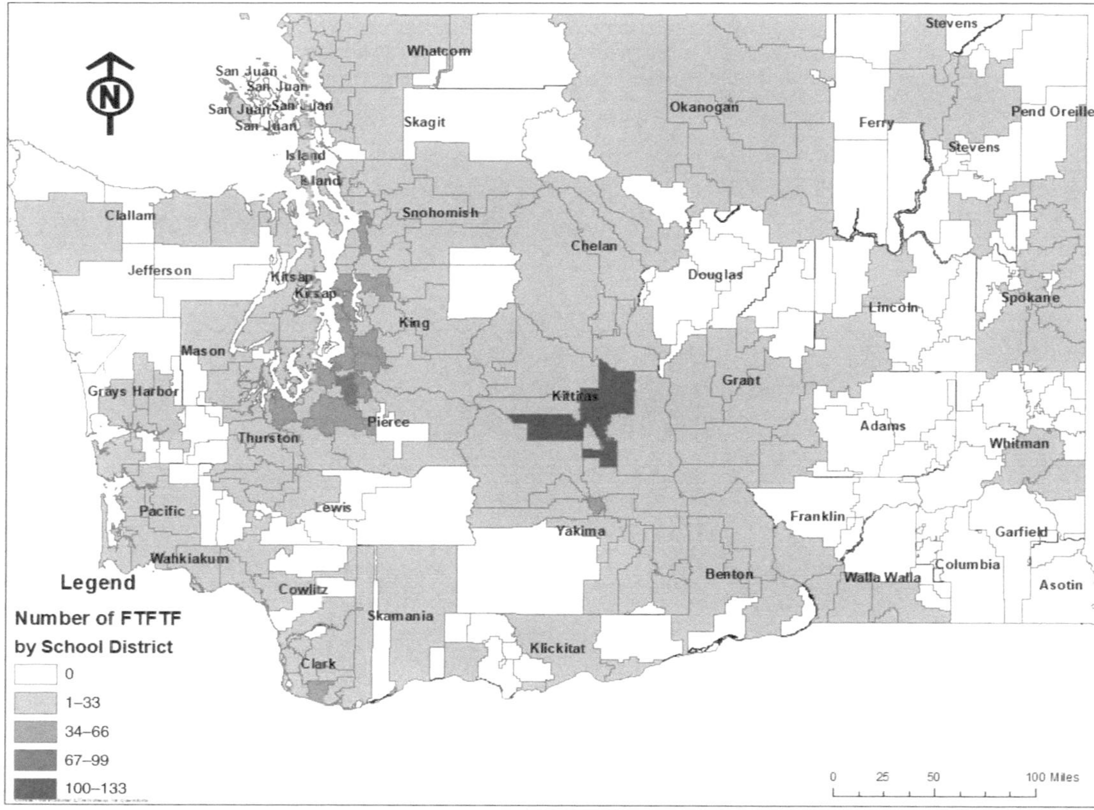


*Figure 15.8* School districts help administrators with recruitment strategies. As expected, part of Kittitas County yields the most students because CWU is located there.

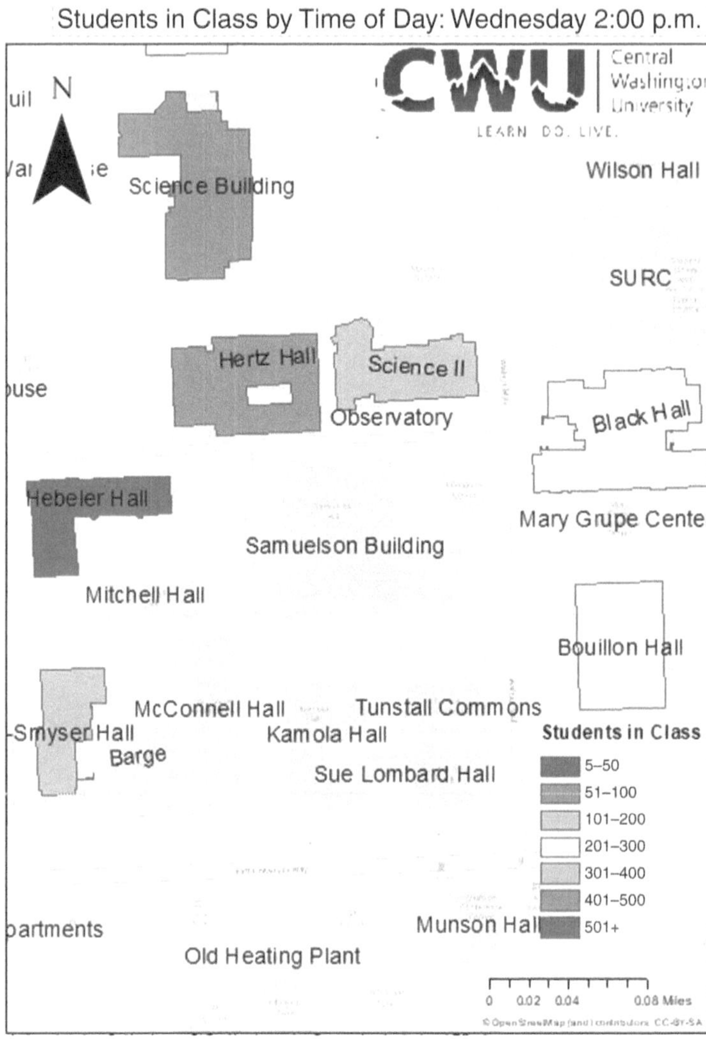


Figure 15.9 Choropleth map of students in class at 2:00 p.m. Wednesday.

be a time saver; if there is a large section of campus or several buildings that required a single location choropleth of students in the area, then a spatial join could be created with the parameter to include any students in class within a predefined distance.

Combining classroom utilization information with date and time information can create powerful overviews, which can assist in planning everything from the pedestrian flow, parking, future building projects, etc. A useful factor to consider in creating helpful campus choropleth maps is building capacity.

A count of students in a building can become more useful for examining the utilization of campus resources when weighted comparisons are used.

The easiest method of weighting is to have the calculations in the dataset before mapping. However, most modern mapping software includes the options needed to create complicated weighting formulas. This allows increased flexibility in designing different weights without having to plan the weighting beforehand (Figure 15.10). Also, if the weighting results in difficulty discerning the data, creating new weights is easier when it is part of the mapping software. More complicated functions such as Dasymetric Mapping can be done using tools similar to the field calculator; Dasymetric Mapping is a cartographic technique for creating population estimates based on several factors and then displaying these using choropleths or other forms of representation (Mennis, 2009, p. 726).

### *Campus Sub-Location Choropleth*

Another method of utilizing maps is at the sub-location level, which is location mapping but zoomed in to a room or floor. Using functions in mapping software that allow one to control what is displayed, Central Washington University can create a campus map that becomes the floor map when zoomed in (Figure 15.11). Using the previously described methods of weighting is still an

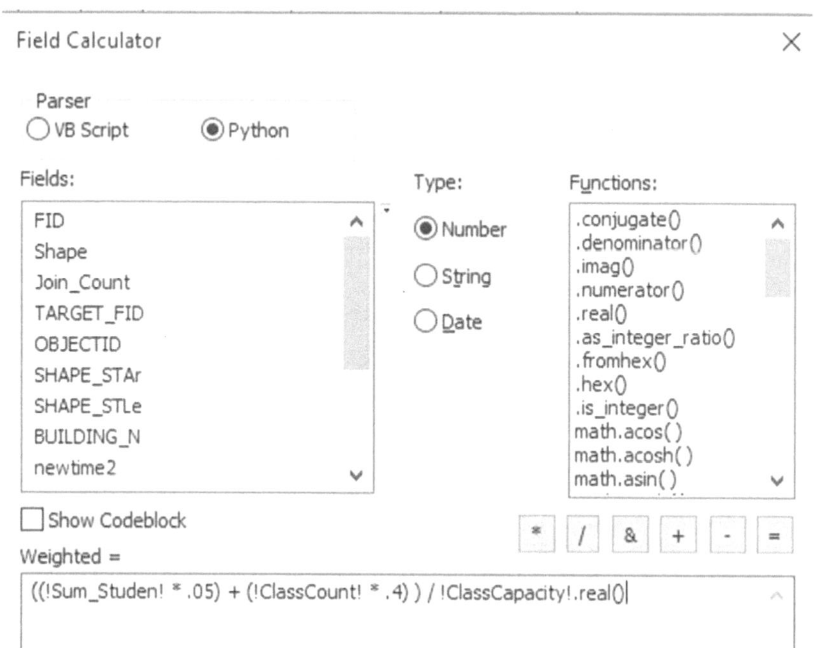


*Figure 15.10* Example of weighting campus data using Python.

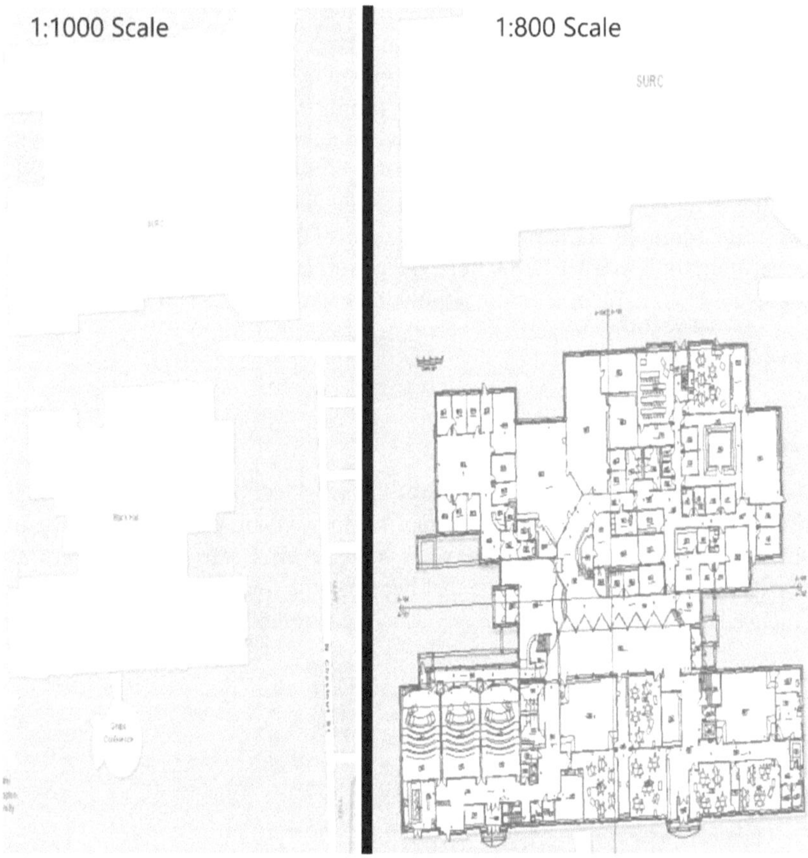


*Figure 15.11* Sub-plan that is only visible when zoomed in.

option on a sub-location choropleth; however, at CWU the primary maps created using this method are classroom space utilization and number of students in the class.

Floor by floor utilization maps can be helpful for tracking classroom use throughout the day. Simple choropleth maps can be created at the floor level. If date and time information has been added to the dataset, videos can be created using tools built into mapping software such as ArcGIS time-lapse. These time-lapse videos can show the classroom use during several days of use, over a brief period; for example, 8 a.m. to 5 p.m. Monday through Friday. This visualization by floor of a building may not be as useful in overall strategic planning but can provide a powerful visual when explaining the underutilization of classroom space. In addition, the visualization of geocoded building and room is a key step in creating accessible tools, so that those with accessibility constraints do not have to engage in extensive pre-journey planning to campus buildings (Tang et al., 2016).

### *Emergency Planning*

Campus mapping can also help campuses prepare for emergencies. There are three primary methods through which Central Washington University integrates emergency planning mapping: choropleth maps (campus and sub-location), overlaying charts, and creating spatial objects. The choropleth methods, as discussed previously for classroom utilization and for such tasks as using weighting in the attribute table, can be applied to emergency planning. Emergency planning could take many forms, such as visualizing capacity of emergency meeting places, response times to emergency procedure drills, etc.

Overlaying charts and icons can often be more informative than choropleth colors. Chart overlays can be used in addition to choropleth maps to provide another level of data for decision-makers. Figure 15.12 demonstrates how emergency response time can be overlaid on top of buildings. Pie and bar charts are the most common charts used to overlay spatial joins. When exploring emergency planning and preparation at the sub-location level, NFPA chemical hazard diamonds can be overlaid on top of rooms to provide awareness of chemical usage across campus. This can be done easily using basic functions available on most mapping programs, through creating points on a map. The identifiable points on a map can then have the icons changed from simple dots to the NFPA diamonds as shown in the map (Figure 15.13). The role of GIS can be essential to emergency management, and "Geospatial Technologies are emerging as one of the most promising frameworks for addressing emergency management" (Bhanumurthy et al., 2015, p. 345). Another prevalent GIS tool that builds upon the examples presented is the use of route analysis, which is considered a valuable tool in in preparing for disaster and responding effectively (Bhanumurthy et al., 2015). Route analysis can be used with Dasymetric Mapping and classroom utilization data to estimate population in a given area when disaster strikes.

### *Semi-Automated Mapping*

There are a multitude of variables that are possible when creating utilization, enrollment, and emergency planning maps. Often several maps are needed to answer questions sufficiently. For example, Semi-Automated Mapping can create maps of campus course enrollment at various times of day, by students of different ethnic and racial groups, by gender, and by major. With planned data prep, making hundreds or thousands of maps can take relatively little time. When an organization takes the time to automate much of the map creation process, it not only frees up personnel but also allows for easier comparisons

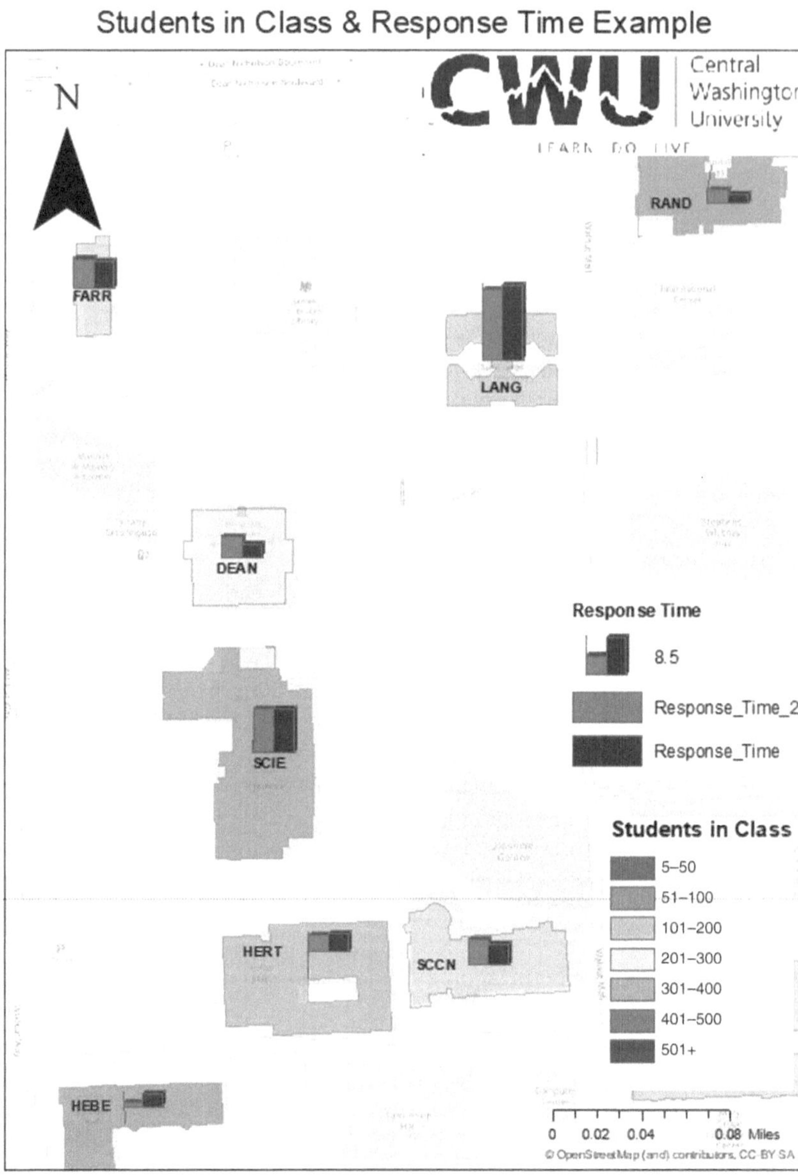


*Figure 15.12* Example of a map that includes student data and emergency response time data.

and new ways of evaluating the data., Through the use of SAS, Python, and ArcGIS ModelBuilder, CWU has created a repeatable process that allows the Office of Institutional Effectiveness to respond rapidly to requests for varying displays of data within maps.

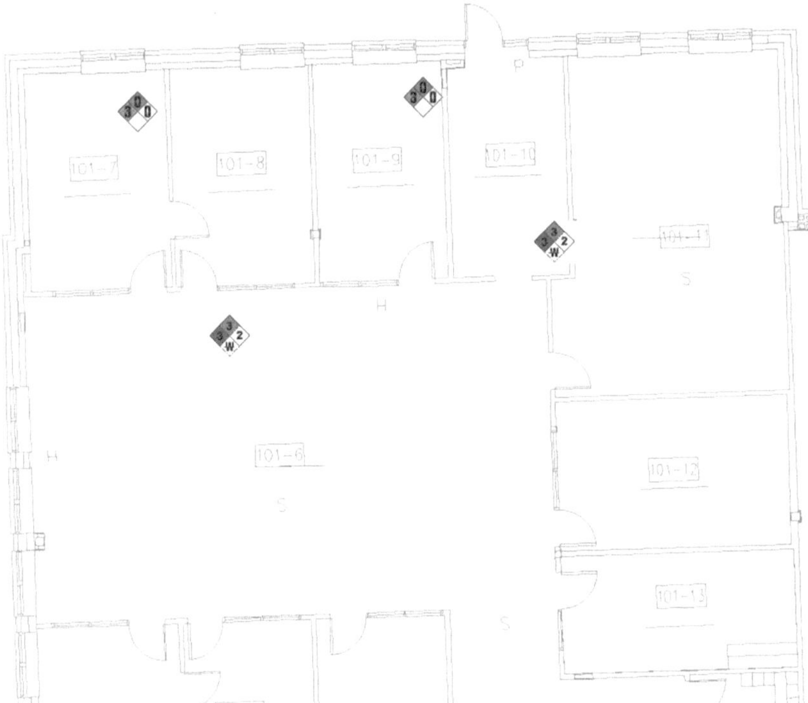


*Figure 15.13* Chemical symbol map at sub-level, example.

### *SAS*

CWU uses SAS for data analysis, which is a software developed by the SAS Institute for Advanced Analytics that can quickly generate and rapidly turn data into maps. At CWU, SAS is integrated with a data warehouse, which combines most data sources on campus into a single accurate system that SAS programs can query. The process that CWU is using can be created through other methods such as R or SQL; however, SAS has easy to integrate Macro and Stored Process options that make automation simple.

### *SAS Macro*

When automating map creation, it is helpful if users are able to easily query data and make immediate changes if needed. Central Washington University accomplished this through SAS Macros. The following commands are simple examples of SAS Macros that are used in automating processes:

```
%Let Term ="1179"; *In the CWU system this is fall 2017;
%Let Term="1179" OR "1181"; *In the CWU system this is fall and Winter;
%Let Gender="Female"
```

The previous commands, when used with SAS programs, allow users to generate a dataset that produces all data to be mapped by the academic term requested. In addition, users are able to select multiple terms and other variables, as used in the example. The created, easy to change dataset can be loaded into various mapping programs for quick analysis and to generate multiple maps.

In order to perform an analysis using mapping software and analysis variables, such as mapping classes in progress by time and day, two other components are required. The first is the building or location name; this is used in spatial joins or reference points in mapping software. The second is the GIS coordinates or Lat/Long of each building or location. The benefit of using SAS is its ability to create formats that can be shared among users at the institution for reuse.

### *Apply SAS Formats*

SAS formats can easily be used to populate Lat/Long data by taking the building name and first creating a format that links to the building name for Latitude and Longitude. The location/building should be one of the columns in the dataset; this column should then be duplicated twice, so three columns display the building/location name. The next step is to apply the Latitude of the building/location to the first duplicate building column and the Longitude to the second duplicate column. The use of advanced formats can save team members a significant amount of time by applying a format and storing it for others to use, as shown in Table 15.1.

### *ArcGIS ModelBuilder and Python*

The ArcGIS ModelBuilder has been useful for automating map productions at CWU. ModelBuilder is a collection of code blocks that can be strung together to assist in automating many ArcGIS functions. Each block contains Python code that interacts with the ArcGIS functions in a simplified interface. The model in Figure 15.14 is the one CWU has made for creating layers that show students in session by time and day.

*Table 15.1* Application of SAS formats

| *Before SAS Format* | | | | |
|---|---|---|---|---|
| *Students_In_Class* | *Time_of_Day* | *Building* | *Latitude* | *Longitude* |
| 200 | 4 p.m. | Bouillon | Bouillon | Bouillon |
| *After SAS Format* | | | | |
| *Students_In_Class* | *Time_of_Day* | *Building* | *Latitude* | *Longitude* |
| 200 | 4 p.m. | Bouillon | −120.538257 | 47.000494 |

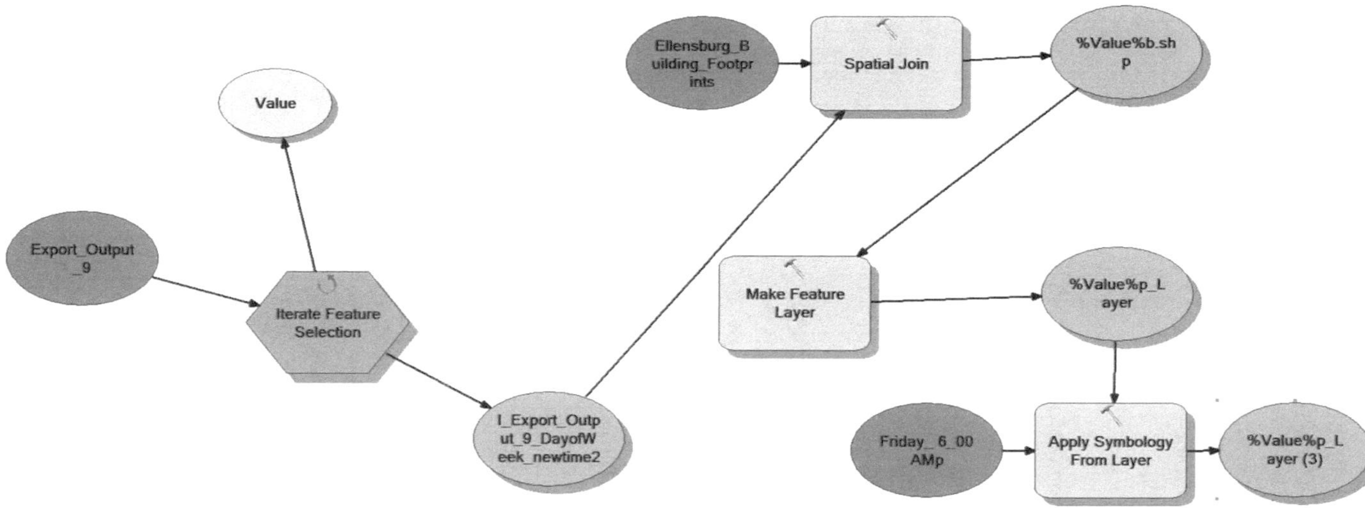


*Figure 15.14* CWU ArcGIS model for Mapping Automation.

This model takes the outputted SAS dataset → iterates over a time and day of the week → selects the relevant data → creates a spatial join with that data → applies the symbology template → and finally creates a layer. This process then repeats for all possible combinations of time and day. The layers can then be exported as a PDF. Another option is to use the data with compatible online services to create interactive maps. Since each function of ModelBuilder uses Python, it is useful to know the basics of Python programming to access the full functionality of ModelBuilder.

### *Python*

Two of the most popular GIS mapping programs, ArcGIS and QGIS, both use Python as a scripting language. Python is currently one of the most popular programming languages, and the integration with popular mapping software allows automated mapping to be completed. ArcGIS includes a Python command terminal to input commands using the various functions directly. Python is a programming language but is often referred to in conjunction with GIS programs a scripting language. Zandbergen states: "Scripting is a programming task that allows you to connect diverse existing components to accomplish a new, related task. Scripting is the glue that allows you to put various existing languages together" (Zandbergen, 2015, p. 4)

At CWU, Python allows the user to automate almost anything ArcGIS can accomplish. This includes complicated proximity maps, spatial joins, and distance calculations, formatting maps, geolocation, and creating datasets. Depending on the combination of features and complexity, some of this can be created with ModelBuilder without any prior experience with Python. However, with knowledge of Python and ModelBuilder, a department can automate its ArcGIS production to produce thousands of maps or to automate the map creation file process entirely by running the Python script in the ArcGIS console.

Another function that works better if coded using Python is the creation of mass PDF files. Using the "arcpy.mapping.exporttoPDF function" and programming logic, instead of creating layers in ArcGIS, individual PDFs can be created. An example of this is creating a PDF file that shows enrollment by time and day of week, using multiple base maps, generating choropleths, but only including certain layers in the PDF function based on the enrollment numbers. The possibilities are endless in terms of what can be accomplished using SAS, ArcGIS, and Python.

CWU can automate some functions of the mapping process by opening SAS, running the program, and then opening ArcGIS Python Console and selecting run. The ArcGIS Python Console then imports the file created in SAS and generates the requested maps. This is what CWU refers to as Automated Mapping. The Automated Mapping process uses campus data and combines it with the analysis software and mapping software. The time commitment to create the variables and programs, and to create initial templates can be minimized.

Besides the initial time to develop automated mapping, another limitation is changing technologies or needs that would make the automated mapping process unviable for future projects. To prevent a net loss of time and effort, any automated mapping projects should be part of long-term strategic planning.

## Conclusion

GIS, when paired with accurate data sources, can be a powerful tool that enhances strategic enrollment and campus management. This chapter presented only a few of the ways in which GIS mapping can be integrated with various aspects of enrollment management to provide key information to decision-makers. With key enrollment management information, decision-makers can make adjustments to overcome weaknesses in recruiting strategies and improve retention. While simultaneously improving enrollment, GIS mapping can be used to enhance the management of campus, including the use of campus space and emergency planning. One of the many ways campus mapping can assist emergency planning is by providing critical information on the storage of chemicals and building occupancy throughout the day.

The ability to map data is not enough given the rapid change of data on a public university campus. The map creation process can be automated through the use of scripting languages such as Python to create the maps and programs like SAS to update data tables. This automation is key to providing the consistently updated information needed by decision-makers without overtaxing the cartographers creating the maps.

## References

AACRAO. (2004). *Essentials of Enrollment Management: Cases in the Field*. Washington, DC: AACRAO Publishing.

Bhanumurthy, V., Bothale, V. M., Kumar, B., Urkude, N., & Shukla, R. (2015). Route analysis for decision support system in emergency management through GIS technologies. *International Journal of Advanced Engineering and Global Technology*, *3*(2), 345–350.

Mennis, J. (2009). Dasymetric mapping for estimating population in small areas. *Geography Compass*, *3*(2), 727–745.

Tang, H., Tsering, N., Hu, F., & Zhu, Z. (2016). Automatic pre-journey indoor map generation using AutoCAD floor plan.

Zandbergen, P. A. (2015). *Python Scripting for ArcGIS*. Redlands, CA: ESRI Press.

## Section V

# Conclusion

# 16 Conclusion

*Cheyanne Manning*

"GIS is waking up the world to the power of geography, this science of integration, and creating a better future" (Jack Dangermond, 2015). Geographic Information Systems (GIS) will be essential to the future of public agencies and nonprofit organizations. The use of GIS allows these entities to visualize spatial information and make correlations with what was previously hidden in their datasets. This analysis tool provides information for better and more effective decision-making, which is especially important in the public and nonprofit sectors. The chapters in this book provided information on the importance of GIS as a way for various entities to make informed decisions and covered a wide range of topics, from hazard analysis, to public health issues, to the need for enterprise storage of accurate GIS data.

## Natural Resources and Hazards

Chapters 2, 5, and 12 investigate how GIS has been used to create methodology, collect data, and analyze patterns regarding natural resources and hazards. Researchers and practitioners alike use GIS to learn about the effects of natural hazards and, increasingly, as a way to help reduce the hazard occurrence and/or disruption level.

Chapter 2 discusses the use of GIS as a way to view and analyze the ever-changing environment post-disaster, with special emphasis on the effects of Hurricane Rita on plant species regrowth. The authors use imagery/data from satellites (also referred to as remote sensing data) in order to view the health of the vegetation over the area. One reason this study was conducted was that there was not an existing model to look at species regrowth after a hurricane. Natural disasters come with little warning and can cause disruption far beyond what we can understand. The use of satellite imagery allowed the authors to look at the after-effects on the environment. Though the authors didn't find the best solution to analyze this problem, they were able to show that it would be beneficial and that this is an existing gap in research.

Similarly, forest fires can also impact communities of people, plants, and animals. Chapter 5 discusses the fire events triggered from the El Niño in Guyana and the effects the fires had on five plant species important to the indigenous peoples in the region. The study was conducted over a five-year period using remote sensing data, with results in GIS showing differences in regrowth between the five species. This chapter looks at how fire can affect critical food sources for indigenous people. Once problems are identified, researchers and practitioners can use the data to help communities, possibly even before they know they will need it. The methodology used in this chapter was created in order to be replicated, with hope that it would be used in pre-disaster planning.

John Muir (Father of the National Parks) once wrote, "the clearest way into the Universe is through a forest wilderness" (Muir, 1938). Trails create openings into nature for human experience, an experience that Muir felt was essential. Not all trails are well documented with distance markers, signage, and maps. Chapter 12 used GIS in order to create an inventory of trails in West Virginia that were previously undocumented. They took GIS a step beyond its general storage capabilities and mapping potential by creating an online application. This application allows users to suggest edits to the state's trails and to recommend locations for future trail expansion. It also allows users the ability to view information about each trail, in order to help with planning their trips.

## Man-Made Hazards

Human-triggered events are common within the disaster realm, from being the primary source (84%) of forest fires to large-scale terrorist attacks (Daley, 2017). Chapters 4 and 8 covered the potential for GIS to be instrumental in planning for hazardous material transportation and as a tool to help protect surface water drinking supplies.

Hazardous material is "any item or agent (biological, chemical, radiological, and/or physical), which has the potential to cause harm to humans, animals, or the environment, either by itself or through interaction with other factors" (Institute of Hazardous Materials Management, 2019). Hazardous material and waste are necessary to the current industrial climate found around the world. That being said, hazardous material and waste need to be transported for proper disposal. Chapter 4 discusses the risk associated with the transportation of these materials and the need for documentation/risk assessment/route planning to ensure the safety of others and that routes are easily accessible to disaster response teams. Chapter 4 also suggests the need for an agency to track these transports with GPS, monitor through a real-time GIS application, and make decisions on transportation with regard to safety.

Chapter 8 discusses using GIS as a way to protect essential surface water. This concern came about after a chemical spill polluted surface drinking water in West Virginia. Polluted drinking water can have lasting effects on a community, with cleanup being costly and long-term. After this incident, the state now requires critical surface water zones to be delineated and managed. These new zones were created in GIS with buffers specific to water flow/pollution issues. Storage tanks in these zones are now required to be inspected and registered with the state, in hopes that future events will be limited. This is a good example of GIS being used for accountability and hazard planning.

## GIS in Education and Nonprofits

GIS has become increasingly popular in its usage in higher education institutions and with nonprofit organizations. Chapters 7, 9, 11, and 15 discuss the ways in which GIS can be used to improve research and analysis in varying situations.

Higher education administrators are a group that do not frequently use GIS for decision-making purposes; Chapter 9 discusses the support GIS can provide to these practitioners if they were to utilize it. GIS can assist in providing spatial analysis on specific problems higher education administrators face. Some of these challenges include: right of way concerns, building/room utilization, transportation routes, grounds-related data storage, storm water management, and HAZMAT sites. Proximity analysis can be used through geocoding addresses in order to look at distance in relation to academic performance and as a way to analyze the potential savings through working from home/online learning. One example in Chapter 9 explains GIS was used in order to look at the rental market availability and the potential for neighborhood value depreciation due to student renters. This chapter also covers GIS as a planning tool for higher education administrators in both long- and short-term planning for their campuses. Both Chapters 9 and 15 cover the significance of using GIS for higher education, with emphasis on the possibilities of analyzing usage and planning for enrollment.

Chapter 15 discusses the use of GIS to view space utilization within academic buildings on Central Washington University's campus in Ellensburg, Washington. This allows higher education administrators a way to look at whether effective utilization is occurring or if there is potential for improvement. This analysis requires accurate enrollment management data to merge with spatial data (in the case of this chapter, classroom data) to view the frequency of classroom usage in various academic buildings. GIS is an important tool to merge these datasets and show the results of the analysis. The results provide information about which spaces on campus are being underutilized and where there are gaps in efficiency. Enrollment management plays a huge role in the success of a university, and being able to analyze aspects of it in GIS provides administrators the information they need to make informed decisions. Chapter 15 also covers the usefulness of GIS in emergency planning; with the capabilities to visualize emergency meeting location capacity, response times for emergency drill, or as a way to analyze previous response/events. The ability to overlay data in GIS allows the user to compare and contrast different variables in higher education situations. This chapter discusses how Python coding, SAS (a data analysis software created by SAS Institute for Advanced Analytics), and GIS can merge mass quantities of various datasets into something that can be viewed and analyzed. The possibilities are seemingly endless for how GIS can help higher education administrators make more informed decisions and create an environment that keeps students engaged and learning.

Chapter 7 evaluates the problems associated with mapping the college opportunity providers for K–12 children across West Virginia. The goal of this study was to "identify the type and distribution of college access provider organizations [organizations that assist in helping students move onto college] as well as the resources and activities they offered to students in their service areas [focusing on traditionally underrepresented groups]" (Alleman and Holly, 2019). The biggest challenge for these authors was that they were not trained to use GIS nor did they have a mentor to help. When their original study was done, there was limited spatial infrastructure built for the state. This lack of detailed data changed the scope of the project, allowing for vagueness and a higher chance of misinterpretation. The authors chose to create a map based on previous research that maps are approachable and can be understood simply. The approachability of maps makes it easier for simple comprehension, without needing to read extensive text to gain an understanding. This isn't always a good thing, though, as "many theorists conceive of mapping as a socially constructed phenomenon that is subject to the same bias, access and exclusion issues, and majority group dominance that has plagued other forms of inquiry and expression historically" (Shepherd, 1995). The chapter ends with discussion around the final project map and how it didn't provide enough information into the coverage and variety of college access providers in West Virginia. This could be in part due to the data quality at the time, the use of a single map to represent the data, or the inability to explain the details of the providers through a map. The authors noted that GIS will be the future into research and administrative decisions; therefore, cartographers/geographers should be well aware of the potential for bias in their maps.

Nonprofit organizations use GIS as a way to analyze and visualize the extent of their efforts. Chapter 11 covered the existing literature for nonprofits and GIS, the roles of nonprofits, and the potential uses for GIS in relation to nonprofits. "Similar to their public sector colleagues, nonprofit workers are expected to meet the increasing demands of their clients while dealing with static or decreasing resources" (Jordan, 2019). This chapter discusses the four areas in which GIS can assist nonprofit organizations: assessment of community need, new or improved service delivery, tool for engagement/advocacy, and fundraising. GIS could be just what is needed for nonprofits who have limited resources and want to reach the people that need their services. The author discusses the cost of GIS as a deterrent, but also notes that there are many free options available that are becoming more user friendly. GIS is an effective tool for nonprofits because it allows for the visualization of important data, increases analysis capabilities, and, with access to open source mapping, has become easier to use.

## Local Government and Collaboration

Chapters 13 and 14 in the book discuss the importance of GIS for local governments and the effectiveness of collaboration. Local governments work with limited resources, similar to public education institutions and nonprofits. Though there are similarities, local governments tend to be more collaborative and reach more people with their efforts.

Chapter 13 covers the important aspect of collaboration for operations and at the policymaking level. Collaboration at the government level is necessary when there is a shared problem or interest. Collaboration using GIS is common, and "many state governments have GIS councils that provide a collaborative government structure" (Smith, 2019). There are large national coalitions for GIS, including the Coalition of Geospatial Organizations. These coalitions have shared interests, with the intent to create policy as a way to improve GIS functionality. Chapter 13 states that a collaborative governance structure is essential for organizations to form effective partnerships and make consistent and informed decisions. The lack of a structure "results in inefficiency, inconsistency, and waste" (Smith, 2019). The author explains that GIS is critical to analyzing areas of drug abuse/use and the number of children entering foster care as a result of it. These results allow the State of Oregon to focus its resources on specific areas to help communities. The author states that the organizations in these areas do not collaborate or share information, but that they would save a lot of taxpayer money with a collaborative governance structure. Smith defines governance structure as "a formal recognition of decision rights—who makes which decisions, how those decisions are made, what triggers the necessity for a decision, who sits at the table, who has a say, etc." (2019). The chapter explains that one of the most effective collaborative governance strategies is that of habitat protection. Habitat protection is usually regionally specific and covers entities such as states, counties, and railroads, the Forest Service, and the Department of Fish and Wildlife, among others. These entities work to create protection measures, including land use restrictions. The ability for them to collaborate allows for more effective resource management and efficiency in decision-making for these sensitive areas. GIS allows these entities a way to analyze protection sites to enable the timely decision-making for collaborative governance. The chapter discusses the formation of the Oregon Geographic Information Council (OGIC) and legislation they were able to get passed in 2017 that allows OGIC to function as a collaborative governance entity representing all public bodies in Oregon (Smith, 2019; State of Oregon, 2017). The author ends by saying that "to effectively address wildfire risks . . . or any of the myriad of other problems with which GIS can play an important and enabling role, we must have consistent, trustworthy data when and where it is needed" (Smith, 2019) This data consistency will only be possible in the form of collaborative governance, where they will need to work together to support their communities and initiatives.

Chapter 14 focuses on the best ways to utilize GIS for county governments. This includes key challenges and opportunities, and how to manage GIS data. The author defines counties as "counties, boroughs, parishes and municipal districts in the United States and Canada that serve as first tier subdivisions of their state or province" and uses "the term *municipality* to refer to second-tier municipal subdivisions" (Babinski, 2019). The author suggests that a framework is necessary to use GIS effectively at the county level. There are risk factors involved with GIS for counties, including: the availability of resources, staffing, deferred maintenance (maintenance that was pushed back to a future funding cycle), and lack of a documented process. Counties have several responsibilities that are delegated to them. These responsibilities include: "regional policing and jails, E911, superior courts, elections, public defense, property assessment, tax collection, regional highways, regional transit, regional parks and trails, regional planning and zoning, regional emergency management coordination, etc" (Babinski, 2019). Chapter 14 discusses the URISA GIS Capability Maturity Model (URISA, 2013) and how it can assist counties in assessing their GIS capabilities and the maturity of their process. These types of analyses allow counties to use public funds effectively and knowledgeably. Public entities and, more specifically, counties want to make sure that public funds are being spent and managed well. There is usually a focus on return on investment (ROI) as a way to analyze spending. ROI in GIS can be difficult, because the majority of costs lies with data collection. The author states that "GIS managers should be rigorous in looking for opportunities to minimize or reduce costs" (Babinski, 2019). This chapter, like Chapter 13, discusses the importance of collaboration. The author explains that a county GIS manager should have a strong relationship with municipalities, tribes, or state/federal agencies, because those relationships not only help with day-to-day activities but also allow for effective GIS data sharing. The author makes note later in the chapter that county GIS should provide its jurisdictions with GIS data sharing coordination involving infrastructure. GIS software can be expensive; Babinski recommends pooling the software licenses for county users and employing software license management to understand patterns of use (2019). Counties play an important role in managing and allowing public access of GIS data. This chapter discusses how counties can more effectively do so and what capabilities are possible.

## Spatial Infrastructure and GIS Applications

There were a handful of discussions throughout the remaining chapters that covered the importance of GIS infrastructure, regulation of data storage, data reliability, and publicly accessible information. These topics are essential to public and nonprofit organizations because they enable efficiency in providing base data to a project/inquiry.

Chapter 3 discusses the change over time to spatial data infrastructure (SDI) initiatives for the State of West Virginia. The state's GIS Technical Center began in 1993 with the goals of increasing the use and availability of spatial data and providing the necessary support to those using GIS.

> Over its lifetime, the Technical Center has seen a paradigm shift from the early dominance of a federally sourced spatial data infrastructure to one

> where local, state, and private sector entities now play the major role in spatial data generation and distribution.
>
> (Harris and LaFone, 2019)

Of this shift, the Technical Center has seen changes to the sources of data, the accuracy of said data, and the technology employed. The biggest discussion in Chapter 3 revolves around GIS data as a publicly available and easily accessibly source. West Virginia's GIS Technical Center has needed to evolve in order to supply GIS data on demand to the public. These changes have been noted throughout GIS research, especially with regard to the source of data, a topic covered in Chapter 6.

GIS and spatial data can now be created in crowdsourced applications like that of OpenStreetMap (OSM). These applications allow anyone to create spatial data, as long as they log in to the system, similar to Wikipedia. This has provided the opportunity for a large quantity of data to become available for a specific area, which, in turn, could assist those in public and nonprofit work. Chapter 6 discusses how these types of crowdsourced applications create hesitation for users because of concern over data quality. This chapter develops an analysis of data and users that were banned by OSM administrators, in order to learn from and avoid damage to data quality in the future. This analysis sample included 994 bans that occurred between 2009 and 2017, where each ban could be treated as a single event. Based on their analysis, Table 16.1 was created.

Their findings show that the highest error percentage lies within nefarious actions: those actions that are intentional. This chapter ends with recommendations of ways the OSM system could intervene prior to error, including pop-up

*Table 16.1* Themes observed in the bans

| *Broader Themes* | *Percentage of Bans* | *Ban Categories (In Order of Prevalence)* |
|---|---|---|
| Nefariousness | 31% | Vandalism<br>Politically motivated edits<br>Sock puppetry<br>Spam |
| Obstinance | 26% | Failure to cooperate with the OSM community<br>Deleting another person's work<br>Edit wars |
| Ignorance | 23% | Misunderstanding of OSM practices or software<br>Copyright violations<br>Erroneous edits |
| Mechanical Problems | 20% | Data imports conducted incorrectly<br>Bots unintentionally corrupting data |

Source: Quinn and Bull (2018)

boxes notifying users that they are about to make a change, locking the ability to edit certain things, and creating restrictions on allowing mechanical edits. This chapter closes with the statement that open source mapping applications will grow increasingly popular, making it essential to decrease the error created using them.

Chapter 10 involves the creation of a Logistical Tracking System (LTS) for UT-Dallas as a way to evaluate and merge their processes. The LTS was utilized for a number of years at the university; this chapter discusses the positives and negatives to its use, along with why it wasn't able to be maintained. The LTS had its beginnings with the idea that the university's building floor plans could be converted to AutoCAD (a drafting software) in order to increase the efficiency of data reporting. While developing the LTS, it was discovered that the university did not have possession of AutoCAD licenses, but GIS resources were being utilized through the social science and geoscience departments. This existing knowledge base, access to students that could use GIS, and the capability of GIS in comparison to CAD led the group to use GIS for the LTS. "The original purpose of the LTS was to improve facilities management and to permit information in government reports to be utilized by OSPA and the Controller's Office" (Valcik, 2019). The LTS stored and analyzed data in many capacities, which made it applicable to administrators across the university.

The LTS was able to:

- Provide a facilities feed for Registrar's scheduling purposes.
- Track chemical biological, and radioactive materials to location.
- Allow for integration of security systems.
- Tracking of telecommunications infrastructure.
- Personnel assignments in facilities.
- Campus resident assignment to facilities.
- Room equipment tracking.
- Safety equipment tracking.
- Tracking of physical plant door keys.
- Storing utility costs for buildings.

(Valcik, 2019)

The LTS was functional with a database developer and GIS analyst, along with student employees that assisted with programming and data entry. The development team had to overcome issues with server/software compatibility, having to write code to merge different systems, and, ultimately, the loss of staff with the abilities to maintain it. The LTS was user friendly and allowed for dropdown menus to reduce error allowance; first responders were able to view live camera feed in buildings through the LTS; and the university recorded a savings of $1,683,205 over the three-year development period (FY 2001–FY 2003). The LTS was customized to the needs of UT-Dallas and, with personnel who could manage it, would still be beneficial to the university. Unfortunately, the university decided to go with another facilities data storage software without the GIS capabilities.

GIS has the potential to provide nonprofits and public organizations with the information to help them run more effectively. This book has described ways in which GIS can prove essential to functionality, from data storage capabilities, to analysis in wide range (e.g. wildfire restoration, student enrollment, hazardous material transportation, etc.), and the capability to create maps that can be easily understood. These chapters have outlined the importance of GIS to nonprofits and public organizations and its ability to not only be interdisciplinary, but also be used collaboratively to reach a common goal. GIS will continue to be a useful tool for public organizations and nonprofits, and it will be up to them how they choose to utilize it.

## References and Further Readings

Alleman, Nathan and L. Neal Holly. 2019. More Than Meets the Eye: The Methodological and Epistemological Hazards of GIS Map Use in the Public Sphere. In Nicolas Valcik. *Geospatial Information System Use in Public Organizations: How and Why GIS Should Be Used by the Public Sector*. CRC Press, Boca Raton, FL. 2019.

Babinski, Greg. 2019. GIS Best Practices for Best-Run County Governments. In Nicolas Valcik. *Geospatial Information System Use in Public Organizations: How and Why GIS Should Be Used by the Public Sector*. CRC Press, Boca Raton, FL. 2019.

Daley, Jason. 2017. Study Shows 84% of Wildfires Caused by Humans. *Smithsonian Magazine*, February 28. www.smithsonianmag.com/smart-news/study-shows-84-wildfires-caused-humans-180962315/

Dangermond, Jack. 2015. ESRI User Conference. *ArcNews*, Fall. www.esri.com/esri-news/arcnews/fall15articles/awakening-the-world-to-the-power-of-geography

Harris, Trevor M. and H. Franklin LaFone. 2019. Evolving Trajectories in Public Sector Statewide Spatial Data Infrastructure: From Data Product to On-Demand Services and GIS Apps. In Nicolas Valcik. *Geospatial Information System Use in Public Organizations: How and Why GIS Should Be Used by the Public Sector*. CRC Press, Boca Raton, FL. 2019.

Institute of Hazardous Materials Management. 2019. "What are Hazardous Materials?" Retrieved June 8th, 2019. www.ihmm.org/about-ihmm/what-are-hazardous-materials

Jordan, Todd. 2019. Service Delivery for United Way. In Nicolas Valcik. *Geospatial Information System Use in Public Organizations: How and Why GIS should Be Used by the Public Sector*. CRC Press, Boca Raton, FL. 2019.

Muir, John. 1938. *John of the Mountains: The Unpublished Journals of John Muir*. University of Wisconsin Press, Madison, 1979.

Quinn, Sterling and Floyd Bull. 2019. Understanding Threats to Crowdsourced Geographic Data Quality Through a Study of OpenStreetMap Contributor Bans. In Nicolas Valcik. *Geospatial Information System Use in Public Organizations: How and Why GIS Should Be Used by the Public Sector*. CRC Press, Boca Raton, FL. 2019.

Shepherd, I. 1995, Putting time on the map: Dynamic displays in data visualization and GIS, in Fisher, P.F. (ed.), Innovations in GIS 2, Taylor & Francis, London, 169–187.

Smith, C.Y. 2019. One Government: The Enterprise Approach in a Silo Environment. In Nicolas Valcik. *Geospatial Information System Use in Public Organizations: How and Why GIS Should Be Used by the Public Sector*. CRC Press, Boca Raton, FL. 2019.

State of Oregon. 2017. Oregon Revised Statues 276A.

Valcik, Nicolas A. 2019. *Geospatial Information System Use in Public Organizations: How and Why GIS Should Be Used by the Public Sector*. CRC Press, Boca Raton, FL.

# Index

Note: Page numbers in *italic* indicate a figure and page numbers in **bold** indicate a table on the corresponding page.